SECOND EDITION

PUBLIC HEALTH

FOR CHILDREN

SECOND EDITION

PUBLIC HEALTH
FOR CHILDREN

Edited by

Diane DeBell

Anglia Ruskin University, Norwich, UK

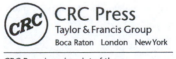

CRC Press
Taylor & Francis Group
Boca Raton   London   New York

CRC Press is an imprint of the
Taylor & Francis Group, an **informa** business

CRC Press
Taylor & Francis Group
6000 Broken Sound Parkway NW, Suite 300
Boca Raton, FL 33487-2742

© 2016 by Taylor & Francis Group, LLC
CRC Press is an imprint of Taylor & Francis Group, an Informa business

No claim to original U.S. Government works

Printed and bound by CPI UK on sustainably sourced paper
Version Date: 20151102

International Standard Book Number-13: 978-1-4822-2748-2 (Paperback)

Visit the Taylor & Francis Web site at
http://www.taylorandfrancis.com

and the CRC Press Web site at
http://www.crcpress.com

Contents

Foreword

Forty years ago, as a junior paediatrician, I worked at Baragwanath, a huge hospital serving the black African township of Soweto on the edge of Johannesburg. There were dramatic differences in disease patterns and severity between our hospital and the hospital for white children in the prosperous city centre. At the white hospital, the children had a similar range of conditions to those I was familiar with in the United Kingdom, whereas the black children in our wards at Baragwanath had preventable conditions that reflected the extreme poverty, mediocre education and family disintegration created by South Africa's political system.

This book is primarily about child public health in Britain, where public policy has been very different from that of South Africa over the past half century—yet, as I now divide my time in retirement between South Africa and England, I am struck more by the similarities than the differences in the problems faced by children in these two very different environments.

Poverty is difficult to define and measure but its effects are all too obvious. It results in food insecurity, unhealthy diets, dental disease and both under and over nutrition. Children in poor neighbourhoods are more likely to attend poor or failing schools. Bullying by peer groups is still a major problem. Sexual exploitation, abuse, unwanted pregnancy, depression, anxiety, substance misuse and antisocial behaviour are all more common in poor families.

It is not impossible to be a successful parent if you are poor, but it is much harder. Parents do not have to be perfect—just 'good enough'; and the good-enough parents take it for granted that they need to plan and space their pregnancies, talk and read to their children, provide experiences and books, support them through the ups and downs of school life, and do their best to prepare them for a successful future as adults. Debate and research continue on how best to help parents who struggle with these tasks, but there is no dispute about their importance from a public health perspective.

The First World War poet Wilfred Owen wrote that 'all the poet can do is to warn'. Warning and informing governments and society about the impact of public policy are not the only tasks of child public health but are arguably the most vital. Health professionals are good at identifying, describing and measuring problems that go beyond purely biological concepts of illness but, on their own, they often despair at the difficulty in bringing about meaningful change. This book brings together experts from a range of disciplines and shows how a deeper insight into societal problems can help us to make a difference both in public policy and in the lives of individual troubled children.

Sir David Hall
Emeritus professor of community paediatrics, University of Sheffield and
Honorary professor of paediatrics, University of Cape Town

Preface

In early 2007, when UNICEF published its first 'report card' of child well-being in rich countries, there was something of a sharp intake of breath across the four countries of the United Kingdom. Using a multidimensional overview of the state of childhood, UNICEF was indicating UK child health and well-being as the poorest amongst 21 industrialized nations when measured on overall health factors.

How could this have happened? From 1997 (a decade earlier), the British government had argued a series of policy intentions directly designed to support population health improvement: a public health orientation to services, a recognition of the social and economic dimensions of health determinants, and a reorientation of service delivery designed to eradicate antiquated departmental and professional boundaries. Indeed the Chancellor's comprehensive spending review in January 2007 reported improvement in reducing child poverty.

Yet, UNICEF in 2010 again reported the United Kingdom as one of the most unequal countries in which to be born. Among the Organisation of Economically Advanced Countries (OECD) the UK in 2010 was ranked thirteenth of twenty-four countries for education, eleventh for health and nineteenth for material well-being. It is the sixth richest country in the world, yet more than one in three households with children (39%) have less than the Minimum Income Standard, which is required to meet the national living standard (food, clothes and shelter only). By 2015, a Joseph Rowntree Foundation report had confirmed this profile as continuing.

This profile applies to whole populations (all age groups) within all four countries of the United Kingdom. When we focus on child health alone, we find that the picture is even more alarming. In effect, we are a nation that is storing up health problems that will have consequences for our next generation of adults. The recent public health agenda for children and young people in Britain was triggered by David Hall and David Elliman in what is now referred to as Hall 4. They formalized and popularized population analyses of child health. Their work continues to inform social medicine across the four countries of the United Kingdom and abroad.

And in 2003, Mitch Blair and his colleagues set an important conceptual lead by specifying a focus on the meaning of child public health, a focus that needs to be foregrounded in the public health agenda for Britain.

It would be fair to say that the shift in 1997 to a public health orientation in health and social care delivery systems set the stage for the possibility of a social model of medicine in the United Kingdom. Yet, there has been slow progress toward achievement. That slow progress has had much to do with engrained habits of working, repetitive service reorganizations, government anxiety about the costs of redistributive approaches to the underlying causes of poverty; and an uncertainty about what is meant by a public health orientation to population health when we think about the work of clinicians and practitioners. And how do we set priorities for child health?

In this book, we examine the health and well-being of children in Britain and we do so by revisiting the full range of public health practice from analysis to action, in other words, from the work of epidemiology to the community interventions that seek to improve health. We do this by locating the child in the family, the school, and the community. These are the three locations that children inhabit as they grow and develop from birth to emergence into adulthood.

Within this profile of thinking, we also encounter questions about resource distribution and service planning. Where should we invest in services that can improve child health and which services should we prioritize and how? How should we design programmes that maximize interprofessional skills? What is the evidence base that we need in order to make such decisions? And what are the factors that most impact child health?

Yet services are only part of the full picture. Child health is affected by language, culture, gender, ability/disability, immigration or refugee status, housing, adult carer health, consumer behaviour, nutrition, sanitation, clean water, transport systems and the ecology of the immediate environment. And child health does not emerge in single focus. It is the constellation of factors in the material and the psychosocial environments that interact to affect a child's ability to grow and develop well or poorly.

This is the second book we have published with the intention of advancing the public health practitioner's approach to child health. Each chapter is the beginning of an important debate and should be read in those terms. If this book triggers widespread argument and further research, it will have achieved its purpose.

Acknowledgements

In 2005, Paul Farmer published *Pathologies of Power* and thereby signalled an international step change in collaborative approaches to public health analysis and action. I read his monumental volume on a family holiday in Tuscany in 2005 and instantly knew that public health practice was experiencing a breakthrough. At the same time, Michael Marmot and his research teams in the UK had been developing our understanding of population health by means of radical new insights.

Public health perspectives on childhood development, however, have been fewer and slower to impact our understanding of population health. Nevertheless, the Harvard Center on the Developing Child is now taking an international lead in public health studies of the early years.

In the UK, Mitch Blair and his colleagues published the formative *Child Public Health* in 2003. And the monumental work of David Hall (and David Elliman) commanded the field throughout the United Kingdom until at least 2004. Practitioners across child health fields still refer to "Hall 4" as a shorthand for research-based child health practice.

In 2007, we published *Public Health Practice & the School-Age Population.*

This new revised volume, *Public Health for Children Second Edition*, rests on the bedrock of these analysts and it also relies on research teamwork. This new volume focuses on public health questions and service planning for children (from birth to adulthood), mainly in Britain but with reference to other OECD countries. It is designed for public health practitioners.

The teams with whom these writers work provide us with important and large scale population analyses of the how and the why of public health practice. And their work is collaborative. It is a model for public health practitioners across the world.

We acknowledge the vast plenitude of experience that the writers in this volume bring to this work.

The formative thinkers about child public health in the United Kingdom are David Hall (and David Elliman) as well as Mitch Blair. Their work has been fundamental in shaping this book and their personal friendship has been critical.

This new volume introduces new contributors and it widens our scope to include childhood from birth.

I owe special thanks to these colleagues and to the book's contributors. I also owe special acknowledgement to Naomi Wilkinson who shepherded both of these volumes through to publication.

Contributors

Jane V. Appleton, RGN, RHV, PGCEA, BA (Hons), MSc, PhD
School of Health and Social Care
Oxford Brookes University
Oxford, UK

Simon Bradford, PhD, MPhil
Department of Clinical Sciences
Brunel University
Uxbridge, UK

Margaret Buttigieg, BA (Open University), RGN, RHV, PGCEA
MAB Consulting
Nottingham, UK

Sarah Cowley, DBE, PhD, BA, RN, RHV, HVT
King's College London
London, UK

Diane DeBell, PhD, MA, BA (Hons), Phi Beta Kappa, FRSA, FCMI, MRSL
Anglia Ruskin University
Cambridge, UK

Maggie Fisher, RGN, NDN, RHV, Cert Ed, BA (Hons) Ed, PG Diploma Infant and Child Mental Health, and PG Diploma in Social Innovation
Institute of Health Visiting
London, UK

Simon Forrest, PhD, MA (Ed), PGCE, PGCAP
School of Medicine, Pharmacy and Health
Durham University
Durham, UK

Leslie Gelling, PhD, MA, BSc (Hons), RN, FHSCE, FRSA
Anglia Ruskin University
Cambridge, UK

Yvonne McNamara, MPhil, PGCE, Dip Counselling, BA (Hons)
Liverpool John Moore University
Liverpool, UK

Dinah Morley, PhD, MSc, BA (Hons)
YoungMinds
London, UK

Tina Moules, PhD, MSc, CertEd, RSCN, SCN
Anglia Ruskin University
Cambridge, UK

Theresa Nash, MSc, PGCEA, Higher Dip, BSc (Hons), HV, RN, SN Cert, FP Cert
School of Nursing, Faculty of Health, Social Care and Education
Kingston University and St George's University of London
London, UK

Niamh O'Brien, MSc, BA (Hons)
Faculty of Health, Social Care and Education
Anglia Ruskin University
Cambridge, UK

Dawn Rees, MA, CQSW, FInstM, FRSPH
Office of the Children's Commissioner and Leadership Development Consultant
London, UK

June Thoburn, CBE, LittD, MSW, BA (Hons)
University of East Anglia
Norwich, UK

PART 1

THE CHILD IN TWENTY-FIRST CENTURY BRITAIN

Background and context

DIANE DeBELL

INTRODUCTION

Amy, age 14, and her brother Nathan, age 16, are adoptive children although Nathan is, in fact, his father's birth child from a former relationship. This is a family-held secret. Nathan is currently serving a custodial sentence and Amy has been able to maintain some contact with her brother via letters delivered by her adoptive father. This young sister and brother have always been close. Since Nathan's arrest, Amy has been distressed and angry at home and at school. Her relationships with teachers at school are poor and she frequently truants. She is currently under threat of expulsion and she has few friends. Her relationship with her mother is poor.

(DeBell 2003, p. 10)

This young girl is failing at school but no one knows why. She is the child of a complicated family profile and a judicial system that neither recognizes nor takes responsibility for its effect on the emotional lives of prisoners' children or siblings. Amy's teachers are not aware that she has a close family member in prison nor do they have experience of the damaging effects the stigma of imprisonment can have on a child. Amy's attempts to keep her brother's imprisonment a secret mean that not even the school nurse knows the nature or cause of her distress. Amy is perceived to be a problem at school and at home.

Does this compilation of circumstances describe a child health problem? And, if it does, how do we understand it in terms of child public health, in terms of preventable illness, in terms of health promotion and in terms of public health practice?

The answers lie within our definitions of child health and well-being. For example, in contemporary Britain we now collectively agree that child emotional and mental distress is, in fact, a health problem. Indeed, child and adolescent mental health is probably the most pervasive health problem in twenty-first century Britain. Meltzer et al., for the Office of National Statistics, estimated in 2005 that 1 child in 10 experiences a mental health problem at some point during their school years. This is the most recent estimate. The charity YoungMinds has placed that figure at double the estimate of Meltzer et al. (see Chapter 8).

Yet we often have difficulty thinking about *health* in terms other than physical and endogenous descriptions. To take this one step further, social definitions of health continue to sit uneasily with medical dxefinitions.

> Health matters have for too long been viewed as somehow separate from the societies in which they are in fact embedded.

(Coburn 2003, p. 338)

Child public health practice, in keeping with Coburn's observation, starts from the position that each individual child's physical and mental health is a consequence of multiple factors within the settings in which the child lives – the home, the school and the local community and neighbourhood. Furthermore, the child's health is affected by a range of government policies arising from disparate government departments. In Amy's case, Home Office policies on family visiting and contact affect her ability to remain in contact with her brother. Teachers and school nurses play an important part in public health practice for school-age children, but the complexities of a child's family life as an influence on health require considerable cross-boundary thinking.

> The social environment is a public health issue because it has such a big impact on health and because public health workers can do so much to improve it. Unlike most health professionals, who are restricted to helping individuals on a case-by-case basis, public health workers can change institutions and laws that organize the social environment at a population level.

(Donald 2006, p. 242)

The questions that follow are twofold:

1. Is child health enabled or is it compromised by the economic, social, material and political environment of Britain today?
2. Whose responsibility is child health protection and improvement?

And thus the over-riding child public health question:

- Is Britain a toxic environment for children growing up in the twenty-first century?

When we think about child public health, our starting point is generally the measurable and observable morbidities. This is the traditional work of epidemiology. This necessary stage of measurement means that interventions are, in turn, more likely to be focused on those facets of preventable child ill-health about which we can hope to make a positive difference at the population level (from dental caries to sun protection; from nutrition and exercise to road safety and cycle helmets; from accidental injury to child protection).

But for public health practitioners, it is also the social and political context, not only the clinical profile, that matters when we think about how to prevent ill-health in children and young people of school age. In other words, it is the population-level information that helps practitioners in their work with individual children and families.

A NEW CHILD PUBLIC HEALTH: WHO IS THIS BOOK FOR?

Child public health is emerging – or perhaps re-emerging – as a speciality of both public health and paediatrics, and as a broadly based interdisciplinary movement.

(Blair et al. 2003, p. 3)

In their comprehensive work of 2003, Blair et al. provide us with the grounding we need to understand causality and risk, concepts that are fundamental to the work of public health practitioners, who, in turn, seek to develop strategies and interventions to improve and protect child health. But Blair and his colleagues do not seek to conceptualize childhood nor to differentiate children by age. In this book, we focus our attention on the child (from birth to transition into adulthood at age 16 or 18 years).

The developmental period from neonatal to school age has long been a focus of investment and research; the school-age years less so. Yet both are critical. Increasingly, there is division of expertise in the training of professionals for work with the pre-school and the school-age years.

Important work in the neurosciences as well as focus on the social and economic formation of family life in the pre-school years is a feature of new public health thinking.

In addition, the school years are a long period of growth and development during which children, young people and their families often experience changing social circumstances and diverse family formations, and they experience school-led transition points as the child moves toward eventual entry into adulthood and independence.

Many diverse health and social care professionals are involved with child health during the school years. But so too are education professionals, housing and local authority officers, youth and community workers, the criminal justice system, voluntary and charitable bodies and local community groups. This book is for these readers. It also provides a rich resource for service managers and service commissioning bodies. Furthermore, the contributions in this book indicate many areas of need for targeted research into the issues that affect pre-school and school-age child health.

This book provides a basis for debate, research and, particularly, for frontline practice. This book is organized in parts that foreground the three settings in which children grow and develop – the family, the school and the local community/neighbourhood. But it also opens in Part I with analysis of the legal issues affecting child health and the implications of difference and diversity for child health in the United Kingdom. The final part of the book specifically addresses two core health issues – child and adolescent mental health and the challenges linked to involving children and young people in decision making about their own health needs.

This book is designed to stimulate discussion and debate, to provide a practical agenda for thinking and for argument amongst its readers and to foreground the health improvement and protection needs of children and young people.

THINKING ABOUT THE SCHOOL-AGE YEARS

This book starts from the premise that our collective understanding of school-age childhood health has been largely under-represented in those critical debates that inform public health thinking at all levels – from epidemiological description to theories of cause for ill-health (health determinants); from intervention designs to measures of their effectiveness and ultimately, the public health policy direction of current government thinking. We are not arguing a *failure* of focus, but rather the need to look closely and specifically at the school-age years in public health terms.

To do that we need to think about what we mean by childhood during these years. In developmental terms, this age span (from school entry age to 16–18 years) is the period of transition from full dependence on family and carers to a presumption about transition into adult rights and responsibilities. These school-age years (about 20% of the UK population or 11.2 million fall into this group*) are a time of dramatic physical and emotional development. And for too many children, these years are not a happy and healthy period of life.

The illnesses, disease, long-term conditions and thus the morbidities of the school-age years are largely preventable, yet they are frequently below the radar of mainstream public health planning. Furthermore, when ill-health is not preventable, many of its adverse *consequences* for individual children *are* preventable. The full picture concerns more than health-care services alone, and child health improvement is dependent on multisectoral analyses and inter-professional service development.

For example, the recently identified child *obesity epidemic* in both Britain and the United States is an example of the way child health tends to be observed in single-issue focus rather than in terms of a complex set of socio-economic and environmental factors that can affect the health of all children and young people of school age. Overweight in children is exacerbated by poverty and by poor regulation of the food industry. It is not simply a matter of individual and family behaviours. We are only at the starting gate in our understanding of the obesogenic environment.

In other words, the factors behind a rise in childhood obesity are preventable, but only by first identifying the multiple causes, including consumer behaviour; the food industry's role in food production, distribution and advertising; the public sector's investment decisions about food for children at school, in hospital and in care and the nature of legislation needed to govern the food industry. And even these initially indicative issues do not include those factors that govern child physical activity – access to pleasurable exercise, safe play areas and the school environment. Nor do they reflect the historic shift in the relationship between body weight/ stature; the measure of calorie expenditure in contemporary labour and the cost, supply and availability of food within any particular developed country.

THINKING ABOUT CHILDHOOD

The very concept of childhood is a culturally bound phenomenon. When we speak of contemporary childhood in the developed countries, we tend to oscillate between overly sentimental terms that deny agency, and thus deny voice to this sector of the population on the one hand, while on the other hand, we can quickly find ourselves resorting to blame or ridicule (of the family, of the child) – most notably from the pre-adolescent period. Defining a balance between

---

* Because data are not maintained specifically for school-age children and young people, we have extrapolated this estimate (for age 5–18 years) from diverse sources for the year 2006.

protecting children and allowing them agency is fraught with cultural as well as political confusion. For example, children are not citizens because they are disenfranchised, yet they are frequently and incorrectly referred to as *citizens with rights*. In the United Kingdom, the concept of children's rights is highly circumscribed, despite Britain's ratification of the U.N. Convention on the Rights of the Child (1989).

The language of social policy and of healthcare is a language imbued with presumptions about progress. For example, when we speak of the present in developed countries, we tend to comfort ourselves that, in general, the conditions of our lives and the directions of government health and social care policy are improving, are 'for the good'. However,

> … it could be argued that if one applies a holistic definition of health, young people now are no healthier than they were a century ago.

> **(Hall 2006, p. i)**

In this book, we take a hard look at two related issues: (1) what is the state of child health in Britain today and (2) what is the function of child public health practice in improving and protecting the health of all children?

No one would seriously argue that a desire to maximize child health is not an a priori good. Yet, a close look at the history of child health in the United Kingdom, as elsewhere, reveals a strangely haphazard approach to children's health once past the neonatal and early years period. Several milestones thus far in the twenty-first century indicate a promising shift in this relative neglect of a more holistic and more comprehensive focus on children's health and well-being:

* *Child Public Health* (Blair et al. 2003)
* *Health for all Children* (Hall and Elliman 2003)
* *The National Service Framework for Children, Young People and Maternity Services* (Department of Health and Department for Education and Skills 2004)
* *The Every Child Matters framework* (Department for Education and Skills 2004)
* *The Children Act 2004*
* *Health Behaviour in School-Aged Children Study 2009/10 Survey* (Currie et al. 2012)
* *Lancet study of 34 countries: Health Behaviour in School-Aged Children* (*Lancet* 2014)
* *Children and Families Act 2014*

We argue in this book that the health of children and young people has not been systematically studied from the perspective of a population cohort. Instead, we have multiple studies of single health issues or of child health and social care delivery systems for specific child health matters. This work is essential but it needs theorizing in terms of public health practice and it needs intensification of attention on the pre-school as well as the school-age years.

Yet, we may be at a point of change in that profile. The moment is opportune for the development of an integrated approach to child public health. Blair et al. (2003), Hall and Elliman (2003), Cowley (2002, 2007) and DeBell (2007) have set the stage for just such a programme of work. And this book takes those arguments and insights as a starting point for investigating and then setting an agenda for the next stage of public health practice.

The linkage between social inequalities and health disparities is well established (Marmot et al. 1991). Less well described are the connections between social inequalities during childhood and adolescence and adult health status (Sawyer 2012). Additionally, little is known about changes in social inequalities during early life, and virtually nothing is known about how these changes might affect social gradients in non-communicable diseases (NCDs) later in life.

(Santelli et al. 2015)

In addition, from a policy perspective, the four countries of the United Kingdom have each begun to focus separate attention on the health implications of the settings in which children live. Specifically, policy in each country has begun to focus on the child from the perspective of service delivery systems and of child health issues (e.g. the recent emergence of public health concerns about childhood obesity, sexual health, risk behaviours linked to alcohol and illicit drug use, child and adolescent mental health and child vulnerability). Furthermore, we see an emerging recognition of the impact that social and environmental factors have on the child's experience of growing up in Britain today.

Population health has a troubling blind spot (as does health promotion at times) to work in the political economy that sheds light on the forces that drive health determinants.

(Raphael and Bryant 2003, p. 416)

Children are a population group in need of coherent and systematic attention but, from a public health perspective, the field is still relatively new and fresh.

To address these questions, we consider concepts of childhood alongside the function of public health practice in its efforts to improve and protect the health of children. The studies in this book focus on the four countries of the United Kingdom at the outset of the twenty-first century in its European context. But we also refer to North American models of public health practice, and we do so with reference to international comparators where appropriate or helpful.

CONTEMPORARY CHILDHOOD

We no longer presume that child labour is an acceptable feature of either the formal or informal economies in developed countries. We also argue for a child's human rights alongside adult human rights, and we have statutes to protect children from, at least, physical abuse or harm but also from demands that they 'earn their keep' by labour. To that degree, we formally seek to protect our children. Yet, children of school age in twenty-first century Britain grow up in an adult culture in which they are largely unprotected from the pressures of consumerism (advertising, publishing, purchasing pressures). Children in Britain share this profile with children in virtually all developed countries.

Furthermore, we infantilize children, while at the same time presuming that their access to adult culture is appropriate. We extend young people's financial dependence on the family into the post-schooling years while at the same time we complain of 'yob cultures' – implying the young person's responsibility to *behave well*, to behave *as an adult*. Our perspectives on child health and our concepts of childhood are contradictory and confusing. We sexualize the child's public and private environment, yet we are squeamish about providing access to effective education about sexual health.

David Hall wrote of school-age children in Britain in March 2006:

An alarmingly high proportion of our young people grow up in disrupted and unsupportive families and attend schools where bullying of all kinds is a daily occurrence, gang membership is the key to safety and mediocre education is delivered by an endless succession of supply teachers.

They live in an obesogenic environment – the lack of facilities for sport and leisure, the disappearance of family mealtimes and home cooking and the emergence of fast food all contribute. They are exposed to a constant emphasis on the desirability of early sexual activity and subtle advertising encourages the huge increase in alcohol consumption by young people. The end product of this toxic mixture is a mixture of physical and mental ill-health which is outwith the experience of mainstream medical care.

(Hall 2006, p. i)

THINKING ABOUT PUBLIC HEALTH PRACTICE

Preventable diseases can be prevented; curable ailments can certainly be cured; and controllable maladies call out for control. However, investigators tend to shy away from posing the questions in their full generosity. To confront the big picture seems like an overpowering challenge.

(Sen 2005, p. xii)

The health economist and Nobel laureate Amartya Sen has written extensively about the reticulated relationships between social and economic rights, and health and well-being. Because Sen is a health economist, he faces no explicit professional demand to look at the humanity of his subject – only to the implications of measurement. Yet his work is deeply humane. He refers to the destructive forces in international health economies as *unfreedoms*.

We have become accustomed to the presence of international child poverty, malnourishment, boy soldiers, child sexual exploitation, poor education systems, child homelessness and family breakdown.

Effective interventions to improve child health are the business of all professionals who work with children, not simply health-care workers, but we have significant difficulty in establishing what it is that makes an intervention effective – what works to improve and protect child health.

Furthermore, the very concept of public health practice resides in a concept of multiprofessional responsibility (Pencheon et al. 2006). Indeed, in Britain we can track the emergence of child public health as a concept for the organization of health and social care services and of other public services and voluntary agencies from the very end of the twenty-first century. And in only a decade, the terminology of public health has become a core part of UK practice (our downstream activities) in community nursing, in paediatrics, in housing, social care, education, youth and community work and in a plethora of child therapies, and it is now embedded in a range of government policy documents (upstream activities).

Any 'look' at the wider history of public health leads us to considerations of both a social agenda for health issues and of matters that require political action. As Kate Billingham wrote in 1997, public health is a way of 'seeing' health problems (see Chapter 5).

Essentially public health is a distinctive way of seeing health problems: public health nurses and doctors ask different questions about their practice, requiring them to look beyond individuals to populations, such as the following:

Why is this happening?

How often?

What is the social context?

Who else should be involved?

What works and what doesn't?

They also make different connections: between one individual and another, between individuals and communities, between individuals and social structures, between the stories that people tell them and the epidemiological evidence, between health services and other agencies, between medical and social models of health and between health and social policies … [they] tend to have a commitment to a set of values based on equity, justice and work for social change at local and national levels.

(Billingham 1997, p. 271)

THEORIES UNDERPINNING CONTEMPORARY PUBLIC HEALTH

Public health practitioners work from a social perspective on population-level approaches to health and well-being. And in order to make a difference, such perspectives are inevitably driven by political argument. For many public health practitioners, the political push behind their work may be sufficiently muted as to be unconscious. Indeed, public health practitioners tend to work within *the present*, with little knowledge of the history or politics that inform their daily work. One purpose of this book is to provide context of this kind to support the multiprofessional and multidisciplinary work of public health practitioners.

Public health practice has a political dimension, whether that is implicit or explicit within individual workforce planning. It is also based within concepts of social justice. Unlike basic scientific medical research, public health practice is embedded in social interpretations of medical data. This means, for example, that arguments premised on social justice have to be proved. It is insufficient to cite social justice as uncontested territory. It is necessary to make the case and to expose the contradictions we find both in human behaviour and in social and economic policies deriving from national governments.

A number of theorists in Britain (e.g. Wilkinson 1996; Bartley 2004; Marmot et al. 2004, 2010) are now articulating arguments about the causes of ill-health (socio-economic, psychosocial, life-course and political economic explanations). Most of these, with the exception of life-course theories, do not yet specify child health separately from analyses of national and local population health comparators.

However, with the contemporary shift in public health focus from conventional analyses of disease and disorder incidence to a strengthened focus on the social determinants of health, not only have analysts highlighted the vast inequalities in health but also recent work has particularly focused on the damaging political and economic systems that govern people's lives and their health.

Poor health tends to cluster in poor communities.

(Coburn 2003, p. 338)

For example, when epidemiologists measure health at the neighbourhood level within a national population, they find that countries with highly competitive economic structures (e.g. relatively unrestrained market economies) have far greater divergence in health outcomes than do societies based on a social imperative to equalize income (Kawachi et al. 1996; Levins 2003). These analyses coincide with, but also go beyond the theories of Marmot (2004) and Wilkinson (1996), the predominating theorists behind British health policy at the outset of the twenty-first century. The implications of such arguments press us to think about the determinants of public health from perspectives that question political economies and national government policy direction (Hofrichter 2003).

In other words, we are beginning to see debates about health inequalities and about social cohesion that challenge more deeply our recent presumptions that income differentials alone are the key determinants of poor health. These debates will matter for child public health practitioners as we move further into the twenty-first century.

UNDERSTANDING THE SUBJECT

This book is written in a context of debate about (1) the definition of health; (2) the determinants of poor health and (3) the priorities for child health in the United Kingdom and across national borders.

As with any centennial moment in history, the twenty-first century has had about it a tone of 'new' perspectives and 'new' insights into what constitutes health and well-being, and how health might be improved. When we think of children, for example, it is helpful to move to the most current health debates. Contemporary debates tend to articulate health determinants in terms of the relative importance of three factors: genetic inheritance, personal lifestyle behaviours and structural factors, including family income differentials. These are the three key determinants of health that are used to justify and to explain the vertical relationship between local and national service delivery and policy-planning decisions as they affect population health.

It is worth our while to think about each of these in turn. For example, the genetic profile is only a single component in any explanation of health status and it matters, not only in terms of itself alone but also in terms of the larger social environment. Skin pigmentation is a useful illustration. This entirely trivial genetic marker matters primarily because of social responses to skin colour within cultures. And a genetic susceptibility to cancer, in turn, is only important if the environmental factors are in place to trigger it (Levins 2003, p. 379). In other words, our predilection for seeking 'cause' often leads us to over-simplification of concepts of cause.

Health-related behaviours, in contrast, are the primary areas in which public health practitioners seek to intervene, but individual human choices are always made from alternatives and within contexts of opportunities. 'Choice' is heavily inscribed by information, knowledge and opportunity.

England, for example, largely (though not wholly) positions its health policy in terms of a focus on individual lifestyle and health-related behaviours (Department of Health 2004) and also on measures of cost-effectiveness (Wanless 2001). And the current direction of debate about the *obesity epidemic* amongst children is a salutary example of what is often referred to as the dangers inherent in context stripping. In other words, weighing and measuring children at school is a valuable tool for epidemiological data gathering. But we need to ask a question about resource distribution, given the multiple factors that need to be addressed by public health practitioners if we are to reverse the current trend in childhood obesity.

In *Child Public Health*, Blair et al. (2003) signal the shortcomings of context-free public health initiatives by constructing a scenario for public health practice in its efforts to address childhood obesity (pp. 237–242).

MAKING A DIFFERENCE

In other words, most contemporary debates are about what causes ill-health. It is the field of health determinants that draws greatest attention from critical analysts. How to improve poor health is, however, an altogether more difficult matter.

In addition, we are only at the starting gate when we ask ourselves what we mean by *health and well-being*. The definitional problems behind these concepts are culturally as well as historically shaped. *Every Child Matters: Change for Children* (Department for Education and Skills 2004) and *Healthy Lives, Healthy People* (Department of Health 2013) provide us with the closest definitional response we have yet achieved, but it is the implementation of appropriate interventions that causes us significant challenges.

This book is a close examination of the *practice* of public health and it orientates the concept of *practice* as one step beyond epidemiology. In other words, we examine the work of practitioners who are seeking to discover which/what kind of interventions will improve and protect the health of babies and children. We take as a given the remarkable achievements of more than a century of epidemiology in its ability to identify the locations and the causes of ill-health.

We are fortunate in being able to take such achievements for granted in the developed countries. It is not the case that epidemiology plays such a sophisticated role as a support for health system design in transition economies (e.g. many of the countries emerging from the post-Soviet period) or in the developing countries.

This book is about public health practice that relies on the findings of epidemiology as its starting point. By *public health*, the contributors mean to include (1) the principles that underlie the discipline of public health; (2) the theories that seek to explain the causes (determinants) of ill-health within populations; (3) the practices that seek to develop effective interventions for the improvement and protection of health and (4) the policies that steer public health practice at any particular historical point and in any particular geographic area.

The conundrum that arises from that perspective, however, is the question of how we link epidemiology, which is a classic system of measurement of disease and disorders, to children's health needs, which often do not necessarily start from 'ill-health'. How do we position children's health needs in terms of exogenous rather than endogenous descriptors.

The great public health pioneers of Europe and North America, for example, have always been concerned with finding the causes of ill-health – what we now refer to as the determinants of health. In so doing, they have also been concerned with how to bring about social and environmental change that can remove those causes.

John Snow was a London general practitioner, whose practice was at the centre of a cholera epidemic in 1854. More than 500 people died in 10 days within a 250 yard radius of Broad Street. By plotting the geographic area, John Snow deduced that the Broad Street pump was the transmission point for infection, and he removed the pump handle (Blair et al. 2003, p. 8).

In John Snow's case, his deductive reasoning led him to an experimental action that stopped the spread of infection. In contemporary terms, it is in the understanding of what makes a public health intervention effective that we discover the most difficult challenges for contemporary public health practitioners. And we find that the contemporary field of public health practice abounds with such examples of health and social care workers experimenting with interventions at just such a local level. Yet we have too little knowledge of the effectiveness of these experiments. We know too little about 'what works'.

The difficulty, however, is in proving the effectiveness of any particular intervention. We need to know if X intervention actually caused Y to change. A further difficulty lies in transferring practice from one location to another and in ascribing outcomes to specific actions (the external validity question). Indeed, there is a kind of swashbuckling heroism in the work of these early public health practitioners.

LOOKING TO HISTORY

In Europe, public health pioneers emerged in response to urban industrialization in the eighteenth and nineteenth centuries and were, from the outset, concerned with finding the causes of ill-health. Their desire, individually and collectively, was always and continues to be a determination to bring about change that can remove the causes of ill-health – social, material, environmental, even political causes of preventable illness, disease or early death. The great public health pioneers have always been change agents. And change agents of this kind are inevitably at the forefront of controversy, and particularly so when change requires large-scale investment or population interventions that run counter to dominant social patterns of behaviour.

For example, the nineteenth century sanitation movement was not achieved without struggle. The cost of engineering drains for entire national populations has always been and continues to be high – vide the contemporary developing world. Conquering the spread of preventable infectious disease by means of universal vaccination was no less radical a step in the work of public health specialists. Indeed, Edward Jenner (1749–1823) enabled the revolutionary development of an effective smallpox vaccination by using entirely unethical means – if assessed by contemporary guidelines. And, arguably, the eventual success of vaccination to protect against infectious diseases relied on the mid-twentieth century rise of welfare state economies in developed countries. Indeed, we still measure general child health within a national context in terms of a nation's ability to ensure vaccination rates.

Now, at the beginning of the twenty-first century, we talk mainly about health inequalities, and the field of debate for the past decade has been focused on understanding the determinants of health and of ill-health as they appear to be a consequence of social and material inequalities within and across national borders. That material deprivation is damaging to health is not in itself a matter of dispute, nor are socio-economic inequalities new. However, why such health inequalities appear to have become increasingly intractable and what needs to be done are matters of considerable debate. For example, the 'war on poverty' and on child poverty is by now familiar. However, national governments do not generally address the issue in terms of income redistribution. Such thinking is mainly absent from the twenty-first century geopolitical thinking. The main exceptions are Cuba, some parts of South America and, to a degree, the Nordic European countries.

But in the twenty-first century, can we realistically identify the mechanisms that produce compromised health as an outcome of material inequality? Do we understand why material deprivation is so intransigent, not only in the developed countries but also particularly in developing and transitional economies, which are, in fact, the homes for roughly 85% of the world's child population? Furthermore, what are the practical interventions that public health practitioners identify that they believe will make a beneficial difference to child health? And how are such interventions designed, how are they practised and what evidence do we have that particular interventions are effective? In the chapters below, these questions are approached with a view to indicating for us some of the challenges that contemporary public health practitioners are encountering, particularly in the four countries of the United Kingdom.

FEATURES OF PUBLIC HEALTH THINKING

Epidemiological measurement, a discipline now more than a century old, is fully capable of identifying the locations and profiles of mortality and morbidity. What such measurement cannot do is tell us how to reverse the profiles of damage, which can be traced to the complex interaction between location, social relationships, material wealth or want and individual decision making about health-related behaviours. Indeed, national political policy direction combined with the operation of macro-economies by nation states can itself be a cause of ill-health or early death (see Hofrichter 2003).

In the United Kingdom, as is the case internationally, it is material poverty that has become the primary focus of attention in health-improvement debates. Where children are concerned, the current child public health policy position has derived largely from life-course theories of health inequalities, which result in arguments for targeted investment in maternal, neonatal and pre-school investment in child health. The Sure Start programmes in the United Kingdom (relatively recent) and Head Start in the United States (dating from 1962) are powerful examples of government policy based on a theory of health inequalities – in these cases, life-course theories. Cowley's work below (Chapter 5) explores these questions in considerable depth.

But the school-age years, in contrast, have trailed behind as a public health subject in terms of financial investment and human resource in both the United Kingdom and the United States.

It is worth thinking about this from a public health measurement perspective. In simple terms, there are two points of measurement that historically have been able to capture a population profile of health status – records of births and deaths (in those countries where these are registered). Thus, we derive *average life expectancy* as an indicator of a whole population's health status.

Of course, no individual is a statistic, nor indeed is a total community's life expectancy inextricably linked to a statistic. These are indicators of underlying health factors and it is the underlying factors that we need to extricate from our explanatory models. What can happen in simple figures of mortality, for example, is the accidental omission of the school-age childhood stage – given our collective assessment of health in terms of neonatal survival (birth to age 5 years) and in terms of adult health as related to mortality and morbidity rates.

Furthermore, the most difficult health field to understand via measurement is the area of long-term conditions and complex illness. These are health problems in which people do not generally feel ill in the sense that acute events are about 'illness'. In the school-age years, however, long-term conditions can be difficult to manage in terms of healthcare, because of developmental changes in the child's height and weight over more than a decade of growth. Long-term conditions are also complicating factors in the child's emotional and intellectual development and in the child's adaptation to his or her environment.

Furthermore, long-term conditions also generate social and environmental challenges in the settings children inhabit – the family, the school, the community neighbourhood. Since the mid-1980s, Britain has moved, more or less efficiently, towards principles of inclusive education, which means that the school setting is theoretically required to accommodate child health needs. This represents a radical conceptual change about child health, ability and disability in educational planning in less than three decades. Yet the consequences for the child in the school setting are not yet resolved and these issues are explored in Chapter 7.

MAKING HEALTHY CHOICES: WHAT DOES THIS MEAN FOR CHILDHOOD?

At the same time, a parallel policy focus on individual *lifestyle* choices about health behaviours has become a pronounced explanatory system and a particular focus of government policy in Britain in the past decade. What constitutes *choice* about health-related behaviours is not, however, straightforward.

Indeed, most practical health-promotion initiatives focus precisely on the design of interventions that are believed to have a capacity to change health-related risk behaviours (e.g. seat belt legislation, tobacco control, sexual health education, 'five a day' vegetables in nutrition), and are believed to have a capacity to change individual decision making about health-related behaviour choices.

This focus on health-sustaining behaviours has become a focus for contemporary government policies in most developed countries.

It is important to note that transfer of responsibility for health from the state to the person can be argued to be a way of reducing the financial burden of ill-health on government budgets. In other words, the balance between enabling or supporting *healthy decisions* amongst the populace on the one hand and investing government funds in health-improvement interventions on the other hand is complex. In addition, every intervention to improve population health must itself be tested for effectiveness. This is a research burden representing considerable cost even before factoring in both the financial and the political costs of funding population-level interventions.

On the other hand, it is also valid to argue that helping to *enable* people to make personal choices that sustain their own health is an indication of a mature democracy. But *choice*, as we have already noted, is heavily inflected by material and psychological factors that reside outside notions of individual agency. We might even go further, with some confidence, and suggest that children are much more severely constrained in matters of choice than are adults.

THINKING ABOUT SOCIAL POLICY

One of the tasks of this book is to analyse the mechanisms (their theoretical underpinnings) that drive a contemporary health policy that is specifically designed to improve the health of babies, children and young people. What presumptions do we make that lie behind our health and social care policies and our public health interventions?

Any 'look' at the history of public health leads us to considerations of both a social agenda for health issues and of matters that require political action, a way of 'seeing' that encourages us to act.

This book is organized into five parts as a means for exploring these issues. Part I (Chapters 1 through 4) sets the context for public health practice for babies, children and young people. Chapters 2 and 3 investigate the legal context for health in the four countries of the United Kingdom and the issues arising from difference and diversity between children. Chapter 4 places child protection in a public health context.

Parts II (Chapters 5 and 6), III (Chapter 7) and IV (Chapters 8 and 9) locate child health within the three settings in which the child experiences growth and development – the family, the school and the local community and neighbourhood.

Part V (Chapters 10 and 11) investigates two of the key health issues affecting contemporary children and young people.

SUMMARY

This book explores public health practice with babies, children and young people. It brings together insights and debates from across diverse disciplines in order to ask questions about the health of our children and young people and about our strategies and practices for improving and protecting their health. Blair et al. in 2003 commented that 'child health is emerging – or perhaps re-emerging – as a speciality of public health' (p. 3). In this book, we have expanded these early observations by Blair, by Cowley and by DeBell (2007).

What do we know? What questions do we need to ask? How do we work across professional, departmental and interest-focused boundaries in order to improve child and adolescent health?

In just over a decade, the principles of public health have become a core part of practice in community nursing, in paediatrics, in housing, social care, education, youth and community work, the youth justice system and in the work of voluntary and charitable bodies (our downstream activities). And public health is at the heart of government policy across a range of departments (our upstream activities). In 2013, public health services in England moved to local authority management and resourcing. From October 2015, local authorities were given full responsibility for children's public health.

Public health practice is inter-professional work at its most demanding, and it involves all these actors working together – not an easy agenda. Pencheon et al. (2006) refer to the 'eternal verities of public health, in disease prevention, communicable disease control, health protection, and health promotion' (p. xxxi). This book explores these concepts but it does so by placing the baby, child and young person in a social, economic and political context.

Many practitioners tell us that they are still unclear about what a public health approach actually means. Billingham in 1997 referred to is as a way of 'seeing'. And by this she was referring to the connections that public health practitioners make between the individual and the population.

It is, if anything, a reflection of the challenges we confront that inter-professional working can, at times, be so very difficult. How to improve and protect the health of children and young people is a challenge that this book addresses, and to achieve that means highlighting, indeed repeating the inter-professional agenda.

The book is divided into five parts, three of which locate the child in the main settings in which children grow up and develop – the family (Chapters 5 and 6); the school (Chapter 7) and the local community and neighbourhood (Chapters 8 and 9).

KEY POINTS

* This book is about public health practice and children from birth to adolescence.
* Public health practice arises from a way of 'seeing' the child or young person within a context and an environment, as part of a population profile.

- During the early years and the school-aged years, the child experiences a long period of growth and development in which we need to make connections between the child's experiences at home, at school and in the local community or neighbourhood.
- Public health practice involves finding strategies to protect and improve health, and for families, children and young people. Public health practice involves inter-professional development and cross-agency working at its most demanding.
- Public health practitioners ask themselves difficult questions about their practice. How can I design effective interventions? Who do I need to include in my work? How do I know what works? And, is what I am doing making a difference?

REFERENCES

Bartley M. (2004) *Health Inequality: An Introduction to Theories, Concepts and Methods.* Cambridge and Oxford, UK: Polity Press.

Billingham K. (1997) Public health nursing in primary care. *British Journal of Community Health Nursing* 2: 270–274.

Blair M, Stewart-Brown S, Waterston T, Crowther R. (2003) *Child Public Health.* Oxford, UK: Oxford University Press.

Coburn D. (2003) Income inequality, social cohesion, and the health status of populations: the role of neo-liberalism. In: Hofrichter R (ed.). *Health and Social Justice: Politics, Ideology, and Inequity in the Distribution of Disease. A Public Health Reader.* San Francisco, CA: Jossey-Bass, pp. 335–355.

Cowley S. (ed) (2002) *Public Health in Policy and Practice: A Sourcebook for Health Visitors and Community Nurses.* London: Ballière Tindall.

Cowley S. (ed) (2007) *Public Health in Policy and Practice: A Sourcebook* (2nd edition). Edinburgh, Scotland: Elsevier.

Currie C, Zanotti C, Morgan A, et al. (2012) Social determinants of health and well-being among young people. *Health Behaviour in School-aged Children (HBSC) Study: International report from the 2009/10 survey.* Copenhagen World Health Organization Regional Office for Europe.

DeBell D. (2003) *Starting Where they are Project: Supporting Young People with a Prisoner in the Family.* London: Action for Prisoners' Families.

DeBell D. (2007) *Public Health Practice and the School-Age Population.* London: Hodder Arnold.

Department for Education and Skills. (2004) *Every Child Matters: Change for Children.* Nottingham, England: DfES Publications.

Department of Health. (2004) *Choosing Health. Making Healthier Choices Easier.* London: Department of Health.

Department of Health. (2013) *Healthy Lives, Healthy People.* London: Department of Health.

Department of Health and Department for Education and Skills. (2004) *The National Service Framework for Children, Young People and Maternity Services.* London: Department of Health. www.dh.gov.uk/PolicyAndGuidance/HealthAndSocialCareTopics/ChildrenServices/ChildrenServicesInformation/ChildrenServicesInformationArticle/fs/en?CONTENT_ID=4089111&chk=U8Ecln (accessed 17 January 2007).

Donald A. (2006) Facilitating community action. In: Pencheon D, Guest C, Melzer D, Muir Gray JA (eds). *Oxford Handbook of Public Health Practice* (2nd edition). Oxford, UK: Oxford University Press, pp. 240–246.

Hall DMB. (2006) Foreword. In: DeBell D, Tomkins A (eds). *Discovering the Future of School Nursing: An Evidence Base for Practice.* London: McMillan-Scott, p. i.

Hall DMB, Elliman D. (2003) *Health for All Children* (4th edition). Oxford, UK: Oxford University Press.

Hofrichter R. (2003) The politics of health inequities: Contested terrain. In: Hofrichter R (ed). *Health and Social Justice: Politics, Ideology, and Inequities in the Distribution of Disease. A Public Health Reader.* San Francisco, CA: Jossey-Bass, pp. 1–56.

Kawachi I, Kennedy BP, Lochner K, Prothrow-Stith D. (1997) Social capital, income inequality, and mortality. *American Journal of Public Health* 87: 1491–1498.

Levins R. (2003) Is capitalism a disease? The crisis in US public health. In: Hofrichter R. (ed.) *Health and Social Justice: Politics, Ideology, and Inequities in the Distribution of Disease. A Public Health Reader.* San Francisco, CA: Jossey-Bass, pp. 365–384.

Marmot M. (2004) *Status Syndrome.* London: Bloomsbury Publishing.

Marmot M, Allen J, Goldblatt P, et al. (2010) *Strategic Review of Health Inequalities in England post-2010 (The Marmot Review).* London: University College London.

Marmot M, Stansfeld S, Patel C, et al. (1991) Health inequalities among British civil servants: the Whitehall II study. *Lancet* 337: 1387–1393.

Meltzer H, Green H, McGinnity A, et al. (2005) *The Mental Health of Children and Young People in Great Britain 2004.* London: Office for National Statistics.

Pencheon D, Guest C, Melzer D, Muir Gray JA. (2006) *Oxford Handbook of Public Health Practice* (2nd edition). Oxford, UK: Oxford University Press.

Raphael D, Bryant T. (2003) The limitations of population health as a model for a new public health. In: Hofrichter R (ed.). *Health and Social Justice: Politics, Ideology, and Inequities in the Distribution of Disease. A Public Health Reader.* San Francisco, CA: Jossey-Bass, pp. 410–427.

Santelli JS, Baldwin W, Heitel J. (2015) Rising wealth, improving health? Adolescents and inequality. *Lancet* 385: 2088.

Sen A. (2005) Foreword. In: Farmer P (ed.). *Pathologies of Power: Health, Human Rights, and the New War on the Poor.* Berkeley, CA and London: University of California Press Ltd, pp. xi–xvii.

Wanless D. (2001) *Securing our Future Health: Taking a Long-Term View. An Interim Report.* London: HM Treasury.

Wilkinson RG. (1996) *Unhealthy Societies: The Afflictions of Inequality.* London: Routledge.

Wolfe I, Thompson M, Gill P et al. (2013) Health services for children in Western Europe. *The Lancet* online http://dx.doi.org/10.1016.S0140-6736(12)62085-6. Accessed 28 August 2015.

WEBSITE

YoungMinds (2007) www.youngminds.org.uk (accessed 5 February 2007).

ACTS OF PARLIAMENT

These acts are published by Her Majesty's Stationery Office in London and can be accessed from the UK Parliament website (www.publications.parliament.uk).

The Children Act 2004
Children and Families Act 2014

Children and young people's health: A legal context

2

LESLIE GELLING

INTRODUCTION

Even the briefest consideration of children's and young people's health would be incomplete without an analysis of the many complex legal and ethical issues. The provision of health and social care and the requirements of the law have become inextricably linked to the extent that legal issues are central to the work of all health and social care practitioners. Most importantly, arguments about who should be involved in decision-making and who can give informed consent, or refuse consent, have been central to the legal and ethical debate and, therefore, the practice of health and social care practitioners.

The law, especially family law, does not exist in a static state. Rather, it reflects changes in social and cultural attitudes (Bainham 2005). In addition, it is important to consider the many rapidly changing demographic factors. For example, during the past half-century there has been a gradual erosion of family networks and the very nature of what constitutes a family. This has been influenced by a growth in the acceptability of divorce, remarriage and co-habitation outside marriage. Such cultural changes, together with greater appreciation of the fundamental human rights of young people, have changed the whole of the climate in which young people live in developed countries. This change has impacted upon the children, their families and those caring for them.

There can be no doubt that the relationship between the legal capacity of young people and the obligations placed upon those with parental responsibility have been fashioned within the context of medical decision-making:

> This is not really surprising since the health of children is self-evidently the most basic and essential consideration in protecting their welfare.

(Bainham 2005, p. 309)

This chapter considers the legal issues and how they relate to young people's health in general but this will inevitably result in a detailed consideration of how young people are involved in decision-making and the role they might play in giving or withholding informed consent. It is important to note that this chapter will not examine the requirement for informed consent to participation in research, which raises many additional complex theoretical, legal and practical dilemmas that are outside the remit of this chapter.

BACKGROUND

First it is important to review the background to the current legal situation in the UK by considering the historical perspective. In doing so, the reader will develop a better understanding of how we have got to where we are today. Although health and social care practitioners grapple with this complex and challenging legal framework every day, this is undoubtedly preferable to where we were at the start of the twentieth century or earlier.

The rights of children and young people* have moved a long way since young people were considered the property of adults and were treated and used as the adults saw fit. This frequently meant that young people were uneducated, had to work to bring much needed income into the household, experienced poor levels of health and were not involved in any decisions about any aspect of their lives. In recent years young people's rights have developed alongside those of consumers of health and social care services but young people have frequently been left off the agenda (Freeman 1993). For example, there was no reference to young people in *The Patient's Charter†* and although *The Health of the Nation‡* stressed the importance of infant and child health, it did so with the aim of achieving success in attaining targets rather than assuring individual rights for young people (Moules 2006).

In considering the background to the current legal situation it is evident that there are still wide ranging opinions that range from a Liberationist view, which propose that young people should have equal rights with adults and have greater decision-making capacity than widely believed in today's society. And, in contrast, a paternalistic view, which argues that young people are incompetent to make decisions for themselves and require adults to protect them and, hence, make decisions for them. In reality and within legal restraints, most young people are treated as being at some point between these extremes. This chapter provides the briefest introduction to the key legal requirements that are relevant to young people's health and their rights.

Involving young people in decisions about their lives is now accepted as an integral component in the delivery of health and social care. This approach is believed to promote self-esteem, increase compliance and, therefore, promote improved health. The notion of rights for young people is, however, a relatively new concept that has its roots in the 1924 *Declaration of Geneva§* in which it states that 'mankind owes to the child the best it has to give'. The Declaration was based on six core principles with an emphasis on protection of the young person with little

* To avoid unnecessary repetition, the term *young people* will be used to mean 'children and young people' for the remainder of this chapter.
† Launched by the National Health Service (NHS) in 1991 and updated in 1995, *The Patient's Charter* was an attempt to set standards for patient care. The Charter was all about the quality of services offered in NHS hospitals and community health organisations. *Patient's Charter: Services for Children and Young People* was not published until 1996.
‡ Between 1992 and 1997 *The Health of the Nation* strategy was the central plank of health policy in England and formed the context for planning of services delivered by the NHS.
§ The *Declaration of Geneva*, also adopted by the League of Nations in 1924, resulted largely from the efforts of the British child's rights pioneer Eglantyne Jebb.

regard for their right to participate in decision-making (Moules 2006). This demonstrated a paternalistic attitude, common at the time, in which adults were believed to be the defenders of young people who were incompetent to make decisions for themselves (Freeman 1983). The Declaration reflected the social circumstances at the time with an emphasis on ensuring that young people were fed and not allowed to go hungry. Clear in the Declaration was the require-ment that all decisions about a young person's health care should be controlled by adults and seldom, if ever, involve a young person in the decision-making process.

The *Children and Young Person Act 1933**[*] took this one step further in the UK and made it a criminal offence not to take the necessary action to protect young people from harm or to take any action that might cause harm to a young person. The Act imposed a minimum standard of medical care on those with parental responsibility. Again, the emphasis was on what was required of parents rather than on the rights of young people.

In the 1950s, the United Nation's *Declaration on the Rights of the Child*[†] further widened the debate on the rights of young people. Despite this, the Declaration still failed to acknowledge that young people had the right to act in an autonomous manner and the focus was again on the adult's responsibility to ensure welfare and protection (Freeman 1983; Moules 2006). This Declaration did, however, take the discussion about the rights of young people further forward by placing the debate firmly in an international context and placing obligations on members of the United Nations.

In the 1960s, there was greater recognition that protecting society from juvenile delinquency and the aim of helping young people were essentially complementary. It was also increasingly uncommon to classify young people into one of two groups, the deprived and the depraved (Bainham 2005). The *Children and Young Person's Act 1969* was heavily influenced by these changing views and moved the focus slightly from only protecting young people to assisting them to become members of society.

The *Family Law Act 1969* set a presumptive standard that young people aged 16 and 17 years old in the UK are presumed to be competent unless it could be demonstrated otherwise. This is based on the assumption that 16 and 17-year-olds were competent if they could understand and retain information and were able to weigh up that information and the likely consequences of any decision they might make. Considering age in this way demonstrated a growing apprecia-tion of the need to treat young people as having different levels of competence. It was no longer acceptable to treat all young people, from newborn to 17, in the same way.

In a landmark decision, in 1980 the Department of Health and Social Security for the UK issued a notice making it lawful for doctors to give contraception and advice to girls under the age of 16. Most importantly, this was allowed without involving the parents and without obtaining their prior consent. This decision was justified on the grounds that the doctors would be acting in the young person's best interests by protecting them from the harmful effects of sexual intercourse. Victoria Gillick, the mother of five girls under the age of 16, sought assur-ances, from her area health authority, that her daughters would not receive such treatment without her permission. This resulted in considerable legal argument during which Victoria Gillick initially lost her case, then had the decision overturned in the Court of Appeal and ulti-mately lost again in the House of Lords[‡].

[*] See www.swarb.co.uk/acts/1933CaYPAct.shtml.
[†] See www.unhchr.ch/html/menu3/b/25.htm.
[‡] Victoria Gillick v West Norfolk and Wisbech Health Authority and Department of Health and Social Security.

The House of Lords held that young people, under the age of 16, could give consent to contraceptive advice without their parent's knowledge or consent providing they could demonstrate sufficient maturity and intelligence to understand the proposed treatment. Although the focus of this legal case was on contraceptive advice and treatment, the resulting legal ruling applied to all medical treatment and was a landmark decision acknowledging the right of young people to take some control of their own health care and introduced the concept of 'Gillick competence', assessed using the following Fraser Guidelines[*]:

- That the young person understands the health professional's advice
- That the professional cannot persuade the young person to inform his or her parent or allow the doctor to inform the parents that he or she is seeking contraceptive advice
- That the young person is very likely to begin or continue having intercourse with or without contraceptive treatment
- That without receiving contraceptive advice or treatment, the young person's physical or mental health or both are likely to suffer
- That the young person's best interests require the health professional to give contraceptive advice, treatment or both without parental consent

The test of Gillick competence became widely used but there was, and remains, considerable debate about what the concept actually means and what level of competence is required to make important decisions about one's own health. The debate was inevitable because competence varies enormously and is dependent on multiple complex factors, including the nature of the proposed treatment, peer pressure and the family environment (Hendrick 2006). It is clear, however, that the rights of young people received a major boost In the UK as a result of the decision made by the House of Lords. The test of Gillick competence had enabled a large number of young people to participate in decision-making about their own health care.

The United Nation's *Convention on the Rights of Children* (1989)[†], ratified in the UK in 1991, has been described as the most authoritative and comprehensive landmark statement of the fundamental rights of young people until that point in time (Bainham 2005). Unlike so many other Conventions and legal provisions, this Convention was universally welcomed and it was signed up to more rapidly and by more countries than any other international instrument (Hendrick 2006). The Convention was the world's first international legal instrument to focus on young people's rights and was based on the following three core principles:

1. Young people have special needs which set them apart from adults.
2. The best environment for a child's development is within a protective and nurturing family.
3. Governments and the adult world in general should be committed to acting in the best interests of the child.

As these principles suggest, the aims and general obligations of the Convention were prevention, protection, provision and participation. In line with the fourth 'p', Article 12 of the Convention set out to assure respect for a young person's views:

> . . . the child who is capable of forming his own views (has) the right to express those views freely in all matters affecting the child, the views of the child being given due weight in accordance with the age and maturity of the child.

(Article 12)

---

[*] Lord Fraser overturned the Gillick ruling in the House of Lords in 1985 and suggested criteria for best practice for health and social care practitioners.

[†] www.unicef.org/crc/

There is, however, a clear and obvious conflict between Article 12, which stresses that young people should be heard, and Article 3, which stresses protection and care with an emphasis on the rights of parents and guardians. Requiring that young people should be heard need not necessarily influence the final decision. Indeed, it could be argued that nothing the young person might say will influence the final decision if the adult does not believe it to be in the young person's best interests. Unlike the later European Convention on Human Rights, this Convention did not result in significant changes to English law but it did establish the important principle that the young person's voice should be heard.

When the *Children Act 1989** was passed, coming into force in October 1991, it was hailed as a *children's charter* because it appeared to give young people the absolute right to provide informed consent and informed refusal. The Act pulled together much of the complex and technical law that had grown up during the preceding decades (Bainham 2005). This new legislation replaced existing law governing the custody and the upbringing of young people and the public law applying to Social Services. In addition, the *Children and Young Persons Act 1969* and the *Magistrates' Court Act 1978* were significantly amended in the UK. More than any preceding legislation, the Act highlighted a young person's right to autonomy and acknowledged their independent status. In doing so, the Act legitimized young people as individuals rather than as objects of concern (Hendrick 2006). Importantly, young people were now allowed to challenge, through the courts, decisions made about their care. For the first time it seemed that young people would truly have a say in decisions about their own care. In reality, however, this has been extremely rare because courts are able to filter out cases in which they believe the young person lacks the necessary understanding of the situation. This filtering process was contrary to the objectives of the Act and again placed the onus of responsibility for decision-making with those possessing parental responsibility.

The Act attempted to strike a balance between the role of the state, the rights of young people and the responsibilities of parents. To do this, the Act was founded on three fundamental principles. The first, the welfare principle, emphasized the need to ensure that the interests of young people should be the paramount consideration. The second principle, the primacy of the family, was based on the belief that the best place for young people to grow up is within their family and that the state should only intervene when it is absolutely necessary. The third and final principle, the young person's voice, set out to enhance the young person's legal status and their capacity for independent action. This was to be achieved by giving young people greater rights to have their views taken into account when making decisions about their health care. This final principle potentially marked a further move away from the prevailing notion of paternalism, a notion that had been enshrined in much of the preceding legislation. As with the United Nation's *Convention on the Rights of the Child*, however, this right to express their views and to have them taken into account only stretched as far as it was deemed not to be interfering with the young person's best interests by those with parental responsibility.

The welfare principle was the main consideration in the Act and was described as the only consideration in any court decision. The Act broke new ground in that it incorporated a statutory checklist of factors that a court should consider when applying the welfare principle. It was not long, however, before the courts demonstrated a willingness to place greater emphasis on the notion of protection and less on hearing the views of young people. In doing so, the courts undermined the clear intentions of the Act (Hendrick 2006). Most clearly, the young person's right to refuse treatment was not upheld by the courts. The Act has also been

* See www.opsi.gov.uk/acts/acts1989/Ukpga_19890041_en_1.htm.

criticized for not achieving all that it might have done, for privatising the family, for not obliging parents to involve young people in decision-making and for not providing sufficient protection for young people (Fortin 2003; Hendrick 2006; Moules 2006). Such criticisms might help to explain why the child protection framework has required so much amendment in the *Children Act 2004**.

The *European Convention for the Protection of Human Rights and Fundamental Freedoms*[†] was ratified as the *Human Rights Act 1998*[‡], implemented in October 2000. The Act resulted in major change in the way cases would be argued in court (Bainham 2005). Although the provisions of the Act altered very few decisions, there had to be greater consideration of the young person's human rights, including the right to be involved in decisions affecting the young person's life.

The Green Paper *Every Child Matters*[§] outlined proposals for information sharing systems in the UK, holding basic information on all young people with practitioners able to indicate that they were providing a service to a young person and, where appropriate, that they had a concern about a young person. The *Children Act 2004* provided the legal framework to enable practitioners to share early information to ensure that young people and families are getting benefit from services such as education and basic health care and to enable them to get the support they need at the right time. In particular, the Act contained provision for the creation and operation of a secure professionally maintained information child index that might be set up at local, regional or national level or a combination thereof. In doing so, the Act provided a legislative foundation for whole-system reform to support this long-term and ambitious programme. One of the key provisions of the Act included the appointment of Children's Commissioners[¶] in each of the four countries of the UK and the establishment of structures to promote interagency cooperation and greater protection for young people. Central to the Commissioner role is the aim of ensuring that the voice of young people is heard. It is clear that although protection has remained the primary concern, the right to have one's voice heard has also been growing in significance.

Considering the complex legal and ethical background is important for health and social care practitioners because it affects every aspect of their everyday practice and every young person's health care. It also demonstrates that current legal provision has shifted the balance from paternalism to inclusion of young people in the decision-making process while retaining the paramount requirement to protect the young person.

YOUNG PEOPLE'S RIGHTS

The whole issue of young people's rights has always been extremely complex. As demonstrated above, much legislation has set out to clarify the rights of young people but this has not always been the outcome. Rather, legislation has highlighted a clear conflict between a young person's rights and the obligations placed on others to provide protection.

Possessing a right requires action or restraint from others and justification for rights are based on either legal or moral principles (Gillon 1985). Legal rights are created by national governments which are based on what is considered right and wrong according to the law.

---

* See www.opsi.gov.uk/acts/acts2004/20040031.htm.

[†] See www.conventions.coe.int/Treaty/en/Treaties/Html/005.htm.

[‡] See www.opsi.gov.uk/ACTS/acts1998/19980042.htm.

[§] See www.everychildmatters.gov.uk/_files/EBE7EEAC90382663E0D5BBF24C99A7AC.pdf.

[¶] Independent of Government, the Commissioner's remit is to promote awareness of views and interests of children.

Moral rights are based on moral principles that are intrinsically specified as *good* by a particular civil society. Universal moral rights are those that apply to all humans and stem from the one fundamental right of all 'men' to be free (Hart 1970). This places an obligation on all people to respect others' autonomy. Special moral rights are those possessed by some but not by others and usually result from prior actions such as promises or contracts. The essential difference between legal and moral rights is that legal rights can be abolished and are subject to change, according to the will of the government of the day. It has been argued that these are the only true rights that exist (Bentham 1970). It is these legal rights that can be enforced. In contrast, moral rights are intrinsically agreed as a collective *good* and are not, therefore, subject to change. The preceding section demonstrated changes to the legal status of young people's rights, marking a theoretical bridging of the gap between legal rights and moral rights.

The rights of young people have only been high on the agenda within the UK in recent years, given a particular boost by the Gillick case and the *Children Act 1989*. English law has been paternalistic or protectionist in orientation and it has been argued that this has resulted in a focus on safeguarding the welfare of young people above any consideration of their rights. The concept of young people's rights is extremely complex and cannot be looked at in a one-dimensional way (Bainham 2005). Any consideration of young people's rights should include elements of both protection and self-determination:

> It can be cogently argued that the welfare of children dictates that they are allowed a degree of self-determination or qualified autonomy.

(Bainham 2005, p. 100)

These concepts should not be considered as existing at the two extremes of a continuum. The concepts do, however, result in potential conflict between a young person's right to self-determination and their right to be protected.

The nature of young people's rights has been a matter of considerable controversy and theoretical debate. Bainham (2005) highlights three influential British theories on rights for young people that merit brief consideration here. Neil MacCormick explored 'Will theory' and 'Interest theory' (MacCormick 1984). 'Will theory' was based on the notion that to possess a right one has to be able to exercise individual choice over enforcement by others. The essence of this theory is the pre-eminence of the right-holder's will over the will of others. The 'Interest theory' focuses on the protection of an individual's interests by imposing duties on others. The critical difference between the two theories is that the 'Will theory' involves the capacity for individual autonomy whereas in the 'Interest theory' it is sufficient for the existence of a right that there is an identifiable interest and a corresponding duty (MacCormick 1984). This suggests that the 'Interest theory' is more relevant to a consideration of young people's rights than the 'Will theory' because law dictates that although young people's opinions should be taken into account, it is the will of others, those with parental responsibility, who will ultimately make or legitimize the decision.

In the second theory John Eekelaar, like MacCormick, focused on the interest theory of rights but places particular emphasis on the need to ensure that an individual's interests are capable of being isolated from the interests of others (Eekelaar 1986). When considering the rights of young people this is extremely complicated because a parent has the legal power to make decisions for a young person and this power is exercised in the young person's best interests or based in the welfare principle. This is problematic because the young person's interests will not always be identical to the parent's interests. Eekelaar argues that because no young person can claim parental independence, a young person's principle right should be to have the best medical decisions made for them by someone with parental responsibility. This paternalistic approach is also extended to young people who are perceived to be competent because Eekelaar suggests two limitations that restrict a young person's right to make decisions and have them respected. First, the decision should be compatible with the general law and the interests of others. Second, the young person should not make a decision that is contrary to his or her physical or mental well-being. This again suggests that a competent young person is only allowed to make a decision if those with parental responsibility concur with that decision.

In the third theory, Michael Freeman adopted a more practical approach and focused on the need to ensure that young people have participatory rights (Freeman 1983). It was emphasized that the implementation of legal rights could become an abstract consideration of theoretical principles if the will of others is lacking to put the principles into practice. Freeman produced the following four classifications of young people's rights:

1. Rights to welfare
2. Rights to protection
3. Rights to be treated like adults
4. Rights against adults

Consideration of these individual rights results in multiple conflicts about who should be making decisions and about who has the right to overturn a decision made by a young person. This again marks a leap between the preferred situation and the real world situation faced by families and health and social care practitioners every day.

There is some common ground amongst these three theoretical perspectives. First, young people possess a fundamental human right to be involved in decision-making. Second, this right is restricted by the requirement to adhere always to the welfare principle and the need to protect the best interests of the young person. Third, this right places an obligation or duty on someone with parental responsibility to ensure that decisions are always made in the young person's best interests. These three points emphasize the need to embrace both 'qualified self-determination' and 'limited paternalism' (Bainham 2005). These theories, and others, offer some clarity about young people's rights but there remains much controversy about the basis upon which paternal or court intervention can be justified.

There is greater theoretical merit underpinning the principle that those with parental responsibility should consider what the young person would ideally want for themselves if they were sufficiently mature or competent to make the decision for themselves. In theory, this principle may require someone to balance what they believe the young person might wish in, what they perceive as, their own best interests and what the individual with parental responsibility might believe is actually in the young person's best interests, again demonstrating the potential conflict highlighted previously. In reality, it is more likely that decision-making will reflect the values and beliefs of the legal decision-maker and will be based upon what they perceive to be in the young person's best interests.

The notion of possessing rights implies the existence of legal and moral duties in someone and immediately focuses on rights that exist in the adult world. These rights will often clash with the rights that might be given to young people (Bainham 2005). One of the main problems when considering young people's rights is that they do not exist in a vacuum. They have to be considered alongside the rights and interests of others and in light of many other potential complex factors.

AUTONOMY

Obtaining informed consent to treatment requires the application of both legal and ethical principles that are founded on the central principle of respect for autonomy. Respecting a young person's autonomy or right to self-determination risks causing tension between the young person and those with parental responsibility. As already demonstrated, it can sometimes be difficult to decide when a parent's legal right to make a decision should yield to the young person's right to make their own decisions (Henricson and Bainham 2005). This is further complicated because the extent to which a young person's rights are upheld may depend on the views of the adults around them. There is a danger that an existing power relationship between an adult and a young person could result in even a well-reasoned argument being dismissed by the adult. This clearly presents a dilemma for health and social care practitioners who are obliged to encourage the young people's views to be heard but ultimately have to concede that parents probably know the young person best and are better placed to judge their competence to make important decisions. Parents may also feel uncomfortable about the notion of involving young people as active participants in decision-making (Diduck and Kaganas 2006).

Thus far in this chapter it has been demonstrated that there are three basic possibilities for making decisions, within an appropriate legal framework, about a young person's health:

- Decisions made by parents
- Decisions made by the young person
- Decisions made by outside agencies, including courts, usually to resolve disagreement between or within the above parties or when health and social care practitioners might disagree with the above decisions

These points demonstrate that, irrespective of who might be involved in the decision-making process, someone must have the final say. If at all possible, the young person's right to make autonomous decisions should be respected or they should at least have their opinions taken into account.

There are, however, a number of reasons why young people may not have their opinions taken into account (Hendrick 2006). The greatest obstacle arises from unfounded prejudices about young people's abilities and the belief that it is unwise, unkind or a waste of time to listen to young people, especially when considering complex medical or health issues. This belief has been demonstrated to be false and evidence has been provided to indicate that young people are able to make complex decisions and plan for the future (Fortin 2003). Other reasons limiting the involvement of young people in decision-making might include:

- Lack of time and resources to facilitate decision-making
- Lack of confidence, on the part of health and social care practitioners, in communicating with young people
- Lack of skill in communicating with young people
- Language barriers between the young people and adults
- Failure to recognize non-verbal communications
- Tension between adults and young people
- Need for adults to feel in control

Respecting autonomy and gaining freely given informed consent from young people is theoretically important but can also be beneficial to all involved for three main reasons

(Hendrick 2006). First, health and social care practitioners will be protected from legal action. Second, it will have beneficial therapeutic effects because it helps to secure the individual's co-operation and trust. Finally, individuals are responsible for their own decisions which promote self-esteem. Practitioners are required to be familiar with legal requirements to ensure lawful practice but they also need to be aware of the multiple benefits of promoting autonomous decision-making. Balancing these can be problematic and requires careful consideration of each situation.

AGE OF CONSENT

Defining what constitutes a 'young person' or a 'child' is a legal concept that requires detailed consideration of multiple social factors. Furthermore, as demonstrated elsewhere in this chapter, such definitions can be changed. In the *Children and Young Person's Act 1969* the status of childhood was redefined with the age of majority being reduced from 21 to 18. This is fraught with complication because young people vary considerably in their legal capacity to make certain decisions and to take certain actions with the result that a young person's competence is determined by the context in which it is being considered.

It is important that young people are not forced to make decisions against their will because respect for autonomy is not an absolute principle but is a matter of degree (Hendrick 2006). If the treatment is complex and carries serious risks, respect for autonomy might be about letting them express their opinion but the final decision will be made by the individual with parental responsibility. If the treatment is relatively minor the young person's wishes can determine the final decision in many instances. In determining a young person's competence to participate in decision-making their age will undoubtedly be taken into account.

Like the Children *and Young Peron's Act 1967,* the *Children Act 1989* defined children as those under the age of 18. These young people can be further divided into three broad age-based groups: those aged 16 and 17; those under 16 years of age and considered Gillick competent; and those under 16 years of age and not considered Gillick competent. It is generally agreed, and in accordance with the *Family Law Act 1969,* that 16 and 17-year-olds are competent to make decisions about their health and to give informed consent to treatment. Despite this, courts retain the right to their protective role and can veto this consent if it is deemed contrary to the young person's best interests. Parents do not have the same right to veto but they can act as a proxy consenter if the young person is deemed incompetent to do so.

The right to give informed consent should also carry the right to refuse to consent to an investigation or treatment but this is not straight forward in this age group. Although a young person might be considered competent, their right to informed refusal can be overruled by the courts, by their parents or by someone with parental responsibility. In such circumstances, health and social care practitioners can obtain proxy consent that overrides the young person's refusal to consent. Again, it must be demonstrated that such decisions are made in the young person's best interests. Overturning a young person's decision in this way might be lawful, but it fails to demonstrate respect for the young person's right to self-determination.

The right of a young person under the age of 16 to consent was established in the Gillick case (discussed earlier in this chapter). Young people demonstrated to be Gillick competent and meet the Fraser guidelines are assumed to be able to consent for themselves but, as with older children, they are unable to refuse consent to treatment if the decision is perceived to be against their best interests. The result is that they can be treated against their wishes. In such circumstances, the courts have stressed the need to ensure that the young person's wishes are considered but the degree to which the young person's wishes influence the final decision is unclear.

Proxy informed consent is required for young people under the age of 16 and deemed not to be Gillick competent. Again the core principle is that all decisions are made in the young person's best interests. In most cases, this will be unproblematic but if health and social care practitioners believe that a parent's decision, or the decision of the person with parental responsibility, is not in the young person's best interests they can apply to a court to have the decision overturned. Making such a decision risks causing considerable distress to all involved, including the young person, and risks damaging the relationship between the family and the health and social care practitioners.

In all circumstances it is necessary to assess a young person's level of competence, which requires consideration of their ability to understand their choices and their willingness to make a choice based on that information. It should not be assumed that all young people wish to make choices about their health care and it is important that they are not pressurized into making decisions. To do so risks causing greater distress than removing the young person from the decision-making process. For example, a young person may be torn between what they might wish to do and a desire to please their parents. Such situations require careful management by practitioners, who need to balance legal requirements and the need to ensure that the young person receives the best possible care.

PARENTAL RESPONSIBILITY

Parental responsibility is central to the *Children Act 1989* in which it describes the legal authority parents have over young people and replaced the phrase 'parental rights' with 'parental responsibility'. Parental responsibility is defined as

> All rights, duties, powers, responsibility and authority which by law a parent of a child has in relation to the child and his property.

(Section 3(1))

The concept of parental responsibility emphasizes the duties of parents rather than their rights. This duty is to take all possible actions to protect the young person from possible harm.

The Act has been criticized because it does not go into detail about what parents can or cannot do. Instead, it has been argued that the Act exhibits 'misplaced complacency over the existing state of family values' and emphasizes the privacy of the family (Fortin 2003). It is further argued that detailed legislation would have been more useful to parents and health and social care practitioners and failing to provide such detail has resulted in continuing uncertainty about what constitutes parental responsibility.

Despite this, it is generally agreed that those with parental responsibility can make decisions about many aspects of a young person's life, including giving informed consent to medical treatment or a health care intervention. Although the scope of parental responsibility is broad it is not absolute and is subject to two main restrictions (Hendrick 2006). First, the welfare principle requires that those with parental responsibility act always in accordance with the young person's best interests. Second, parental responsibility diminishes as the young person matures and becomes more capable of making independent decisions.

Even this, however, is not straight forward because detail is lacking about how competence might be judged, especially in complex situations where competence might be temporarily or intermittently reduced.

Situations may also arise where those with parental responsibility disagree on the decision to be made. As in all other situations, it is the welfare of the young person that should be of paramount importance. Even the application of this principle, however, is not always sufficient to resolve a dispute. For the sake of all concerned, especially the young person, it is essential to make every effort to try and resolve any dispute that might arise. When resolution is not possible it may be necessary to resort to arbitration through the courts but this should always be a last resort.

CONFIDENTIALITY

The principle of confidentiality is one of the oldest in medical and health care ethics and has become one of the central principles in professional codes of practice. The strict requirement to ensure confidentiality is justified on two main grounds, the utilitarian and deontological arguments (Hendrick 2006). The utilitarian argument focuses on the need to ensure that patients feel they can trust health and social care practitioners with information they may reveal. If they feel they cannot trust practitioners they may not be willing to reveal sensitive information or may be deterred from seeking assistance at all. If either situation should occur the young person's health may be adversely affected. Deontologists believe that confidentiality should be respected because it is inherently right to do so irrespective of welfare considerations. This latter argument fails to recognize the need to balance the young person's right to have their voice heard and their right to be protected from danger.

Confidentiality is a universally accepted principle although there is no specific statute in English law to define or enforce it, although Article 8 of the *Human Rights Act 1998* protects respect for private life. Despite this, it is generally accepted that a formal level of confidentiality exists between a patient and health or social care practitioner. This right to confidentiality is owed as much to a young person as it is to any other person, if they are sufficiently mature to form a relationship of confidence with another person. It is important to distinguish between a young person's competence to give informed consent to treatment and their right to confidence.

There are circumstances when the duty of confidentiality is not absolute (Bainham 2005). The right to have one's confidence respected can be breached for two main reasons, to protect a patient's best interests and in the public interest (Hendrick 2006). In all circumstances a decision to breach a confidence must be justified. The disclosure of confidential information in the patient's best interest is paternalistic and limits the young person's autonomy in an attempt to protect a young person's health, their safety and their welfare. For example, if it is suspected that a young person is being abused then breaching confidentiality is a legitimate action because it is acting in the young person's best interests. This situation is more complicated if the young person is Gillick competent and does not wish an aspect of their health to be discussed with a parent.

Disclosure of confidential information in the public interest is more complicated because its scope is much less certain. It can be invoked to justify any breach of confidence if it is thought to be in the public's best interest. In case law, it is required to demonstrate a *real* and *genuine* risk of danger to the public to justify a breach of confidence.

In English law there has been no authoritative ruling on when a young person is entitled to have information kept confidential from parents. In general, however, there is agreement that competent young people have the same right to confidentiality as adults (Bainham 2005).

The situation is much more complicated when considering the rights of incompetent young people. If young people are to be able to retain some control over their person health information, they also need to have access to that information (Hendrick 2006). If young people do not possess control of their health information they also are unable to make truly informed decisions about their own health care.

CONCLUSION

The law has become so important in the provision of health and social care for young people that it is now central to the practice of all health and social care practitioners. In every aspect of their working lives, practitioners have to grapple with the application of legal requirements while always trying to ensure that the young person receives the best possible care. This chapter has explored just some of the legal complexities.

KEY ISSUES

- Any consideration of young people's health would be incomplete without an analysis of the complex legal and ethical issues, especially concerning decision making, informed consent and informed refusal.
- Legal and ethical issues are central to the everyday practice of health and social care practitioners.
- Young people should, as far as possible and within current legal frameworks, be involved in decision-making and providing informed consent to health and social care investigations and interventions.
- If a young person is unable to be involved in decision-making, through lack of competence, proxy decisions can be made on their behalf.
- The welfare of the young person must always be the principle that guides decision-making.

REFERENCES

Bainham A. (2005) *Children: The Modern Law*. 3rd edition. Bristol, UK: Family Law.
Bentham J. (1970) Anarchical fallacies. In: Melden AI, ed. *Human Rights*. Belmont, CA: Wadsworth.
Diduck A, Kaganas F. (2006) *Family Law, Gender and the State*. 2nd edition. Oxford, UK: Hart Publishing.
Eekelaar J. (1986) The emergence of children's rights. *Oxford Journal of Legal Studies* 6: 161–182.
Fortin J. (2003) *Children's Rights and the Developing Law*. 2nd edition. London: Lexis Nexis Butterworths.
Freeman M. (1983) *The Rights and Wrongs of Children*. London: Frances Pinter.
Freeman M. (1993) Laws, conventions and rights. *Children and Society* 7(1): 37–48.
Gillon R. (1985) *Philosophical Medical Ethics*. Chichester, UK: Wiley.
Hart H. (1970) Are there any natural rights? In: Melden AI, ed. *Human Rights*. Belmont, CA: Wadsworth.

Hendrick J. (2006) Legal and ethical issues. In: Moules T, Ramsey J, eds. *The Textbook of Children's Nursing*. 2nd edition. Cheltenham: Nelson Thornes.

Henricson C, Bainham A. (2005) *The Child and Family Policy Divide: Tensions, Convergence and Rights*. York, UK: Joseph Rowntree Foundation.

MacCormick N. (1984) *Legal Right and Social Democracy: Essays in Legal and Political Philosophy*. Oxford, UK: Oxford University Press.

Moules T. (2006) Children's rights. In: Moules T, Ramsey J, eds. *The Textbook of Children's Nursing*. 2nd ed. Cheltenham, UK: Nelson Thornes Ltd.

Difference and diversity as determinants of health: Ethnicity, gender and disability

3

SIMON FORREST AND THERESA NASH

INTRODUCTION

This chapter explores the ways that difference and diversity can be seen as contributory determinants of children's and young people's health and wellbeing. The reader will gain an understanding of why we should be concerned with difference and diversity when it comes to adopting a public health approach to thinking about working with children and young people, the historical and policy context for the concern and also some of the ways that difference and diversity are associated with the inequitable patterning and distribution of health within contemporary British society.

This chapter focuses on the following tasks:

- Defining the concepts of difference and diversity and charting their emergence as important in public health analysis, planning and action
- Describing the UK policy context
- Exploring three important dimensions of difference and diversity
  - Ethnicity
  - Gender
  - Disability

WHAT DO WE MEAN BY DIFFERENCE AND DIVERSITY?

Awareness that there are population sector differences in the ability to gain access to health services and to positive health outcomes is not a preserve of contemporary political and academic life. However, our attention to these differences, and our understanding of their importance for health and the mechanisms by which they have influence for better or worse has increased quite dramatically over the modern period. In fact, more than a century has passed since the vulnerability of some groups to poorer health and higher mortality was first observed. And, in striking resonance with contemporary analysis, the connection between health inequalities and the social, economic and environmental deprivations experienced by these minority groups was initially elaborated in the nineteenth and early twentieth centuries (Trask 1916; Engels 1987; Acheson 1998; Marmot et al. 2010).

This broader and evidence-based understanding of how socio-economic position relates to health inequality has set the context for thinking about how aspects of difference and diversity affect health. An important concept to grasp here is that difference and diversity are historically and socially specific constructs. This means that what constitutes difference, how and which groups of people are categorized as different and how these differences are responded to is context bound.

Societies are not stable and unchanging entities in which a limited variety of diverse groups are simply waiting to be discovered by increasingly subtle investigative technologies. The very investigative technologies with which we explore society are, at least to some extent, the means by which we construct groups, and even where differences within society are apparently self-evident, like the differences between men and women, how we define those categories, how we impose them and how we regard people within them reflect ideological, political and cultural investments and assumptions about what constitutes norms and hence what (or whom) is different from the norm.

This means that alongside understanding some of the categorical ways that we can conceptualize difference – for example, the major topics dealt with in this chapter gender, ethnicity and disability – we also have to always be mindful of how children and young people understand and experience their place in a social world and ways that they are different or similar to others. This is not to assert that children and young people do not belong to groups or that they cannot be categorized as different from one another in terms of dimensions like ethnicity, gender and (dis)ability, but that the homogenizing of individuals through grouping can unhelpfully smooth over the realities of lived experience in which children and young people develop a sense of identity that is similar to or different from others, more or less strongly according to the particularities of specific social interactions, circumstances and contexts. In terms of public health practice, this means that their encounters with health and other professionals and their understanding of public health messages are all contexts in which their sense of difference and diversity may be more or less accentuated according to a whole range of factors.

THE EMERGENT NATURE OF DIFFERENCE, DIVERSITY

Approaching a consideration of child public health from this perspective involves us in exploring some of the influences that have contributed to the emergence of increased awareness of difference and diversity within the field, and which represent social sites where children and young people may experience a sense of their difference and diversity from others.

As we have already suggested, advances in behavioural and disease epidemiology have a constructive role to play in the development of increasingly sophisticated ideas about difference and diversity. The capacity to access more data about the health of the nation, and our ability to subject it to more subtle and complex interrogation, has enabled public health analysts to identify ways of characterizing vulnerability to disease or ill-health by factors that are associated with the increasing fragmentation of society into groups. It is possible to talk about differences and diversity in health not only by gender and age, but also by locality, ethnicity, sexual orientation and (dis)ability. Moreover, increasing subcategories of the population can be created by exploring the interactions between these dimensions of difference.

These changes in how we describe groups within a population have been linked to changes in the nature of public health practice *per se.* In the UK and other rich developed countries, this has been particularly marked in relation to children and young people where public health has widened its scope in terms of both the topics with which it is concerned and the variety of agencies engaged in this work (Blair et al. 2003). The effects of broadening both the *what* public health is and the *who* is involved in securing and promoting it have inevitably increased the potential for identifying different and more diverse target groups and settings.

Changes in public health have, of course, not taken place in isolation. The trend towards a *rights-based* inflection in the development of public policy has also sharpened attention to difference and diversity. In recent years, the UK has enshrined in its own statutory law a commitment to global and regional declarations on human and children's rights (Council of Europe 1950, 1961; United Nations 1989; *Human Rights Act 1998*). The effect of spelling out the rights of the individual and pledging to ensure that these are equitably available naturally causes a spotlight to fall on those groups and individuals who are denied the entitlements associated with these rights. This *rights-based* agenda within public policy both sets the tenor for public health practice and has a very direct influence on it by committing the UK Government to take steps to ensure that the health of all children and young people is protected and promoted.

The rise of *rights-based* inflections within public policy can also be connected with the increased emergence of social movements that aim to achieve recognition and equality for a wide variety of groups. Putting human rights on a legal footing gives extra political leverage to individuals and groups who feel militated against or denied entitlements that they are due. Some of these have had a very direct bearing on public health practice. To take one example, the political movements among gay men in the wake of the emergence of the HIV/AIDS epidemic, seeking equal recognition of their identity and acknowledgement of their particular vulnerability to HIV. These illustrate a sense of the way group identity can be galvanized through threats to individual health and well-being.

One potential effect of the mobilization of minority groups is the destabilization of norms in the wider population and the creation of more awareness of forms of diversity and difference. The emergence and success of the gay rights movement have contributed to the liberalization of thinking about sexual identity as a whole as well as the fragmentation and multiplication of sexual identities since the 1980s (Forrest and Ellis 2011). You might also consider the way that poorer health outcomes for groups such as women and children have been associated with threat to or losses in human rights in contexts such as Afghanistan creating a clear link and hence mobilising demands for equal rights and recognition of difference and diversity (Amowitz et al. 2002).

Awareness of the political dimension to the emergence of difference and diversity alerts us to the wider historical processes of struggle against stigmatization and oppression that often form their backdrop. This is particularly important because there is a tendency to lose sight of the fact that the history of many forms of difference and diversity reveals associations with negative experiences for minority groups so defined. For example, when we talk about ethnicity as a dimension of difference in public health, there may be a risk of regarding it as fairly neutral. We see it as a term that emphasizes socially constructed differences between people associated with their group and individual origins, shared social background, cultures, traditions and sense of identity (Brady 2003). It is also the case as disciplines such as anthropology show us, the concept may represent a conflation of ideas about culture, genetics and social relationships which unhelpfully glosses over the history of discrimination and racial prejudice (Dressler et al. 2005). The relatively recent replacement of *race* by ethnicity as the preferred lexical construct for dealing with these forms of difference between people reminds us that, when we talk about ethnic minorities in the UK and across Western Europe as a whole, we are generally talking about people whose experiences of their ethnic difference has largely been associated with a history of colonialism, nationalism, racism, the exploitation of the labour of poorer nations by richer nations and, more particularly in recent times, the flight of people from persecution, poverty, unrest and war.

Understanding this history enables us to track its effects on contemporary debates about health issues. For example, the migration of people to Western European countries from the poorer East and South often stimulates debate about the relationship between nationality and entitlement to health services and the extent to which immigrant people are identified as a potential source of disease or demand on health services. Pejorative and generalizing views of immigrants as posing a risk to indigenous populations and placing a burden on health services can enter the public realm and thereby configure debate in ways that limit effective political and strategic action on health (Schmidt and Spies 2014).

Finally, changes in the nature of social institutions and cultural practices also influence our understanding of social diversity and difference. Among the most significant of these changes are those that have taken place in the nature of the family and childhood. While we can still talk about *the family* in public health analysis and practice, the term now refers to a wide range of social, economic and relational arrangements between people. Families not only comprise men and women and their biological offspring, but they also comprise same-sex couples, single parents, non-biological parents and a variety of re-formed families (blended families) who parent both their own biological and other children. The nature of childhood has altered too. Whereas it once referred to a relatively short period of life ending around the early teenage years, it has now expanded and diversified such that it extends into the teenage years and beyond, thus resulting in the creation of whole new social groups of young people (Office of National Statistics [ONS] 2012).

THE POLICY CONTEXT

Our objective here is to provide a sense of the UK public policy context around difference and diversity with a focus on public health for children and young people. You might find it useful to read this in conjunction with the details of the policy context which have been dealt with elsewhere in this book.

One of the peculiar features of this context is that there is no one policy which we can consider when we think about where difference and diversity among children with respect to health and well-being is represented in the public sphere. Our approach is therefore to provide a sense of the ways that difference and diversity crop up in policy and to illustrate these with a number of examples.

An underlying feature of health policy as a whole has been the attention to the link between social and health inequalities, especially since the Black report of 1980. One effect of this link has been to provide an impetus to looking at the ways that difference and diversity between population groups is associated with, contributes to or is a product of the wider structural social problem. The concern with health as a problem of inequalities reflects the rise of concern about human rights mentioned earlier in this chapter. An important policy development that reflects this link between difference and diversity on one hand and inequalities and rights on the other hand is the *Equality Act* (2010).

The Act brought together a number of already existing bodies, each responsible for aspects of equality including race and disability, into one entity – the Equality Commission – which is designed to oversee and monitor implementation of a wide range of powers and responsibilities incumbent on individuals, employers and organisations to both protect and respect difference and diversity.

The *Equality Act* is important because it defines some of the key references for our current understanding of difference and diversity. It also gives individuals the power and the right to challenge organisations that do not respect individual rights or treat them fairly as a consequence of having so-called *protected characteristics*. It also places responsibility on organisations to promote equality and understanding and to tackle prejudice. The protected characteristics identified by the Act are

- Age
- Being or becoming a transsexual person
- Being married or in a civil partnership
- Being pregnant or having a child
- Disability
- Race including colour, nationality, ethnic or national origin
- Religion, belief or lack of religion/belief
- Sex
- Sexual orientation

The Act provides people with protection from discrimination in a wide range of situations including at work, in education, as a consumer, when using a public service, buying or renting property and as a member or guest of a private club or association. This right extends to people who are associated with someone who is discriminated against because of a protected characteristic.

If the *Equality Act* can be seen as setting out a broad prospectus, then another important approach, which reflects these concepts and definitions but places them in the context of public concern with population and group differences and needs in terms of health, can be seen in the reconfiguration and conceptualisation of Public Health within England. This is reflected in the White Paper of 2010, *Healthy Lives, Healthy People: Our Strategy for Public Health in England*.

The White Paper sought to move responsibility for public health from central to Local Government. It framed five key areas of activity. Two have a specific salience for children and young people: a focus on improving maternal health in order to reduce infant mortality and the numbers of low birth-weight babies with the intention of giving children the best start in life. A focus on driving up educational attainment; reducing risks to mental health; and reducing unhealthy lifestyles has special relevance for children and young people.

What is significant here is that difference and diversity surface in references to specific health needs and are directly associated with population groups. For example, the White Paper referred to the importance of tackling childhood obesity while noting that rates were higher in some black and minority ethnic groups as well as among children from lower socioeconomic groups.

It is clear then that the general direction of travel of public policy has a number of dimensions that are relevant to children and young people. The general thrust of policy is towards recognition that access to health services and positive health outcomes is inequitable in the UK and that dimensions of difference and diversity are associated with these inequalities. The major underlying concern is with the stark (and increasing) differences between children and young people that are linked to their socioeconomic backgrounds. In addition, ethnicity, disability, social marginalization and exclusion, gender and sexuality are also recognized to varying degrees as relevant dimensions of difference and diversity in the efficient and effective targeting of public health activities. In this context, policy aims tend to cluster around the following:

• Ensuring that access to health and to services is equitable
• Recognizing that children and young people from marginalized and minority groups (e.g. ethnic minorities, disabled children, those in care and young prisoners) are often disadvantaged in terms of the quality of their health and their access to health services
• Acknowledging that disadvantage is rooted in a number of factors, including some that are directly within the influence of public health as part of the broader public sector offer

Examples include challenging discriminatory practices within health and social care services and practices by health and social care professionals as well as ensuring accessible and acceptable health provision for people from minority groups.

EXERCISE

Drawing on what you know about the policy context here and in earlier sections of this book, use the matrix below to analyse how public policy might affect children's and young people's health if changed in various ways.

	Impact on children and young people			
	All children and young people	Impact by gender	Children and young people from ethnicity minorities	Children and young people with disabilities
Expanding early years provision to all two-year-olds				
Access to free swimming and reduced PE				
Increased concern about child sexual abuse				
Reduced public services (libraries, parks and youth projects)				

KEY POINTS FOR REFLECTION AND CONSIDERATION

You might find it helpful as you complete this matrix to consider the following questions:

* What evidence would you draw on to assess the impact of any change in public health policy when you think about the health and well-being of children and young people?
* How might any change in public policy align with the spirit of recognition and protection of equality and difference and diversity expressed in the *Equality Act*?

CHILDREN, YOUNG PEOPLE, ETHNICITY AND HEALTH

Data derived from the 2011 Census report indicated that around 14% of the population of England and Wales describe themselves as being part of a Black or Minority Ethnic group (BME). This has risen from around 8% in 2001. The largest BME group described themselves as Indian (2.5%) followed by Pakistani (2%). The group comprising Indian, Pakistani, Bangladeshi, Chinese and Other Asian make up 7.5% of the population. African, Caribbean and Black British people comprise about 3.3% of the population and people of mixed ethnicity about 2%.

There has been significant growth in the group described as 'White Other' to stand at around 4.4% of the population. It has been suggested that this reflects migration, including from Eastern Europe. Data from the ONS show that the Polish population in England and Wales grew by half a million between 2001 and 2011. While this represents the single largest source of growth, the 'White Other' category also includes people described as White French, White Australian, White Argentinian and White American. The 2011 census for the first time included two new categories: Gypsy or Irish Traveller and Arab. These account for 0.4% and 0.1% of the population, respectively.

Analysis of the 2012 census has yet to reveal the age profile of the population by ethnicity but data from 2001 showed that the younger population was more ethnically diverse than the older population. However, age distribution is not similar across all ethnic minorities. Trends reflect waves of immigration such that the population of people categorizing themselves as Irish, for example, have the oldest age structure, followed by people from the Caribbean. People from Africa and the Far East tend to be younger than the population as a whole. The 'Mixed' group have the youngest age structure with half being under the age of 16 years. The Bangladeshi, 'Other Black' and Pakistani groups also have young age structures: 38% of both the Bangladeshi and Other Black groups were aged under 16 years at 2001 and 35% of Pakistanis also fell into this age group. This was almost double the proportion of the White British group where one in five (20%) were under the age of 16 years. Ethnic diversity within the UK also has a strong geographical character with around 45% of all 'non-white' people living in London (Office for National Statistics 2001).

In recent years, increasingly detailed research on ethnicity has emerged. It has identified and explored the epidemiological, behavioural and social aspects of differences in health status and service use between and within ethnic groups (see for example, Health and Social Care Information Centre [HSCIC] 2005; Neale et al. 2005; Wardle et al. 2006). With regard to children and young people, evidence has emerged of an association between some conditions and diseases and ethnicity.

For example, children from Indian, Pakistani, Bangladeshi and Chinese backgrounds have been found to be less likely to report acute sickness than other ethnic groups. Indian and

Pakistani boys are more likely to be overweight than boys in the general population. African-Caribbean and Pakistani girls are more likely to be measured as obese than girls in the general population (Office for National Statistics 2004a).

Explanations for the inequitable distribution of ill-health among children and young people from ethnic minorities are the subject of some disputes, although there seems to be consensus that the effects of ethnicity cannot easily be disaggregated from other social factors, particularly socio-economic disadvantage.

It has been suggested that aspects of ethnic heritage, genetic predispositions, behavioural norms within communities, the impact of racism and inequalities in uptake and experiences of health-care and socio-economic status may all be influential factors. In some areas the picture is becoming clearer, however, with one recent systematic review showing a strong relationship between experience of racism and mental ill-health (Priest et al. 2013). Furthermore, problems with disaggregating ethnicity as a single influencing factor reflects limitations in both the data available for analysis and the theorizations of socio-economic status and ethnicity that are being used (Smith et al. 2000).

Research on service uptake among ethnic minority groups also suggests links with socio-economic status, although ethnicity does seem to emerge as a factor in its own right in some studies. Evidence suggests that Indian and Pakistani children are more likely to have visited their general practitioner in the preceding fortnight than children in other ethnic groups, and that they and Bangladeshi and Chinese children are less likely to have attended an outpatient clinic in the preceding quarter. Such results would be more meaningful if other factors such as perceptions of health status and the orientation of services were also taken into account (Cooper et al. 1998, 1999; Saxena et al. 2002; Szczepura 2005).

What evidence there is on this score suggests that health status varies by ethnic group, and that, while children from Asian ethnic groups report better health, African-Caribbean children report worse health than the population in general (Saxena et al. 2002). However, both health needs and perceived susceptibility may vary by gender at least as much as by ethnicity, and gender may be more influential than ethnicity in determining the views of young people with regard to some health issues, particularly sexual health (Connell et al. 2004).

Parents' and carers' roles in assessing the health status of children and young people, and in facilitating their access to health services, are poorly understood. Yet some research suggests that they play a major role in deciding when young people access health services, which services they then access, and in organizing appointments and accompanying young people to the majority of consultations. How this affects consultations, confidentiality and young people's preparedness to disclose their concerns has not yet been the subject of investigation (Jacobson et al. 1994).

Qualitative studies on attitudes to health and service uptake among young people provide some illumination on the range of factors that may inform differences in service use but they rarely adopt any specific focus on ethnicity. A body of work on the accessibility and acceptability of health services with a focus on general practice suggests that, although satisfaction with services is high, health professionals are generally perceived as providers of advice on biomedical problems rather than on disease prevention. In addition, significant minorities of young people experience problems in consultations with health professionals, particularly. These range from ambivalence about whether they are given enough consultation time to difficulties with expressing personal concerns. Young people also report problems associated with confidence that they are being taken seriously. And young people also express serious reservations about achieving privacy in the reception areas of surgeries and about the maintenance of patient confidentiality (Atkinson et al. 2003; Churchill et al. 2000; Jacobson et al. 1994; Malik et al. 2002).

REFUGEE AND ASYLUM-SEEKING CHILDREN

Accurate data on the numbers of children and young people who are or have sought/are seeking refuge or asylum in the UK are very difficult to obtain. This is partly because of ways in which these statuses are defined and the processes of documentation that, in all probability, lead to an under-estimation of the population itself (Blinder 2013). Nonetheless, it is thought that children comprise at least a quarter of all asylum seekers, around 6000 annually and, additionally, around 3000 unaccompanied children arrive in the UK each year (The Refugee Council 2015).

These figures only capture *documented* asylum seekers. Recent estimates suggest there were 155,000 irregular or undocumented migrant children living in the UK at the end of 2007. The majority of these (85,000) were children born in the UK while about 70,000 children were born abroad but came to the UK alone or as dependants. This latter figure would include children who have been victims of human trafficking on false papers.

Many child and young refugees are at risk of having been exposed to infectious disease but have not been vaccinated or have uncertain medical histories. They may be or may have been malnourished and may have witnessed or been subject to violence and torture. Girls and young women may have been subject to female genital mutilation and/or domestic violence (Burnett and Peel 2001). Research has shown that a disproportionately high number of child refugees display signs and symptoms of severe trauma and experience mental and emotional ill-health. This not only includes various forms of depression, anxiety and agoraphobia but is also manifest in problems impacting on their ability to integrate with other young people and society more widely, including problems with peers, hyperactivity, depression and conduct disorders (Fazel and Stein 2003; Boguic et al. 2012). Access to mental health services for refugee and asylum-seeking children is poor (Reed et al. 2012).

It can be difficult to respond to these complex and sometimes acute needs because of language barriers and cultural differences that can hamper intercultural communication. Refugee children and young people may not be clear about their entitlements or what services are available to them or how to access services. The importance of interpreters and the advocacy and social and emotional support provided by appropriate cultural organizations based in the community has been highlighted. In addition, web-based resources are playing an increasingly significant role in supporting refugees and asylum seekers as are professionals who work with them in health and welfare services.

Poverty at all stages of the asylum process, whether as an initial applicant, a refused applicant or a refugee compounds children and families' vulnerability. Many families have been recognized as destitute, particularly those refused asylum but are unable to return to their country of origin. These families generally have no status, few rights or resources, and are perceived to be a growing challenge to the National Health Service (NHS) (Faculty of Public Health [FPH] 2008).

The Children Society Study (TCS 2012) has documented the realities of destitution: children growing up in households without food, heating or toys; mothers driven to prostitution in order to survive; young people in care who are cut off from any help at age 18; and pregnant women who cannot afford nutritious food, housing or access to additional healthcare needs (TCS 2012). Poverty has a profound impact on both maternal and child health. Compounding problems include difficulties of access to primary care registration. Language barriers are also specific health-care problems for children. The dangers to child health include malnourishment and communicable disease risk (TB, Hepatitis, HIV). This is particularly the case if children have travelled from refugee camps where nutrition and sanitation are poor or from countries with limited health-care resources or where health-care systems have collapsed.

Once in the UK, delays in processing applications for residence mean that families can live in severe poverty, often for many years, resulting in poor child nutrition, family breakdown and/or domestic violence and thereby increasing child vulnerability. The *Study* (TCS 2012) also notes that children are particularly vulnerable to becoming destitute, including those who leave care, some of whom may have been victims of trafficking. Those children escaping trafficking (domestic servitude, labour exploitation, benefit fraud or sexual exploitation) often have no documentation and are therefore refused support. This further compounds their vulnerability and isolation. Increasing numbers of unaccompanied children are accessing third sector care services and are forced to engage in survival strategies that include: sleeping on the streets, low paid work (TCS quoted £1.50/hour), transactional sex (for food, shelter or money), begging or stealing. Children in such circumstances report a range of health problems: frequent coughs, chest infections, exhaustion, inability to eat when food is available and self-harm. Education is severely disrupted by frequent moves, lack of rest, inability to concentrate or to learn effectively. Coupled with this profile of challenges, maintaining personal hygiene can be difficult (e.g. accessing sanitary towels, nappies and laundry services).

CHILDREN, YOUNG PEOPLE, GENDER AND HEALTH

Areas of major gender difference include susceptibility to accidents and resultant disabilities. Research suggests that over three times as many road traffic fatalities involve boys as girls between the ages of 15 and 19. A gender differential, albeit smaller, is also reflected in other accidents among 2- to 15-year-olds with boys particularly prone to accidents. This figure may reflect the greater involvement of boys in sports and outdoor activities.

Cancer is relatively rare among children. However, cancers account for 23% of all deaths among girls between the ages of 5 and 15 years. Scrutinized year, data from Cancer UK suggest that there was a slightly higher proportion of boys (55%) than girls (45%) aged 0–14 years old among the 1574 new cases of cancer between 2009 and 2011 (Cancer UK 2014). There are some gender differences in the kinds of cancers that affect children and young people, with leukaemia and bone and brain tumours occurring more often among boys than girls.

Obesity also has a gender dimension among both children under 10 and teenagers. In both age groups, the trend between 1995 and 2006 was for a rise in the proportion of both boys and girls described as obese and then a fall between 2006 and 2010. Among boys in the age group 2–10 years old, the trajectory was from 9.7% to 17.4% and back down to 15.3% measuring as obese. Among girls, obesity levels during the same period moved from 10.6% (1995) to a high of 17.4% and then down to 13.9% (2010). The data for those children in ages 11–15 years old showed that there was a shift among boys from 13.9% in 1995 to 24.5% in 2006 and back to 19.9% in 2010. The same pattern was observed among girls from 15.3% to 26.7% to 16.6% (HSCIC 2012).

Problems of overweight and obesity are linked to exercise and diet but also to self-image and nutrition choices, which are highly gendered. Young men tend to see themselves as fitter than do women and boys are less likely to see their diet as important to their well-being. The influence of self-image is also discernible in the prevalence of eating disorders, notably those associated with attempts to lose weight, which are more prevalent among girls and young women than among boys. There is emerging evidence, however, that not only are eating disorders rising among young men but that recognition and appropriate service responses are lagging behind (Räisänen and Hunt 2014). Work on the link between diet, weight, eating disorders and attitudes towards food suggest that there are distinct gender differences in views about and motivations for eating behaviours, with girls more likely to cite emotional reasons for over or undereating and boys more likely to cite social reasons. Young people in the UK seem well aware of the social link between feminine physical beauty as associated with being thinner and masculine attractiveness with being heavier, more muscular and taller (MacKinnon et al. 2002).

In the past, there were marked and clear differences in trends for health-related behaviours between boys and girls. However, recent data for smoking, drug use and alcohol consumption (as examples) suggest both consistent decreases in these behaviours over the past decade among girls and boys and convergence in the proportions of girls and boys who engage in health risk behaviours as well as the frequency and nature of risk behaviours (HSCIC 2014). For example, in 2013, the prevalence of regular smoking was down to around 8% among 15-year-olds and the long-standing difference between girls and boys that had seen more girls than boys smoking since the mid-1980s had disappeared. Data relating to frequency, number and timing of cigarette smoking also became similar across the sexes. However, there are some indications of a slight increased prevalence among 14-year-old girls to smoke compared with boys.

A similar pattern has been observed for drug use with overall reporting of 'ever having taken drugs' decreasing from around 30%–16% in the decade between 2003 and 2013. There have been no differences in type of drug(s) being used or the frequency of use when analysed by gender. Only with respect to questions relating to having ever been offered cannabis do any gender differences endure with a slightly higher proportion of boys (20%) than girls (17%) providing an affirmative response. With regard to alcohol use, the same overall tendency to a decrease in 'ever having used' has been observed among 10- to 16-year-olds. There appear to be no significant differences in use or frequency of drinking between boys and girls although boys reported that they were more likely than girls to drink beer, lager or cider (87% of boys compared with 60% of girls). The reverse was true of wine (49% of girls and 17% of boys) reporting in 2014.

Boys are more likely than girls to suffer from a recognizable mental disorder. Among 5- to 10-year-olds, 10% boys and 5% girls are reported to have a mental disorder. Among 11- to 16-year-olds, the reported proportions are 13% boys and 10% girls. Overall, hyperkinetic and conduct disorders are much more common among boys than girls between the ages of 5 and 16 years and girls are much more likely to report emotional problems between the ages of 11 and 16 years (Office for National Statistics 2005). There are also very distinct gender differences in suicide data, which continue to show much higher levels of suicide among all men compared with women. Among young men aged 15–19 years old, ONS 2005 data reported a rate of 6.4 boys/young men per 100,000 compared with 1.9 per 100,000 for young women. The methods of suicide are also gender differentiated with young men using more violent methods – e.g. hanging, strangulation, suffocation over poisoning and young women opting for the reverse (drugs, poisoning).

We also know that sexual health behaviours have a strong gender dimension with boys and young men much less likely to know about sexually transmitted infections and less likely to know that they are infected than do girls and young women. Boys are also less likely to know about and to seek treatment (Lloyd et al. 2001; Stone and Ingham 2003). Despite these significant differences in health outcomes and behaviours by gender, robust analysis of the reasons behind them is remarkably rare.

An exception would seem to be recent research on boys and young men (a potential gender bias in itself), which has found that beliefs about and the acceptability of risk-taking among boys and young men plays a part in some aspects of their susceptibility to accidents. Their tendency towards *physicality* might also account for their disproportionate representation in conditions like hyperkinetic disorders. This work also points to the need for a subtle and sophisticated model of gender that can take into account both individual factors and social norms when service provision is being considered. For example, services may be practically and qualitatively more acceptable and accessible to girls and young women while boys and young men may perceive expressions of concern about health issues and the use of services as signalling weakness and/or a failure to cope that conflicts with their understanding of masculinity (Lloyd et al. 2001; Tyler and Williams 2014).

CHILDREN, YOUNG PEOPLE, SEXUALITY AND HEALTH

In addition to gender, sexuality is an important dimension of diversity among young people, with particular significance for public health practice. For some time there has been a focus on the promotion of sexual health among young gay men because of their vulnerability to sexually transmitted infections, including HIV. This focus is associated with efforts to develop specialist services, targeted health awareness and informational/education materials. At a more general level, attempts to reach young gay men with better prevention earlier have been given some support by more liberal guidelines on sex and relationships education in schools (Department for Education and Employment 2000).

However, a proper consideration of sexuality from a public health perspective implies much more than thinking about appropriately targeted measures for older, sexually at-risk young gay men. Sexual identity is more diverse and includes young lesbian women and bisexual young people. For many young people, long in advance of their sexual debut, uncertainty about sexual identity can make them vulnerable to mental health problems associated with defining their sexuality and coping with other people's reactions to them (Mustanski et al. 2010). Well and widely reported problems with homophobic bullying (for both gay and non-gay children and young people) are known to have potential for significant impact on young people's mental well-being (Collier et al. 2013). There is an inverse relationship between their willingness to discuss their concerns about sexual identity and ill-health (Ellis and High 2004). Despite making some inroads through activities like the Healthy Schools initiatives, it is evident that there is scope for public health practice to adopt a wider and more active approach to challenging heterosexism and homophobia within and outside health and social care services.

CHILDREN, YOUNG PEOPLE, DISABILITY AND HEALTH

The *Equality Act* (2010) defines a person with a disability as one who has a physical or mental impairment that has a substantial and/or long-term adverse effect on his/her ability to carry out normal day-to-day activities. While this definition may assist in understanding support, it lacks the depth and more-rounded character of the social model of disability. This recognizes that disability may be a positive personal and social identity, and that society itself (not the disability) creates barriers (segregation and marginalisation) to participation (Shakespeare 2006).

The Family Resources Survey (2010) estimates there to be 952,741 disabled children in the UK, 7.3% of the child population. Slightly more boys (8.8%) than girls (5.8%) live with a disability. This may be an underestimate as a recent research project drawing on multiple longitudinal surveys has found (Plant et al. 2013a). The Millennium Cohort Study (MCS) and the Longitudinal Study of Young People in England (LSYPE) (2013a) are the main sources of reliable data. The MCS surveys (19,000 children born between 2000 and 2001) and the LSYPE (a large scale, representative study of nearly 16,000 young people born in the early 1990s) vary from each other slightly. The MCS uses three of the indicators below whereas the LSYPE uses two of the indicators.

These studies demonstrate the challenges in defining disability yet the importance of a definition in reaching estimates of the numbers of children and young people affected. Plant et al. (2014) conclude that the prevalence of disability varies according to the measure used and estimate that between 11% and 17% of seven-year-olds have experienced a disability as well as 7%–10% of young people. The number of children impacted by disability has grown in the last decade, particularly those requiring intensive medical assistance. As survival of premature neonates improves, those living with life limiting conditions and with an increasing prevalence of ADHD and Autism (Davie 2013) translates into higher percentages of disability in the total population.

Plant et al. (2013b) have also demonstrated the relationship between child disability and the impact of socioeconomic disadvantage. To date, Plant et al. 2014 have confirmed that child disability is associated with family socio-economic disadvantage as indicated by living in a lone parent family and/or living in a workless household. This applies to all definitions of child disability and across all age groups, but risk is particularly high for children with special educational needs (SEN). They suggest that disability may be a stress factor and may cause cumulative disadvantage. Their findings concur with previous research suggesting that disabled children and their families are the 'poorest of the poor'.

Children from the most disadvantaged groups have been found to be three and a half times more likely to have a limiting long-term illness or disability and more likely to live with low income, debt and poor housing than children without disabilities (Spencer and Read 2010; Department for Work and Pensions [DWP] 2004; Blackburn et al. 2010). This has been found to be particularly the case for disabled children from black, minority ethnic and mixed parentage groups and lone-parent households. There appear to be a number of coalescing factors – for example, the maintenance costs of a child with a disability is estimated to be 10%–18% higher (e.g. fuel costs, travel, increased washing, use of continence aides). In addition, the demands of caring reduce the ability of both parents or a lone parent to gain and maintain paid work. Plus a shortfall in state allowances is estimated to be between 20% and 50%. Finally, many families may not be accessing their full benefit entitlement. There is increasing concern in some quarters that this situation is set to become worse in the UK with a shift to a Universal Credit system and a prediction made in 2012 that 100,000 disabled children could lose as much as £28 per week.

The anxiety is that up to 40% of children might eventually be living in poverty in the UK (The Children's Society [TCS] 2012). It has been suggested that 4 in every 10 disabled children already lives in poverty, much higher than previous estimates. TCS has expressed grave concerns about financial cuts being introduced in the Universal Credit system, the latter threatening to push more families into poverty.

Furthermore, the estimated risk of violence, including physical, sexual, neglect and abuse of children with disabilities is three to four times higher than the risk of non-disabled children (Jones et al. 2012). Of particular concern, 97%–99% of abusers of victims with developmental disabilities are known and trusted by the victim (Davis and Modell 2010).

Plant et al. (2014) specified that 34% of children with SEN experienced *relational bullying*. This refers to a spectrum from being called names or being excluded from groups or friends – including text and emails to physical bullying. They also found that physical bullying was high incidence within this group at 27% and included being forced to give away money or possessions. It referred to and included all forms of physical violence (e.g. hitting and kicking). Being viewed as 'different', lack of carer 'support' and a need for 'personal safety education' have also been identified as related factors.

Disabled children also face barriers in accessing quality health services because of the complexity of services required: a lack of co-ordination between agencies; challenges linked to transition into adult services; low priority and lack of participation in decision making

(Mooney et al. 2008). Since 2008, *Every Disabled Child Matters* (EDCM 2011) has called for improved integration; co-ordination across education, health and social care; improved access to service information and identification of disability; and intervention in the early years. This policy expansion has now been embedded within *The Children and Families Act (2014)* Part 3, Children and Young People with Special Educational Needs and Disabilities (SEND). The Act places new legal duties on Local Authorities (LAs) and Clinical Commissioning Groups (CCGs) to improve services. It enshrines the need for both parents and children to be involved in decisions that affect them and requires LAs and CCGs to develop Education, Health and Care (EHC) plans. Once the plans are agreed, CCGs will have a legal duty to commission health services that are detailed in the plans. Additionally, within the 2014 Act, parents will have increasing choice over the use of personal budgets. New statutory guidance was published in January 2015 in order to review this and to review how the EHCs are being implemented (visit www.gov.uk). How successful this legislation will be at improving the complexity of children and young people's lives when they are living with disability will emerge as services begin to respond to the 2014 Act.

CHILDREN AS CARERS

It needs to be noted that a significant burden also falls on young people who provide care for a family member with a disability. See Table 3.1 for prevalence of child disability. A recent report from TCS (2013) illustrates the severe impact that caring responsibilities have on children's education, financial security and future life chances (Box 3.1).

BOX 3.1: Hidden From View: The Experience of Young Carers in England. The Children's Society (2013)

KEY FINDINGS

- 166,363 young carers in England, compared with around 139,000 in 2001. Likely an underestimate as young carers tend to be 'under the radar' of professionals
- 1 in 12 cares for more than 15 hours per week and 1 in 20 misses school because of caring responsibilities

YOUNG CARERS COMPARED WITH THEIR PEERS

- Are 1.5 times more likely to be from Black, Asian or Minority ethnic communities, and are twice as likely to speak English as a second language
- Are 1.5 times more likely to have a special educational need or a disability
- Have an average annual income for their families that is £5000 less than families who do not have a young carer
- Are NOT more likely to come into contact with support agencies
- Have significantly lower educational attainment at General Certificate of Secondary Education (GCSE) level, the equivalent to nine grades lower overall
- Are more likely than the national average not to be in education, employment or training (NEET) between the ages of 16 and 19

Table 3.1 What is the prevalence of child disability?

Measurement	MCS	LSYPE
Frequency of Data collection	9 months, 3, 5, 7 and 11 years	Survey ages 13/14 followed annually for 7 years
Developmental delay at 9 months	12%	Not measured
Long-standing limiting illness	11%	7%
Special Educational Needs (SEN)	17% (4% have a statement)	9.6%
Children with three measurements	1%	
Children with one or more measures	31%	14%

Source: Plant L et al., *Research Summary Four: Are Disabled Children and Young People at a Higher Risk of Being Bullied?* Briefing paper. London: Centre for Longitudinal Studies, 2014. http://www.cls.ioe.ac.uk/page.aspx?&sitesectionid=1203&sitesectiontitle=Trajectories+and+transitions+in+the+cognitive+and+educational+development+of+disabled+children+and+young+people (accessed on 2 March 2015).
Developmental delay – Motor co-ordination and communicative gestures at 9 months.
Long-standing limiting illness – Long-Term health conditions such as Type 1 diabetes or asthma, mental health problems and impairments such as a missing limb or sensory loss.
Special educational needs (as defined by parent, teacher or both) – These include health conditions or impairments that may inhibit learning such as hearing loss; behavioural difficulties such as attention deficit hyperactivity disorder [ADHD]; learning-related conditions such as dyslexia and learning disabilities.

REFLECTIVE EXERCISE

Think about each of the dimensions of difference and diversity that you have been introduced to in the chapter and consider how you employ them to address each of the following scenarios.

1. You are trying to persuade Lianne, an 18-year-old young woman who is expecting her first baby, to stop smoking.
2. You want to refer Mohammed, who is 7-years-old and entered the UK as an asylum-seeker, for blood-tests.
3. You have been asked to undertake a project while on placement in the community to look at how to make a polyclinic more accessible to young disabled people.

KEY POINTS

With regard to (1) you might have thought about whether Lianne is aware of the potential deleterious effects of her smoking on her baby's health, and also what her motives for smoking are. You might want to look into what research tells you about why young people smoke and also why they stop and see if you can identify the gender-specific aspects of the advice for practice (Lynes and Lynes, 2012).

With regard to (2) you probably considered the ways that Mohammed's experiences as a refugee and asylum-seeker might have affected his confidence in other people, his capacity and willingness to communicate his concerns and needs, and other aspects of his mental health and social competency. You might look at practice advice from organisations such as Social Care Institute for Excellence (2010) and assess your skills and competency needs.

With regard to (3) you might well have considered what range of disabilities young people might have and how they impact on physical but also psychological barriers to access. You might want to look at the case studies in the Care Quality Commission report on *Health care for disabled children and young people* (CQC 2012).

CONCLUSION

The purpose of this chapter has been to demonstrate why difference and diversity are important considerations in a public health approach to protecting and promoting the health and well-being of children and young people. This is because dimensions such as gender, ethnicity and disability are all associated with differences in health experience and outcome and are critical to an understanding of how inequalities in health and access to health arise and are maintained. We have also indicated that all health professionals and public bodies have certain responsibilities to consider the ways that difference and diversity may affect health and also to challenge the prejudice and discrimination with which they may be associated. You should now be clear that an understanding of the way that rights inform an approach to difference and diversity is essential to public health effectiveness. And also essential to the capacity of healthcare professionals to carry out their work in ways that are commensurate with statutory, regulatory and moral obligations as well as best practice.

KEY POINTS

- Public health practice needs to take difference and diversity among children and young people into account in order to understand and respond to inequities in access to health services and in order to achieve positive health outcomes for the whole population.
- The public policy context in the UK provides a broad platform for achieving equity in terms of drawing increasing attention to human rights and respect for different needs and for reducing social exclusion.
- Health-specific policy places specific demands on service planners and providers to respond positively to difference and diversity.
- Although this chapter has explored five major dimensions of difference and diversity among children and young people – ethnicity, refugee status, gender, sexuality and disability – it is important to recognize that diversity is not experienced only in these categorical terms but as dynamic aspects of personal and group identity in the context of specific social interactions and settings.

REFERENCES

Acheson D. (1998) *Great Britain Independent Inquiry into Inequalities in Health*. London: The Stationery Office.

Amowitz L, Reis C, Iacopino V. (2002) Maternal mortality in Herat Province, Afghanistan, in 2002: An indicator of Women's Human Rights. *Journal of the American Medical Association* 288(10): 1284–1291.

Atkinson K, Schattner P, Margolis S. (2003) Rural secondary school students living in a small community: Their attitudes, beliefs and perception towards general practice, *Australian Journal of Rural Health* 11: 73–80.

Black D. (1980) *Inequalities in Health: Report of a Research Working Group.* London: DHSS.

Blackburn C, Spencer N, Read J. (2010) Prevalence of childhood disability and the characteristics and circumstances of disabled children in the UK: Secondary analysis of the Family Resources Survey. *BMC Pediatrics* 10: 21.

Blair M, Stewart-Brown S, Waterson T, Crowther R. (2003) *Child Public Health.* Oxford, UK: Oxford University Press.

Blinder S. (2013) *Briefing: Migration to the UK: Asylum, Migration Observatory.* http://www.migrationobservatory.ox.ac.uk/sites/files/migobs/Briefing%20-%20Migration%20to%20the%20UK%20-%20Asylum_0.pdf (accessed on 20 March 2015).

Boguic M, Ajdukovic D, Bremner S, et al. (2012) Factors associated with mental disorders in long-settled war refugees: Refugees from the former Yugoslavia in Germany, Italy and UK. *British Journal of Psychiatry* 200: 216–223.

Brady H. (2003) Describing ethnicity in health research. *Ethnicity & Health* 8(1): 5–13.

Burnett A, Peel M. (2001) Asylum seekers and refugees in Britain: Health needs of asylum seekers and refugees. *British Medical Journal* 322: 544–547.

Cancer UK (2014) *Childhood Cancer Incidence Statistics,* http://www.cancerresearchuk.org/cancer-info/cancerstats/childhoodcancer/incidence/childhood-cancer-incidence-statistics (accessed on 14 March 2015).

Care Quality Commission. (2012) *Health Care for Disabled Children and Young People: A Review of How the Health Care Needs of Disabled Children and Young People Are Met by the Commissioners and Providers of Health Care in England,* London: CQC, http://www.cqc.org.uk/sites/default/files/documents/health_care_for_disabled_children.pdf (accessed on 5 March 2015).

Churchill R, Allen J, Denman S, et al. (2000) Do attitudes and beliefs of young teenagers towards general practice influence actual consultation behaviour? *British Journal of General Practice* 50: 953–957.

Collier K, van Beusekom G, Bos H, Sandfort T. (2013) Sexual orientation and gender identity/expression related peer victimization in adolescence: A systematic review of associated psychosocial and health outcomes. *Journal of Sex Research* 50 (3–4): 299–317.

Connell P, McKevitt C, Low N. (2004) Investigating ethnic differences in sexual health: Focus groups with young people. *Sexually Transmitted Infections* 80: 300–305.

Cooper H, Smaje C, Arber S. (1998) Use of health services by children and young people according to ethnicity and social class: Secondary analysis of national data. *British Medical Journal* 317: 1047–1051.

Cooper H, Smaje C, Arber S. (1999) Equity in health service use by children: Examining the ethnic paradox. *Journal of Social Policy* 23: 457–478.

Council of Europe (1950) *Convention for the Protection of Human Rights and Fundamental Freedoms.* http://conventions.coe.int/Treaty/en/Treaties/Html/005.htm (accessed on 9 January 2007).

Council of Europe. (1961) *European Social Charter.* http://conventions.coe.int/Treaty/en/Treaties/Html/035.htm (accessed on 9 January 2007).

Davie D. (2013) The child with a disability. In BMA (2013), *Growing Up in the UK – Ensuring a Healthy Future for Our Children.* BMA Board of Science. http://bma.org.uk/working-for-change/improving-and-protecting-health/child-health/growing-up-in-the-uk (accessed on 13 March 2015).

Davis M, Modell S. (2010) Children with disabilities: Victimisation, sexuality and communication. *Injury Prevention* 16 A95 doi:10.1136/ip.2010.029215.344.

Department for Education and Employment. (2000) *Sex and Relationship Education Guidance: 0116/2000*. London: Department for Education and Employment.

Dressler W, Oths K, Gravlee C. (2005) Race and ethnicity of public health research: Models to explain health disparities. *Annual Review of Anthropology* 34: 231–252.

Ellis V, High S. (2004) Something to tell you: Gay, lesbian or bisexual young people's experiences of secondary schooling. *British Educational Research Journal* 30(2): 213–225.

Engels F. (1987) *The Conditions of the Working Class in England*. Harmondsworth: Penguin.

Faculty of Public Health. (2008) *The Health Needs of Asylum Seekers: A Briefing Statement*. Faculty of Public Health. http://www.fph.org.uk/uploads/bs_aslym_seeker_health.pdf (accessed on 10 February 2015).

Fazel M, Stein A. (2003) Mental health of refugee children: Comparative study. *British Medical Journal* 327: 134.

Forrest S, Ellis V. (2011) The making of sexualities: Sexuality, identity and equality. In Cole M, ed. *Education, Equality and Human Rights*, 3rd edition. Oxford, UK: Routledge. 101–127.

Health and Social Care Information Centre. (2012) *Statistics on Obesity, Physical Activity and Diet, England: 2012*. London: NHS Health and Social Care Information Centre, Public Health Statistics. http://www.hscic.gov.uk/catalogue/PUB05131/obes-phys-acti-diet-eng-2012-rep.pdf (accessed on 12 February 2015).

Health and Social Care Information Centre. (2014) *Smoking, Drinking and Drug Use Among Young People in England–2012*, London: NHS Health and Social Care Information Centre, Public Health Statistics, http://www.hscic.gov.uk/catalogue/PUB11334 (accessed on 20 March 2015).

Her Majesty's Government. (2010) *Healthy Lives, Healthy People: Our Strategy for Public Health in England*. London: The Stationery Office.

Jacobson LD, Wilkinson C, Owen PA. (1994) Is the potential of teenage consultations being missed?: A study of consultations in primary care. *Family Practice* 11: 296–299.

Jones L, Bellis A, Hughes K, et al. (2012) Prevalence and risk of violence against children with disabilities: A systematic review and meta-analysis of observational studies. *The Lancet* 380(9845): 899–907.

Lloyd T, Forrest S, Davidson N. (2001) *Boys and Young Men's Health: Literature and Practice Review Interim Report*. London: Health Development Agency.

Lynes D, Lynes A. (2012) Strategies to help adolescents stop smoking. *Nursing Times* 108(26): 12–14.

MacKinnon D, Shucksmith J, Spratt J. (2002) *Young People and Health in Scotland: What Matters to Young People about Their Health and Well-Being*: Research in Brief 3. Edinburgh: Health Board for Scotland.

Malik R, Oandasan I, Yang M. (2002) Health promotion, the family physician and youth. Improving the connection. *Family Practice* 19: 523–528.

Marmot M, Allen J, Goldblatt P, et al. (2010) *Fair Society, Healthy Lives: The Marmot Review*. London: The Marmot Review available at: http://www.instituteofhealthequity.org/projects/fair-society-healthy-lives-the-marmot-review (accessed on February 2015).

Mooney A, Owen C, Statham J. (2008) *Disabled Children: Numbers, Characteristics and Local Service Provision*. London: Thomas Coram Research Unit Institute of Education, University of London.

Mustanski BS, Garofalo R, Emerson EM. (2010) Mental health disorders, psychological distress, and suicidality in a diverse sample of lesbian, gay, bisexual, and transgender youths. *American Journal of Public Health* 100: 2426–2432.

Neale J, Worrell M, Randhawa G. (2005) Reaching out: Support for ethnic minorities. *Mental Health Practice* 9: 12–16.

Office for National Statistics. (2001) *Social Focus in Brief: Children.* www.statistics.gov.uk/downloads/theme_social/social_focus_in_brief/children/Social_Focus_in_Brief_Children_2002.pdf (accessed on 9 January 2007) www.strategy.gov.uk/downloads/work_areas/disability/disability_report/pdf/disability.pdf (accessed on 9 January 2007).

Office for National Statistics. (2005) *Mental Health of Children and Young People in Great Britain, 2004.* http://www.hscic.gov.uk/catalogue/PUB06116/ment-heal-chil-youn-peop-gb-2004-rep2.pdf (accessed on 2 March 2015).

Office for National Statistics. (2011) *Ethnicity and National Identity in England and Wales 2011.* http://www.ons.gov.uk/ons/rel/census/2011-census/key-statistics-for-local-authorities-in-england-and-wales/rpt-ethnicity.html (accessed on 11 January 2015).

Office for National Statistics. (2012) *Measuring National Well-being – Households and Families, 2012.* http://www.ons.gov.uk/ons/dcp171766_259965.pdf (accessed on 20 February 2015).

Office of the Deputy Prime Minister/Department for Work and Pensions/Department of Health/Department for Education and Skills. (2005) *Improving the Life Chances of Disabled People: Final Report.* London: The Stationery Office.

Plant L, Parsons S, Chatzitheochari S, et al. (2013a) *Research Summary One: What Is the Prevalence of Child Disability?* Briefing paper. London: Centre for Longitudinal Studies. http://www.cls.ioe.ac.uk/page.aspx?&sitesectionid=1203&sitesectiontitle=Trajectories+and+transitions+in+the+cognitive+and+educational+development+of+disabled+children+and+young+people (accessed on 2 March 2015).

Plant L, Parsons S, Chatzitheochari S, et al. (2013b) *Research Summary Two: Do Families with a Disabled Child Face Greater Socio-Economic Disadvantage? And How Does the Risk of Disadvantage Vary with Age?* London: Centre for Longitudinal Studies. http://www.cls.ioe.ac.uk/page.aspx?&sitesectionid=1203&sitesectiontitle=Trajectories+and+transitions+in+the+cognitive+and+educational+development+of+disabled+children+and+young+people (accessed on 2 March 2015).

Plant L, Parsons S, Chatzitheochari S, et al. (2014) *Research Summary Four: Are Disabled Children and Young People at a Higher Risk of Being Bullied?* Briefing paper. London: Centre for Longitudinal Studies. http://www.cls.ioe.ac.uk/page.aspx?&sitesectionid=1203&sitesectiontitle=Trajectories+and+transitions+in+the+cognitive+and+educational+development+of+disabled+children+and+young+people (accessed on 2 March 2015).

Priest N, Paradies Y, Trenerry B, et al. (2013) A systematic review of studies examining the relationship between reported racism and health and wellbeing for children and young people. *Social Science & Medicine* 95: 115–127.

Räisänen U, Hunt K. (2014) The role of gendered constructions of eating disorders in delayed help-seeking in men: A qualitative interview study. *BMJ Open* 2014;4:e004342 doi:10.1136/bmjopen-2013-004342

Reed RV, Fazel M, Jones L, et al. (2012) Mental health of displaced and refugee children resettled in low-income and middle income countries: Risk and protective factors. *Lancet* 379: 250–265.

Refugee Council. (2015) *Children in the Asylum System: March 2015.* British Refugee Council http://www.refugeecouncil.org.uk/assets/0003/3863/Children_in_the_Asylum_System_Mar_2015.pdf (accessed on 12 February 2015).

Saxena S, Eliahoo J, Majeed A. (2002) Socioeconomic and ethnic group differences in self-reported health status and use of health services by children and young people in England: Cross sectional study. *British Medical Journal* 325: 520–526.

Schmidt A, Spies D. (2014) Do parties 'playing the race card' undermine natives' support for redistribution? Evidence from Europe. *Comparative Political Studies* 47(4): 519–549.

Social Care Institute for Excellence. (2001) *Good Practice in Social Care with Refugees and Asylum Seekers*. London: SCIE. http://www.scie.org.uk/publications/guides/guide37/files/guide37.pdf

Shakespeare T. (2006) The social model of disability. *The Studies Reader* 2: 197–204.

Smith GD, Chaturvedi N, Harding S, et al. (2000) Ethnic inequalities in health: A review of the UK epidemiological evidence. *Critical Public Health* 10(4): 375–408.

Spencer N, Read J. (2010) Prevalence of childhood disability and the characteristics and circumstances of disabled children in the UK: Secondary analysis of the Family Resources Survey. *BMC Pediatrics* 10: 21.

Stone N, Ingham R. (2003) When and why do young people in the United Kingdom first use sexual health services? *Perspectives on Sexual and Reproductive Health* 35(3): 114–120.

Szczepura A. (2005) Access to health care for ethnic minority populations. *Postgraduate Medical Journal* 81: 141–147.

The Children's Society. (2012) *Holes in the Safety Net: The Impact of Universal Credit on Disabled People and Their Families*. Report of the joint inquiry led by Baroness Tanni Grey-Thompson for The Children Society and Disability Rights UK. http://www.childrenssociety.org.uk/sites/default/files/tcs/holes_in_the_safety_net_disability_and_universal_credit_full_report.pdf (accessed on 20 March 2015).

The Children's Society. (2013) *Hidden from View the Experience of Young Carers in Britain*. http://www.childrenssociety.org.uk/sites/default/files/tcs/hidden_from_view_-_final.pdf (accessed on 15 March 2015).

Trask JW. (1916) The significance of the mortality rates of the coloured population of the United States. *American Journal of Public Health* 6: 254–260.

Tyler R, Williams S. (2014) Masculinity in young men's health: Exploring health, help-seeking and health service use in an online environment. *Journal of Health Psychology* 19 (4): 457–470.

United Nations (1989) *Convention on the Rights of the Child*. www.ohchr.org/english/law/pdf/crc.pdf (accessed on 9 January 2007).

Wardle J, Brodersen NH, Cole T, et al. (2006) Development of adiposity in adolescence: Five year longitudinal study of an ethnically and socioeconomically diverse sample of young people in Britain. *British Medical Journal* 332: 1130–1135.

ACTS OF PARLIAMENT

Human Rights Act 1998
Children and Families Act 2014
Disability Discrimination Act 2005
Equality Act 2010

The changing landscape of child protection

4

JUNE THOBURN

Jenny and Tommy Brown (a teenager and an infant in need of additional services)

Tommy was born when his mother Jenny was 16. She was the youngest of three children, had a mild learning disability though remained in mainstream education with a Statement of Special Educational Needs. She had an apparently normal childhood until she became rebellious after her father left home to live with another woman and her mother began to suffer from depression. Jenny, in turn, began to truant from school, 'clubbing' with young people, and on occasion she came home drunk.

When she became pregnant at the age of 16 she refused to say who Tommy's father was but said that she was pleased she was pregnant, gave up smoking and followed all advice given. Jenny and Tommy lived with the maternal grandmother for six months and Tommy was given good care by his mother and grandmother and he thrived. When he was eight months old Jenny began to see her former friends and returned to clubbing and drinking. Following a row with her mother, she and Tommy moved into a bedsit with her new boyfriend, Max Williams, a man in his thirties who had regular but low paid work as a cleaner. Jenny became pregnant again, and home conditions for Tommy deteriorated, causing concern to the GP, health visitor and midwife.

Jenny confided in the health visitor that, although Max was generally good with Tommy, sometimes he lost his temper and shouted at her and at Tommy. She said that this was made much worse because the one bedroom flat was very damp, the neighbours were rowdy and kept Tommy awake at night, and they desperately needed to move before the new baby was born. With the agreement of Jenny and Max, the health visitor made a referral to Children's Social Services for an assessment of the family's needs for additional help, focusing particularly on the need for more suitable housing and for support in caring for Tommy in the later stages of the pregnancy.

The changing fortunes of the 'Brown/Williams' family are used in this chapter to illustrate how health and social services may become involved in the lives of children and their families when they have additional needs.

INTRODUCTION: CHILD PROTECTION IN ITS PUBLIC HEALTH CONTEXT

In an important series of papers on child maltreatment published in *The Lancet* (2008), internationally respected practitioners and researchers from across health and social welfare were in general agreement about the factors likely to cause harm to children. They also agreed that the incidence of child maltreatment is very considerably higher than reported in the published statistics and that the decision to define some behaviours as abusive and requiring protective action by the state varies over time and place. In other words, *child abuse* and *child protection* should not be used (as they often are) interchangeably to refer to a broad range of public health and corrective measures.

As an obvious example, to smack a child is an assault in some countries but in others (including the four nations of the United Kingdom) it is a permitted form of discipline. That said, the characteristics of children and families who may need additional (*nonuniversal-track*) services that come under the broad *child protection* heading, are generally similar across time, across national boundaries and across service settings*.

The prioritisation of types of need and the configuration of services do, however, differ considerably in different contexts, not least with respect to the wealth or poverty of a country and its people, and the readiness or otherwise to devote national resources, when they are available, to both universal and *targeted* services. These differences are reflected in the discourses around societal values, family needs and rights, family strengthening provisions as well as what is considered to be *abuse* or *maltreatment* requiring state intervention in family life.

This chapter focuses on developing the understanding of child maltreatment and approaches to meeting need for both voluntary and more coercive services in the four UK nations[†]. It makes reference to how these fit into the context of other Anglophone nations with whom we share a common literature and, to some extent, research base as well as Western Europe and the Nordic countries whose post-war welfare systems are more similar to those in the United Kingdom.

Irrespective of political and welfare systems, the right to privacy and to family life is enshrined in the United Nations Convention on Human Rights and the UN Convention on the Rights of the Child (UNCRC) (United Nations 1989; Reading et al. 2009). Both have contributed to a broad consensus on the respective roles of the individual and the state. The latter provides for periodic inspections of compliance by the signatories (i.e. all nations except the United States, Somalia and Taiwan).

---

* The generic terms *service* and *agency* are used in this chapter to include health trusts, primary care services, schools and various local government departments.
† Where data and legislative provisions are cited, they are for England.

> **Using language respectfully when we communicate with clients and between professionals**
>
> An important question about which there is no agreement is how we should refer to the families and children needing additional services. For example, if parents are not to be referred to as *perpetrators* or *child abusers*, what term is appropriate? The term in the England legislation is *child in need* (or family member of such a child) or child/family *in need of a targeted service*. Other phrases often used are *vulnerable* children/families; families under stress; struggling families; children/families in especially difficult circumstances (used in UNICEF reports). These are used interchangeably in this chapter. The term *service user* (with connotations of *customer* and voluntariness) that is used in much social care literature does not fit well in all situations since there is often an element of coercion or social control (of parents or older children). A sense of coercion is never far away even when the parents or children ask for a service and work cooperatively as members of the team around their family.

THE CHANGING DISCOURSES OF *CHILD ABUSE* AND *CHILD PROTECTION*

In this contextual overview, I make no apology for locating recent changes in their historical context. In a recent *Memoir*, Olive Stevenson (author of the minority report on the death of Maria Colwell) commented *It is irresponsible not to look back and ask – how did we get here, what has been learned and what has been lost?* (Stevenson 2013, p 98). See Table 4.1

An immediate problem is created by the terms *at risk, child protection* and *prevention* as they beg the question – protection from/prevention (at risk) of what? The question has recently come to prominence again in England with lobbying for a clearer definition of a criminal offence of child neglect (Action for Children 2013).

Prior to the post WW2 establishment of welfare states across much of Western Europe, including the United Kingdom, the emphasis was on rescuing children from (mainly parental) cruelty, or on providing care for homeless, abandoned or orphaned children. Otherwise, the family was generally left well-alone.

But since the creation of social services departments (in England the specialist Children's Departments followed the ground-breaking *Children Act 1948*), the emphasis has increasingly been on helping parents and children who are experiencing stressful circumstances and on encouraging self-referral. This help was initially provided by out-of-home care when requested at

Table 4.1 The emerging language of child maltreatment

Nineteenth and twentieth centuries — New concepts and language
- Child cruelty/abandonment (eg NSPCC) (nineteenth century)
- Battered child syndrome (1960s)
- Non-accidental injury (1970s to the present)
- Failure to thrive (1970s)
- Munchausen's by proxy/fabricated illness (1970s)
- Sexual abuse/ritual (satanic) abuse (1980s to the present)

Twenty-first century — The most frequent concerns
- Chronic physical and emotional neglect (often associated with addictions)
- Emotional/psychological abuse (including exposure to domestic violence)
- Trafficking/grooming/online abuse by adults
- Child on child abuse (bullying, gangs)

times of stress (alongside the only occasionally used *child rescue* services). Hence, most children were 'received into care' at the request of parents rather than 'taken into care' via court action.

Since the *Children and Young Persons Act 1963* (Section 1), there has been a duty placed on local authorities to provide assistance to children in their own homes. Initially, this was under the guise of *prevention* but the ambiguity over 'prevention of what?' was resolved by Part 3 of the *Children Act 1989* when the language changed to the more positive 'family support'. The originators of the 1989 Act (referred to in more detail below), influenced and were influenced by those working on the UNCRC (United Nations [UN] 1989). Unsurprisingly, the English legislation and the UNCRC are very similar in tone and content, and unlike much other UK health and welfare legislation, the Act and the accompanying statutory guidance remain largely unchanged to date, though some 'tweaking' and clarifying has occurred. Similar legislation has since been passed across Europe. In essence, the statutory duty (largely placed on public social work or social welfare agencies) is to achieve a balance between supporting children in their own families, but using clearly defined legal or administrative powers to act decisively to protect children from harm that arises from parental acts of commission or omission.

> The terms *social services*, *social care* and *social work* may be understood differently in different contexts. In this chapter, I use social care, social care services or children's social services as the broader terms to include all aspects of child and family social welfare services. The social work service is that part of the social care service for which a registered social worker holds the case accountability or a team leader/monitoring role. Although social workers have a lead role in managing and providing social care services, a wide range of professionals and para-professionals may be employed in or formally attached (out-posted) to public or third sector children's social care agencies.

The family support provisions also recognize that children may need protection from harms other than those for which their parents can be held responsible. The statutory agencies are required to provide appropriate services to all family members to ensure that children identified as *in need* of additional services are able to have a 'reasonable standard of health or development'. These are defined in terms of physical, emotional, cognitive and behavioural development and children are to be protected from any impairment of their health or development irrespective of the factors that may be resulting in actual or likely harm.

This brings us back to the changing discourse of what is understood in a particular place and time (and in the United Kingdom now) by the terms *child protection, child abuse* and *safeguarding children*. Until Kempe's work on 'the battered child syndrome' became known to professionals in the United Kingdom (Kempe et al. 1962), the overall term was *child cruelty* (as in *NSPCC*) and the first *BMJ* article on the 'battered baby syndrome' was that of Griffiths and Moynahan (1963). To cover specific offences that could lead to prosecution of a parent and/or of a child being compulsorily removed from the family home, the courts were required to follow the making of a 'Fit Person Order'. In the 1970s, the language in more general use changed to either *child abuse* (by parents, people known to them, or strangers) or to *non-accidental injury* (Table 4.2).

The local co-ordinating committees led by Children's Departments (Social Services Departments since the 1960s) that reviewed the cases of children *at risk* were renamed in 1974 as Area Review Committees (ARCs). This change followed publication of the findings from the Maria Colwell inquiry report (DHSS 1974a). Local authorities were strongly advised to set these up but they were not yet required by legislation. They were tasked with devising local procedures for the management of cases of maltreatment and with *approving written instructions describing the duties of all personnel concerned with any aspect of these cases* (DHSS 1974b, p. 1).

Table 4.2 The changing discourse of child protection

- Child rescue/child saving/taking into care/'fit person orders' (pre 1948)
- Prevention of maltreatment/preventive services (1948/1963)
  (Area Review Committees – 1974)
- Family support for children *in need* (1989)
- Area Child Protection Committees (ACPCs – 1988)
  (Child Protection Registers [CPRs])
- Local Safeguarding Children Boards (2006)
  (Child Protection Plans [CPPs])

They were also tasked with increasing awareness of non-accidental injury. (The emphasis at this point was still on physical abuse of infants.) Most local authorities began at this point to use *child abuse registers* listing the names of children considered by multi-disciplinary case conferences to have been abused or neglected or to be at risk of maltreatment.

A PROCEDURAL APPROACH TO CHILD PROTECTION

It could be argued that this was the beginning of a *procedural* approach to preventing and responding to child maltreatment rather than a *professional competence* approach. The dominant professionals were paediatricians and A&E consultants, social workers and police. The agencies that focus more on the practical aspects of child welfare (housing departments and social security staff) had been important members of the co-ordinating committees that then dropped into the background. The ARCs were renamed ACPCs and were put on a mandatory basis in 1988. At this point, children's names began to be placed on Child Protection Registers (CPRs). This change of language (from *abuse* to *protection*) moved the focus from establishing what *had* happened to *what was to be done* by the (protective) services. The earlier emphasis on physical assault was also broadened to include sexual abuse and emotional and physical neglect and also psychological abuse but the emphasis was still on responding to maltreatment rather than its prevention.

The first official government *Working Together* guidance in 1988 was subtitled 'a guide to arrangements for interagency *cooperation for protection from abuse'*. This at least produced clarity, for parents and professionals, that the focus of this work was abuse or serious neglect. It was understood that an element of coercion was part of these administrative processes. And it included the threat of recourse to court and the removal of the child into compulsory care if the child was re-abused or the care of the child did not improve. However, a series of influential DH funded research studies published during the 1980s (summarized in *Child Protection: Messages from Research*, Department of Health [DH] 1995) led to a stronger emphasis in the *Children Act 1989* on family support and working collaboratively with parents and children. A duty was placed on other publicly funded agencies at this time ('any health authority' was specifically mentioned), to assist the local authority in carrying out its duties to provide services to children 'in need' and their families and to do so beyond narrower child maltreatment cases. This consolidated the changes that had already been happening and moved towards a broader public health focus. In this way, growing evidence emerged that only a minority of children and families need a co-ordinated service and not all should be 'caught in the child protection net' (Gibbons et al. 1995). This is a point recently re-stated in *The Lancet* papers (Gilbert et al. 2009).

The next version or *Working Together* (Home Office et al. 1991) came out fairly quickly to take on board what became known at the time as the DH encouragement to *refocus* services with

Returning to our case study above, if the midwife or GP had decided to refer Jenny Brown (a young person with a learning disability, aged only 16 when she became pregnant, and known to have behavioural problems), it is likely that both Jenny as a vulnerable teenager and her baby when born would be assessed as *in need* of additional services. She is, however, in the care of the primary care team who can exercise professional judgement not to make a referral to Children's social services at this stage. They will be aware that the local authority threshold for the allocation of a social work service is high, and also that Jenny is best served by advice from the primary health care team and the support of her mother and older sister.

greater emphasis on earlier intervention to provide assistance to families experiencing stressful circumstances. It included a section on the involvement of parents (and older children) in the protective and supportive services and a requirement to include family members in child protection conferences wherever possible. A parallel guide: *The challenge of partnership in child protection* (DH 1995) emphasized this change of approach. Nevertheless, the emphasis and most of the guidance was still on child maltreatment and child protection procedures.

As with earlier legislative change, a government-funded inquiry following the murder of a child (in this case the Laming report on the death of Victoria Climbié was instrumental in further government activity. Following the *Every Child Matter* white paper (HMG 2004), legislated for by the 2004 *Children Act*, the direction of travel towards a public health approach was emphasized by the change of language. In the 2006 version of the statutory guidance, this was emphasized by the change of title (*Working Together to Safeguard Children*, HMG 2006) and ACPCs became Local Safeguarding Children Boards (LSCBs). Although the actual procedures changed very little and multi-disciplinary child protection conferences retained their central place, CPRs were abolished and decisions had to be taken as to whether a child was in need of a (formal) CPP.

The remit of the LSCBs was broadened to include safeguarding children from all forms of harm or impairment. The duty of all agencies to co-operate with the local authority child welfare services were further strengthened (*Children Act 2004*, Section 10). The latest version of Working Together (HMG 2013) confirms this more inclusive approach.

1. Providing early help is more effective in promoting the welfare of children than reacting later.
2. Early help means providing support as soon as a problem emerges, at any point in a child's life, from the foundation years through to the teenage years.
3. Effective early help relies upon local agencies working together to
   - Identify children and families who would benefit from early help; undertake an assessment of the need for early help; and
   - Provide targeted early help services to address the assessed needs of a child and family which focuses on activity to significantly improve the outcomes for the child. Local authorities, under Section 10 of the *Children Act 2004*, have a responsibility to promote inter-agency cooperation to improve the welfare of children (HMG 2013, p11).

The 2004 legislation also saw responsibility for children's social services transfer from the Department of Health to the Department for Children Schools and Families for national policy and regulatory purposes. At local level, accountability for children's social care services transferred from social services departments covering all age groups to children's services departments thus combining children's social care services with education services. The rationale was that this change would achieve greater emphasis on the needs and rights of children, and would help to avoid the over-emphasis (reported in some child abuse inquiries) on prioritising the views and meeting the needs of parents over those of the children. Arguably this split (at national and local level) between responsibility for the provision of services to vulnerable children and responsibility for vulnerable adults resulted in a step backward in the move toward a coherent public health approach to family support and child maltreatment. In a majority of cases in which children are assessed as in need of additional social care services, at least one parent has a physical or cognitive disability, chronic or acute health conditions or mental health and addiction problems, and there is evidence that the split between adult and children's social care services has made it more difficult to provide timely and co-ordinated services to families struggling with a range of adult, child and relationship difficulties (Brandon et al. 2008; Thoburn 2010; Thoburn et al. 2013).

The broader role envisaged for LSCBs was in line with the legislation, but concerns have been expressed that their wider remit risks blurring accountability between the different health, education and social care services. Also, concerns have been expressed that LSCBs might 'take their eye off the ball' of ensuring the sort of collaborative approach needed for the most serious cases of child maltreatment that may lead to death, serious injury or long-term impairment to wellbeing.

ANOTHER TRAGIC CHILD DEATH AND ANOTHER REVIEW OF CHILD PROTECTION SERVICES

Following the highly publicized death of Peter Connolly at the hands of his mother and associates, the Munro review of child protection was set up to enquire more broadly into the functioning of the child protection services (Department for Education [DfE] 2011). Although the term *protection* rather than *safeguarding* was used, the broad emphasis towards combining family support with protective services continued. The report contains a chapter titled *'Sharing the responsibility for early help'* which highlights, for example, the work of the multi-disciplinary Sure Start children's centres and the nurse–family partnership projects (see Part 2 *'The Child in the Family'*).

The chapter on social work expertise in the Munro report emphasizes the need to move away from procedurally driven practice encouraged by a *target* and *risk averse* culture towards one which emphasizes professional accountability, values and skills and spending more time with parents and children to inform professional judgements. The term *child and family social worker* rather than *child protection social worker* is used to emphasize the importance of high quality services. It recognizes that a child and family may be in need of additional help.

In summary, in the United Kingdom and much of Europe and indeed in many poorer countries, the term *child protection* is now usually understood (at least in professional circles though not necessarily by the media or general public) as protection from a range of harms, including, but not exclusively from abusive acts, neglect or the failure of parents to protect from such harms. Accordingly, child protection services include family support services (sometimes referred to as *family strengthening services*), and they are to be provided wherever possible on a voluntary basis in consultation with parents, wider kin, and older children. This differs from the United States where broader family support and child treatment services are not generally available unless covered by insurance, and then they are usually time limited. The language in England and much of Europe is of *referral* for a service rather than *notification* of possible abuse; *helping* rather than providing an *intervention* or *clinical practice*. It is noticeable that in the latest version of the statutory guidance on working together to secure better outcomes for children, chapter 1 has the title: 'Assessing Need and Providing Help'. It does not say 'investigating maltreatment and providing interventions'.

THE LEGAL MANDATE TO HELP FAMILIES AND SANCTION COMPULSORY INTERVENTION

The legislation referred to here is specific to England, but as already noted, child and family welfare law is broadly similar across EU jurisdictions, following, as it does, the requirements of the UNCRC. Since 1948, the main accountability for children's social services, (covering children living in their own homes and those actually or formerly in public out-of-home care) rests with the local authority.

Referrals for a child and family social work service can be made by family members themselves, members of the community or community professionals. In recent years, health, education and housing services, the police and other public safety professionals and voluntary agencies have all been encouraged to use the *Common Assessment Framework* (Children's Workforce Development Council [CWDC] 2000). It is guidance and a set of tools and schedules intended to facilitate collaborative working and appropriate referrals to children's social services. Anyone (professional or community member) who considers that a child has been maltreated or is likely to be maltreated can make a referral for this to be investigated and all professionals have a duty to do so. However, it is not a criminal offence not to do so as is the case in several other countries – see 'mandatory reporting'.

The Brown family provides a case example.

When Jenny was pregnant with her second child, the primary health care services (the GP, health visitor and midwife working closely together) recognized the vulnerability of the Brown/Williams family and provided an enhanced service, which Jenny was pleased to have. No services (other than health) were involved. Therefore, a multi-agency assessment for an early help service (using the Common Assessment Framework procedures) was not considered appropriate. When Jenny told the Health Visitor about Max's loss of temper, she concluded that Tommy and the expected baby were likely to be considered children *in need* of a targeted family support service, and she hoped that children's services could lend weight to the family's application for supported housing. The parents agreed to the referral in the hope that it would help achieve a housing move.

Following referral, an initial assessment will lead to a decision as to whether any child in the family is a *child in need* of additional services, and whether the particular local authority's threshold for the provision of services has been crossed. The assessment must be conducted by a registered social worker but will involve discussions with the referrer and others working with the family. Whether or not this was mentioned by the referrer, the assessment will seek to discover if there is evidence that a child is suffering or likely to suffer significant harm. Once assessed as *in need* the allocated social worker (in consultation with their team leader) has a duty to ensure that appropriate services are made available. Section 17 of the *Children Act 1989* states that a child is *in need* of additional services if

- He or she is unlikely to achieve a reasonable standard of health or development without the provision of [additional social care] service
- His or her health or development [mental, physical or cognitive] is likely to be significantly impaired without the provision of an additional social care service
- He or she is disabled (disability is tightly defined but a child with a moderate disability may be assessed as *in need* under the first three provisions)
- He or she is aged 16 or 17 and his or her health or development is likely to be seriously harmed unless provided with (Section 20) accommodation

The agreement of parents and older children is required for the assessment and provision of services, unless there is reason to believe that a child may be abused or neglected. The threshold for compulsory investigation and intervention is that there is evidence that a child is suffering or is likely to suffer significant harm (Section 31 of the *Children Act 1989*).

Although all local authorities are under pressure, and seek to keep social work caseloads down to a manageable size, this is a demand-led service. Waiting lists may be possible for specific services, but not for allocation to a social worker caseload once it is decided that there is a child *in need* in the family. *It is not lawful to confine service provision only to those cases where there are concerns about maltreatment.*

There is often confusion about the term *statutory* service, since services are required, by statute, to be provided to children assessed as *in need* as well as those who may be in need of protective services. Social workers and their team managers who *sign off* the assessment are accountable for the professional judgement about whether a child is *in need*. They can be disciplined if their work is considered incompetent in this respect. The local authority, however, has considerable discretion as to which services will be provided, including whether an out-of-home placement is appropriate on a voluntary basis or an application must be made to court for a care or supervision order.

The difference between providing a family support service because a child's 'health or development is being or is likely to be significantly impaired' and providing a formal child protection service because a child is suffering or is likely to suffer significant harm is one requiring professional judgement. Usually, if there is a possibility of significant harm which may be attributable to parental fault, the formal child protection processes will be appropriate (see below). The decision about whether services will be provided with parental agreement under the 'family support'/'child in need' provisions or under a more coercive formal CPP will be arrived at following a multi-disciplinary child protection conference. A relevant factors being considered, alongside the degree of risk and the severity of any abuse or neglect already experienced, will also include the willingness of parents and older children to work alongside the professionals to improve parenting and reduce any identified risks.

In short, there is no clear distinction (except at either end of the continuum) between a family for whom a co-ordinated 'early help' (tier 2) service will keep serious problems at bay; a family for whom a targeted 'in need'/family support service is appropriate; and a family where a formal child protection service is required. In a small number of cases, for example, if a child is sexually assaulted by an 'infiltrating perpetrator' (Cleaver and Freeman 1995) and the mother takes protective action as soon as this is known, a skilled, intensive but short-term service may be what is needed.

However, many families with complex difficulties will need longer term services and will move between lower level family support services and more formal child protection services depending on the extent of stress. For them, there will be protective elements in family support plans, and supportive services will be incorporated within any protection plan. For this reason, in this chapter, the term *formal child protection* is used to distinguish services that are provided under the statutory guidance on working with cases of alleged child maltreatment as differentiated from those where there are protective elements in the child *in need* service provided.

THE CHILDREN AND FAMILIES WITH ADDITIONAL NEEDS

So which parents and children are most likely to have additional needs that will trigger the provision of a targeted social work service? The first point to make is that the stresses resulting from material poverty, poor environments (including inadequate housing or insecurity of tenure) result in increased stress and vulnerability for all except the most resilient families (Sidebotham 2001; Ghate and Hazel 2002). These are not causative factors in that many families living in adverse circumstances manage well enough with the support of primary and acute health services, schools and community support services. However, data on the incidence of referrals for a targeted *in need* service, children with protection plans and children in out-of-home care in different local authorities, closely map onto the indices of deprivation (Dickens et al. 2005).

Over and above the impact of material deprivation, there is agreement amongst researchers and professionals that the following parental characteristics are to be found amongst parents who need additional services if children's short- and long-term welfare is to be safeguarded. Two characteristics they often share are complexity, and parental ambivalence about seeking or accepting help (see e.g. Sidebotham 2001; Sidebotham et al. 2006; Social Exclusion Task Force 2007).

Thoburn (2010, p. 11) in a paper on 'hard to reach' and 'hard to change' families identified the following characteristics found in different combinations in parents and children likely to need additional services. Parents who are more likely than the average to

- Be isolated, without extended family, community or faith group support
- Have been abused or emotionally rejected as children or had multiple changes of carer
- Have a mental illness and/or a learning disability, especially if no other parent or extended family member is available to share parenting
- Have a borderline personality disorder
- Have had more than one partner, often involving an abusive relationship
- Have an alcohol or drug addiction and not accept that they must control the habit for the sake of their child's welfare
- Have aggressive outbursts, a record of violence, including intimate partner violence
- Have obsessional/very controlling personalities, often linked with low self-esteem
- Have been in care as a child or adolescent, and have experienced multiple placements or 'aged out' of care without a secure base (potentially mitigated if they had a good relationship with a carer, social worker or social work team who remained available to them through pregnancy and in early parenting)
- Be especially fearful of stigma or suspicious of statutory services (including those from communities which consider it stigmatising to seek state assistance
- Be immigrants who have experienced coercive state power before coming to the United Kingdom, or because of their own experience of poor services as they grew up

Some children and young people have characteristics which make them 'hard to engage' or 'hard to help/change' and, when combined with one or more of the above parental characteristics are most vulnerable to continuing harm:

- Children born prematurely and/or suffering the effects of intrauterine drug and/or alcohol misuse, which can result in infants being fretful, hard to feed and unresponsive.
- Children with disabilities or other characteristics which make them hard to parent or *unrewarding* in the eyes of parents lacking in self-esteem and confidence.

- Individual members of sibling groups singled out for rejection and/or targeted for abuse.
- Children returning home from care, especially if they suffer the loss of an attachment figure (usually a foster carer). Several recent studies have demonstrated that children who return to a parent following more than a short period of planned out-of-home care are more likely to be re-abused than those who remain in permanent foster care, are placed with relatives or are adopted (Sinclair et al. 2007; Brandon and Thoburn 2008; Farmer and Lutman 2012).
- Teenagers (n.b., those who have suffered from unrecognized or ignored abuse or neglect) who engage in risk-taking or anti-social behaviour (Stein et al. 2009).

NUMBERS AND RATES OF CHILDREN RECEIVING TARGETED SERVICES AS CHILDREN *IN NEED* OR *IN NEED OF PROTECTION*

The Department for Education publishes data on children referred for an *in need* or formal child protection service, and also for those for whom an out-of-home care service is provided (referred to as 'accommodated if the service is provided under a voluntary agreement) or "in care" if there is a court order' (DfE 2013b; DfE 2013c).

During 2012–2013

- Almost 600,000 children were referred in England as possibly *in need*.
- 395,100 (approximately 68% of those referred) began to receive an *in need* service. (Others will have been briefly assessed, and possibly referred to a more appropriate service.)
- 52,000 children became the subject of a formal CPP.

On 31 March 2013

- 378,600 children were receiving a targeted social care service for children *in need* including those who were subject to a CPP (333 per 10,000 children aged 0–17).
- Just over 68,000 (a rate of 28 per 10,000 children) were in out-of-home care (the legal terminology is 'looked after children').

Thoburn (2013) compares service systems and incidence in eight European countries. They find the England rate to be towards the middle of the continuum (lower than New Zealand with a rate of 347 per 10,000 children but higher than the United States (225 per 10,000). The rate of children in England with a CPP within the year (around 28 per 10,000) is considerably lower than the 146 substantiated cases of maltreatment in the United States (Gilbert et al. 2008b). However, these data must be treated with caution as England data does not record substantiated cases of maltreatment (only those with a formal protection plan). It should also be noted that this is because of the high number of suspected child maltreatment reports. In the United States, a service is not always provided even when allegations of maltreatment have been substantiated.

A higher proportion of those receiving services in the United States, Canada and Australia do so under formal child protection procedures than is the case for England and most other European countries. The rate for children entering out-of-home care in the United States is also higher (42 per 10,000 compared with 28 per 10,000 in England in 2012–2013). Almost all children enter care under a court order in the United States following substantiation of an allegation of child maltreatment, whereas almost two thirds of those who began to be looked after in England do so with parental agreement. However, around two thirds of those looked after on a given date in England are subject to court orders, since those entering care on a voluntary basis tend to stay for shorter periods.

AGGREGATED DATA ON TYPES OF MALTREATMENT

There has been little change over the years in the categories of maltreatment resulting in child protection registration. A child protection plan refers to physical abuse, sexual abuse, neglect (including emotional neglect and/or exposure to intimate-partner violence and/or emotional (psychological) abuse. There has also been considerable continuity over the years in formal child protection procedures.

However, the recent change from a child being *registered* as a maltreated child to being 'the subject of a formal CPP' does represent a change of emphasis. It has changed from a focus on identifying parental acts of commission or omission to identifying likely future harm. The purpose is to achieve as much agreement as possible with family members before arriving at a coherent multi-disciplinary and inter-agency plan.

There has also been a shift over the years from abuse to neglect and emotional harm categories and a shift in the proportion of children registered with a CP plan in the different categories. For example, while the 'main concern' for protection plans in 2012–2013 was sexual abuse in 5% of cases and physical abuse in 12% (with 11% under the 'multiple' category including one of these), by far the largest categories were neglect (41%) and emotional abuse (37%).

THE SERVICES

Families with some of the characteristics listed above may cope 'well enough' if they have support from community or specialist health services or additional support from schools or youth or community safety services. It is important to flag up here the importance of family strengths and resilience as well as extended family and neighbourhood support systems and the potential for these to be strengthened by early help (tier 1 and tier 2) services. *Working Together* (DfE 2013a) incorporates the earlier *Assessment Framework* guidance on inter-agency working before targeted services become necessary. It also focuses on social workers assessing whether *in need* or formal protective services are required.

In other words, attention paid to the service and community systems as well as to the strengths and problems of parents and children brings an *ecological*, or *whole systems* approach to the assessment of need and the provision of services (Gill and Jack 2007; Jack 2011).

The statutory duty (*Children Act 1989*, Section 17) is on providing, alongside an assessment, whatever help can relieve immediate pressures before a longer term *package* of support, care and protection is put in place. Such decisions require consultation with parents, older children and others in their wider circle as well as professionals who are already working with the family (Figure 4.1).

The 1989 *Children Act* makes provision for the flexible use of a wide range of services, including financial assistance to assist during a crisis or for longer periods. Such periods may include occasions when relatives step in to provide crisis or respite care or the provision of subsidized day care services or the provision of short or longer term out-of-home care. Services can be provided to any member of the family provided they are of benefit to the child who is assessed as *in need*. By definition, this is also including children on formal protection plans or in out-of-home care.

Examples include the following:

- Holidays for siblings of a child with disabilities instead of or as well as *respite care* for the child him- or herself
- Travel fares to ensure that siblings still at home can spend time with a brother or sister in care
- Financial assistance if a grandparent takes time off work or travels from another part of the country to look after grandchildren if a single parent has to be admitted to hospital, including addiction care

It is not the purpose here to describe these *targeted* services in any detail. There is a strong UK knowledge base on the essential elements of social work practice with families

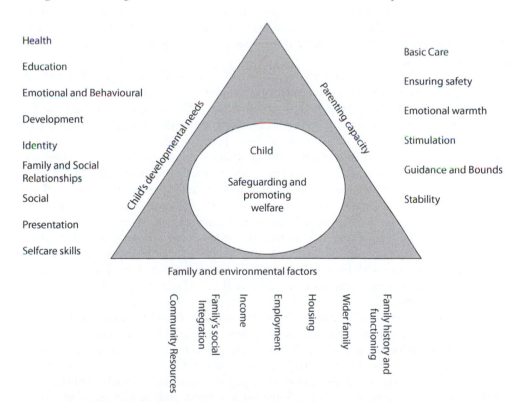

Figure 4.1 The assessment framework.

with complex needs and their children, including those who have been maltreated or need out-of-home care and, in a small minority of cases, placement for adoption. Broadly this includes the knowledge, values and analytic skills for assessment and for helping such as the following:

- Assessment of psycho-social need and of protective and risk factors in the parents, children and wider kinship network and community.
- Assessment of the suitability, motivations and skills of supplementary or substitute carers (volunteers, kinship and unrelated foster carers and adopters) as well as matching carers with families.
- The putting together of effective packages of care, therapy for parents and children (see Chapter 10), of education in the broadest sense (including parenting education) and of support for each family member and the family as a whole.
- The direct provision of a relationship-based psycho-social casework service.
- The co-ordination and active membership of teams set up around individual families or children.

All key practice and research texts on social work with vulnerable children and families emphasize that a reliable, honest and respectful professional relationship is the essential component of services. In almost all cases, a flexible approach is needed which combines elements of practical help, care and control (see Thoburn 2010 for an overview). Although the language has changed over the years, there is much that unites the most frequently used approaches to helping families where there may be child protection concerns. These include 'ecological' (Jack 2011) or 'signs of safety' models of practice (Turnell and Edwards 1997).

Parton and O'Byrne (2000) identify the essential elements of these approaches, both of which emphasize the need to consult parents and children about the services they would find helpful as well as being clear about necessary changes to safeguard and promote the welfare of each child in the family. The forward-looking (enhancing strengths) rather than a backward-looking (problems-based) stance of these approaches can be successful in encouraging family engagement in the work to improve children's and parents' wellbeing. However, Brandon et al. (2008, 2009), use findings from their serious case reviews (SCRs) on child death or serious injury, to emphasize the importance of a detailed psycho-social history. They identify a 'start again syndrome' as a feature of casework with some families and argue that this can contribute to a failure to identify indicators of serious risk. In contrast, some of the *evidence-based* methods imported mainly from the United States and Australia, often originating in psychology rather than social work, are based on social learning theory. Several of these methods bring with them techniques (e.g. *scaling questions* from solution-focused therapy) and a range of tools that can be used in different situations and with a wider range of approaches to practice.

Group-based parenting education interventions (as with Incredible Years, or Tripple P) alongside (Webster-Stratton and Herbert 1999; Lindsay et al. 2008) tend to be used in their 'pure model' at 'universal' and 'tier 2' levels. These are more likely to be used by health and school personnel than by social workers and family support workers. However, many family support workers, especially those employed as intensive outreach workers, have received training in these methods and some aspects and techniques are used as part of broader packages of help when working with more complex families (Thoburn 2010; Thoburn et al. 2013).

The package of support and services to the Brown/Williams family

The health visitor introduced the social worker to the family and together they enabled Jenny and Max to talk about the pressures they were under, their tiredness, and the fact that Jenny found housework and budgeting difficult. With letters of support from the health team, the social worker advocated successfully for the family to be rehoused shortly after Jamie's birth. Financial assistance (*Children Act 1989*, Section 17) was provided to Jenny's mother so she could take time off work to provide day care for Tommy on three days a week. The family was also provided with practical and financial assistance to help with the house move, and a family support worker provided parenting advice, help with sorting out debts, and practical help over the period of Jamie's birth, since Max was afraid of losing his job if he took more than a few days off work. The health team continued to monitor the health of Tommie and Jamie. Three months after Jamie's birth, a *child in need* meeting attended by the parents, Jenny's mother, the social worker, health visitor and family support worker concluded that both Tommie and Jamie were making good progress and stresses between the parents had reduced. The case was closed to social services but the financial support to Jamie's mother continued to allow her to provide day care for both children on two days a week so that Jennie could keep up with her household chores and get some rest because nights were still disrupted.

INTER-PROFESSIONAL AND INTER-AGENCY WORKING

Accountability for the provision and monitoring of targeted services, including the effective operation of the LSCBs and the appointment of the LSCB chair, is placed by law on local authorities and are usually delegated to the lead elected member and the Director of Children's Services. Local authorities also have the broader duty to encourage the development of tier 2/early help support services, and are encouraged to commission such services from the voluntary sector (Morris et al. 2008; Featherstone et al. 2014).

MULTI-DISCIPLINARY TEAMS

With individual cases, collaborative practice (both inter-agency and multi-professional) is almost always essential. Some of this work takes place in multi-disciplinary teams including diverse health professionals, teachers or early years workers, and social workers but also, as in the case of Youth Offending Teams (YOTs) or youth addictions teams, specialist police and youth workers. Sure Start Children's Services are an example of multi-disciplinary teams combining health, social work and education professionals from the statutory and voluntary sectors (Tunstill et al. 2007). Child Guidance Clinics, the precursors of the present CAMHs teams, used to be another example but in recent years these teams have tended to be multi-professional with members from across the health professionals but not inter-agency in that few have social workers act as team members. The work of the Tavistock Clinic is an important exception. More recently, multi-agency safeguarding hubs (MASHs) have been formed to improve the appropriateness and quality of response when families are referred for a 'tier 3' service.

WORKING IN NETWORKS

Most inter-professional and inter-agency work with vulnerable children and families is carried out by professionals coming together in changing networks to provide a service to individual children and families. This *team around the family* approach is now much used with families of children in need and is an extension of *core group* work that was required for many years under *Working Together* provisions and entailed a formal protection plan (see Hallett 1995; Thoburn et al. 2013). Effective working in networks or multi-disciplinary teams can often be helped if single agency teams are *co-located*, for example, a locality social work team based in a housing department or close to a GP surgery.

SYSTEMS AND PROCEDURES AIMED AT SECURING COLLABORATIVE WORKING

Inter-professional working within teams or networks, which may involve joint visits as well as professionals meeting with and without family members, relies on but is not synonymous with *inter-professional collaboration* or *inter-agency co-ordination*. These terms tend to be used interchangeably to refer to professionals and agencies in which each have defined roles and tasks but take steps to ensure the overall coherence of the service provided. The child protection procedures required by the *Working Together* statutory guidance focus more on inter-agency *coordination* rather than joint working as members of multi-disciplinary teams around the family. There are separate sections in the Guidance for the 17 different agencies or service providers whose roles and duties must be co-ordinated (in different combinations according to the needs of the family) to ensure best possible outcomes for vulnerable children.

List of Agencies
Children's Social Services
Schools and Colleges
Early years and child care
Health services
Police
Adult social care
Housing authorities and social housing providers
British Transport Police
Prison service
Probation service
The secure estate for children
Youth Offending Teams
The UK Border Agency
Children and Family Court Advisory and Support Service (Cafcass)
Armed services
Voluntary and private sector agencies working with children
Faith organisations

As noted earlier, the latest version of the guidance continues the direction of travel towards a continuum of better co-ordinated child health, social care and protective services across the service *tiers*. There are specific roles and duties for different professionals who may have a part to play in the helping and protective processes, from assessment through child protection conferences; and from the drawing together and monitoring of formal protection plans to the care given to children who become looked after, in some cases until the age of 26.

LOCAL SAFEGUARDING CHILDREN BOARD

Local authorities are accountable for the effective functioning of LSCBs and the appointment of their Chair, who is now required to be independent of the local authority and of any of the local agencies contributing to its work. The LSCB is tasked with the following:

- Producing and publicising the child protection procedures specific to their areas (based on the *Working Together* statutory guidance)
- Monitoring the Section 27 (*Children Act 1989*) and the Section 10 (*Children Act 2004*) duties of all agencies in their collaboration on individual cases
- Monitoring the Section 11 (*Children Act 2004*) duty of all statutory and voluntary agencies working with children to ensure that checks are carried out on all staff and volunteers who have access to children
- Providing and monitoring the quality of inter-agency and multi-disciplinary training to ensure that all those working with children recognize indications that a child may be experiencing or at risk of experiencing abuse or neglect and are familiar with referral procedures

Each agency required to be represented on the LSCB is also expected to provide joint funding (in cash or in kind). Despite all the duties placed on them, they usually have only a small staff group, mainly involved in providing multi-disciplinary and inter-agency training, and have no direct executive powers to require compliance from any of the member agencies.

It is yet to become clear how they will work with the Health and Wellbeing Boards that are now located within local authorities following NHS reorganisation. The broader public health remit of the Boards also includes monitoring the adequacy and quality of co-ordinated services to vulnerable children and families.

REFERRAL PROCESSES AND SHARING INFORMATION

Much attention is paid in the guidance to mechanisms for ensuring that children receive the appropriate level of service and that there are smooth transitions when case accountability moves between agencies. The England *Working Together* guidance has, over the years, become increasingly explicit that 'child protection is everybody's business'. All those working with children or having contact with them as part of their work, whether public or voluntary sector, have a duty to follow the procedures in their area for notifying children's services if they have reason to believe that a child is suffering or is likely to suffer *significant harm* whether at the hands of a parent or another person. Not to do so, if evidence later emerges that the signs of maltreatment were clear, may result in disciplinary action and, for registered professionals, may result in being removed from their professional register.

However, unlike in many other jurisdictions, the UK nations do not have a system of *mandatory reporting*. In other words, failure to report suspected maltreatment is not a criminal offence. The advantages and disadvantages of mandatory reporting have been debated in the United Kingdom over the years – most recently following the revelations of sexual and physical assault by prominent public figures.

The evidence on the value of mandatory reporting is equivocal, not least because it means different things in different countries. In Sweden, the mandate is to refer any child in need of an additional child welfare service to reduce the risk of maltreatment or impairment. There is no *substantiation of abuse* requirement and therefore less stigma in the eyes of those referred and there is no available information on the numbers of maltreated children. In the United States,

Canada and most Australian States, the mandate is to *notify* or *report* suspected maltreatment, though in some places maltreatment is defined narrowly and in others it includes all forms of possible harm.

The problem with these more inclusive versions of mandatory reporting is that, whilst a physical assault is usually apparent, sexual abuse is less clear and what constitutes serious neglect or emotional abuse, even less so. Professionals tend in mandatory reporting jurisdictions to *play safe* and be more reluctant to use appropriate professional discretion. The higher rate of abuse investigations in these countries (the majority unsubstantiated) has resulted in over-stretched services. Even many of the 'substantiated' cases do not receive a service, and few resources are available for early help services.

When Tommie was four and had just started school, and Jamie was two, the teacher became concerned that Tommie was often late or missed school, often seemed tired and withdrawn and also his clothes were smelly. Jenny told her that the family had a lot of debts and she was frightened when debt collectors came to the door and she had no money. On the positive side, Jenny was going fairly regularly to the Sure Start centre with Jamie and was enjoying doing a basic IT course there whilst Jamie was in play group.

Jenny became very upset at a Sure Start parents' group and told the worker that she and Max were shouting at each other a lot. He had lost his job and was blaming their debts on her inability to manage the money. He also said she was not looking after the children properly. Following the authority's *early help* procedures (the Common Assessment Framework, the Sure-Start worker suggested holding a family meeting between Max and Jenny and all those involved with the family (Sure-Start, GP, health visitor, nursery school, early years teacher, housing support worker and the Sure Start welfare benefits adviser). Max was seeing the GP because of depression and sleep problems and he had also taken up again an earlier cannabis habit. Jenny thought the GP would be the best person to suggest the family meeting to Max, which he did, but Max refused. When, a month later, Tommie arrived at school with grip-marks suggesting that he had been shaken, the head teacher told Jenny she would have to refer the family to children's services.

Next Steps:

… At this point, an allocated social worker would read through the case files on the family; interview Max and Jenny, talk with Tommie together with his teacher, and ask the parents to take both children to the GP to check for any other signs of injury. S(he) would also have discussions with all the professionals who know the family. She would also provide immediate help. This might include assistance in sorting out debts, the allocation of a family support worker, or time spent 'patching up' relationships between Jenny and her mother as the children said they were missing their granny. If the local authority used a locality model of case allocation, the social worker's task could be made easier if she or the team leader knew the family from the earlier referral. Depending on the analysis of the information gained by using the *assessment triangle* domains (see Figure 4.1), the case might be opened as a *child in need* case and a package of services agreed by the *team around the family* (the social worker as lead professional and the others already involved or brought in at this stage to provide specialist help).

Alternatively, the children might be the subjects of a child protection strategy discussion involving, as a minimum, the social worker, the GP and the police child protection unit. The children might become the subject of a formal child protection conference. Depending on the attitudes of the parents and the extent of any harm, the service could be provided under child in need provisions (Section 17) or formal child protection plans.

> If the situation deteriorated further and it became clear that one or both children were suffering significant harm, he/they might be accommodated (*Children Act 1989*, Section 20) and placed with Jenny's mother. The parents would need to agree to this and they might do as an alternative to court action to remove the children compulsorily.
>
> If the harm or likely harm was such that there was a strong possibility that the parents were unable to meet the children's long-term needs, a legal planning meeting might progress to care proceedings. The preferred placement option would be with the grandmother or other relatives but if this were not possible, given the age of the children, placement with an adopter would be the most likely care plan.

The other key issue around the referral stage as well as the helping stages and formal protection procedures is inter-professional communication and data sharing. Alongside the statutory guidance, this has to be understood in the context of international conventions and national legislation on privacy and the protection of personal information. In summary, personal information provided to a statutory or voluntary agency should only be used for the purpose for which it was given, and should remain confidential to the professional or team within the agency that is providing the service (e.g. a school, a social work team, a hospital or CAMHs team or a Sure Start children's centre), unless the person providing the information gives permission for it to be passed on to other named persons, or those fulfilling specific roles. (See HMG 2008, *Guidance on information sharing for practitioners and managers*.)

Critically, an exception to these provisions is that there must be reason to believe that an adult or child is at risk of suffering significant harm if permission is likely to *increase* the risk of harm to a particular individual or to unknown individuals. Each profession has its own code of ethics that guides how these over-arching principles are interpreted, and these codes are broadly similar across the main helping professions. However, those for the police when investigating an alleged crime are somewhat different. In summary, whilst sharing information on a 'need to know' basis to provide appropriate help is to be encouraged, if the service is provided on a voluntary basis, sharing should not happen without the consent of parents or older children. Even when formal child protection intervention is being considered, consent should always be sought whenever this can be done without increasing the risk of harm.

There is therefore a tension between the desirability of sharing information to improve the effectiveness of collaborative working and the requirement to respect privacy and follow ethical codes of practice. In addition to the detailed guidance in *Working Together*, most LSCBs produce their own guidance and protocols on maintaining the confidentiality of identifiable personal information, and the appropriate sharing of information. Some agencies seek to smooth the way for collaborative inter-agency practice and seek to pre-empt any later problems by making a general statement to parents and older children offered a service. In other words, they report at the outset that it is their practice to share information with statutory agencies. This is sometimes made a condition of service provision as with some multi-disciplinary intensive services that are provided to families with complex needs (Thoburn et al. 2013).

When early help services are offered following the *Common Assessment Framework* protocols, parents are asked to agree to the sharing of information with other professionals working with the family, and parents can say if there are specific agencies that should not receive specific information. At a national level, governments have sought to find ways of increasing data sharing, urged by enquiry reports such as the Laming enquiry after the death of Victoria Climbié (House of Commons Health Committee 2003). With the *Contact Point* initiative, the Labour Government went some way down the route of creating a specific identifier and a minimum data set on *all* children. Information (accessible only by specified professionals) was to be made available on the agencies who were providing a service to each child. This was 'switched off' when the coalition government came to power in 2010, on the grounds of effectiveness, rights to privacy and cost. Since then, more modest ideas are being attempted to link identifiable child level data across agencies, as with the 2013–2014 Department of Health led Child Protection Information-sharing project (DH 2014).

Whilst some commentators and writers of SCR reports have called for better systems, and tougher sanctions for those who do not share concerns about possible maltreatment, others have stressed that communication between professionals (backed up by but not replaced by effective, clearly understood and confidential systems for the sharing of written and other records in appropriate cases) should remain the main mechanism for ensuring that the response to each situation is appropriate.

SERIOUS CASE REVIEWS

Following a series of public child death inquiries from the one on the death of Maria Colwell (DHSS 1974a) up to the Laming Inquiry after the death of Victoria Climbié (House of Commons Health Committee 2003), a decision was taken that in most such cases an SCR, rather than a public inquiry, would be held. This change was intended to switch the focus from the allocation of agency and individual professional responsibility (which remains a responsibility for governance bodies for each agency), to ensuring that lessons are learned that contribute to improved practice in the future.

The LSCB must set in motion, monitor and publish the report of an independent SCR in the event of the murder of a child or death resulting from a non-accidental injury, chronic neglect or suicide. In cases of very serious non-accidental injury or neglect likely to result in long-term impairment to health or development and when more than one agency has been involved in the case, the LSCB has some discretion as to whether to commission an SCR.

Initially, only anonymized summaries of the recommendations were published, but an early decision of the coalition government in 2010 determined that the full reports (redacted to protect the confidentiality of any surviving children) should be published. The intention to take the focus off the 'naming and shaming' of professionals has not been realized as was apparent following the recent publication of the SCR reports on Peter Connelly (Jones 2014); and Hamzah Khan (Bradford Safeguarding Children Board 2013). A more nuanced analysis of the findings from these reports is to be found in the series of biannual reports first commissioned by the DCSF/DfE (Brandon et al. 2009). Whilst these remind us that 'hard cases make bad laws' and that making changes following exceptional cases can have negative consequences for the majority, they also identify learning points for each profession working with children across the age range, as well as for inter-agency practice.

THE NEED FOR A HIGH QUALITY, ACCOUNTABLE SERVICE FROM ALL PROFESSIONALS WORKING WITH VULNERABLE CHILDREN

Whilst both a public health focus and insights from SCRs place emphasis on inter-professional and inter-agency working, they also locate high-quality single-professional practice at the centre of effective multi-disciplinary practice. Whether the service is provided by multi-disciplinary teams or practitioners joining together in networks to meet the needs of individual families, parents and children living in stressful circumstances depend on the professional competence of each worker they encounter. And each professional group has its own internal and external quality assurance systems. In the social care domain, social workers and social work managers must be registered with the Health and Care Professions Council (HCPC) and can be disciplined by the HCPC either because of misconduct or lack of competence.

However, this does not apply to Directors of Children's Services, many of whom have a teaching qualification only as an outcome of their frequent dual responsibility for the local authority education services. The same can be the case for family support workers. Since these posts are usually not filled by registered social workers, accountability for decisions about the tasks allocated to them and for the quality of their work, rests with the accountable social worker or social work manager within the authority. This is also the case for nurses and class-room teachers who increasingly work with and supervise support staff.

Because of the high level of discretion that social workers exercise, often working alone in the family home, and sometimes having to take or initiate decisions that have profound consequences, social work teams place much emphasis on regular casework supervision and consultation. Increasingly the term, performance management is used to describe the internal systems for ensuring that any professional service is of an acceptable standard whilst not impeding professional confidence. The Munro report (DfE 2011) regretted that the social work service places too much reliance on the meeting of performance targets and concluded that the fear of blame (e.g. the result of media exposure in high profile cases) was inhibiting the exercise of professional judgement and leading to inappropriate risk-averse practices. Similar reservations have been expressed about paediatricians undertaking child protection assessments and giving evidence in court.

Responsibility for monitoring the quality of services for vulnerable children and families is located with Ofsted, which inspects and reports on the services provided in each local authority. Inspectors make judgements about the overall service provided to children who may be *in need* of additional services, including the formal child protection services. This includes a judgement on the extent to which other agencies fulfil their Section 10 duty to collaborate with children's services, in the provision of *early help*, formal child protection services and services to children who are looked after or who have left care.

Since 1995 when the Department of Health published the influential **Child Protection: Messages from Research**, other relevant DH and DfE studies have been reported in Messages from Research publications. Most relevant to this chapter amongst recent publications are; Family Support: Messages from Research (Quinton 2004); Quality Matters in Children's Services: Messages from Research (Stein 2009) and Safeguarding Children across Services: Messages from Research (Davies and Ward 2013). These report on a range of outputs (i.e. what services were provided and did they reach the *target* population) and, to a lesser degree, did they meet child and adult well-being outcomes?

CONCLUSION: OUTPUTS, OUTCOMES AND THE NEED FOR A PUBLIC HEALTH APPROACH

This chapter cannot even begin to summarize the complex messages from research on outcomes for children and families receiving targeted services other than to state the obvious. On average, children who experience abuse or neglect do less well than those who do not, and adverse effects often persist into adult life, even for those removed through the courts and placed with adoptive families (Neil et al. 2013). Research suggests that abuse by a stranger (a sports coach, for example) is usually less damaging than abuse by a parent provided it becomes known and the parent responds appropriately and speedily. But, the longer the maltreatment continues the more difficult it is to take action to mitigate long-term harm to wellbeing.

It is even more difficult to summarize the messages from research about 'what works' when services can range from a short piece of advocacy and advice to sort out debts and achieve a move to more suitable housing; to episodic support and therapy over many years when a parent has a mental illness; to permanent placement with a substitute family. A two-year old removed from home and adopted, though often considered a *positive outcome*, is an *output* of the casework and legal services that were provided. However, it may not be clear if a successful outcome has been achieved until he or she is in her early 20s. This is because it is recognized that children experiencing trauma and then placed with a substitute family have additional obstacles to overcome before they reach maturity.

A public health approach that encourages families to seek early help, and professionals and community members to make appropriate referrals to sources of assistance and protective action, is therefore the best way forward and is the direction of travel in UK legislation. This approach is also supported by EU institutions, funded research and policy. It is believed to encourage a less *blaming* and more participatory approach to service provision whilst also requiring timely action when coercive intervention becomes necessary.

Given these areas of agreement, there is one key component of public health research and policy that is central to preventive health measures and almost missing from child welfare policy and research. Links between poverty, poor living environments and adverse health outcomes have long been recognized. Poverty and material deprivation are strongly associated with the need for a targeted child welfare intervention. This is illustrated by the higher incidence of protection plans and children removed from home on care orders in the more deprived local authorities in the United Kingdom. Yet, with a few notable exceptions, and mainly led by the charitable sector, child welfare research has focused on individual, family and relationship problems. Far less attention than in the field of physical health has been given to the impact of broader societal and environmental stressors on escalating family problems. This is particularly the case for those who reach the level at which more intrusive remedial or substitute placement services are needed.

REFERENCES

Action for Children. (2013) *The Criminal Law and Child Neglect*. http://www.actionforchildren. org.uk/media/5178586/criminal_law_and_child_neglect.pdf (accessed on 23 March 2014).

Bradford Safeguarding Children Board. (2013) *A Serious Case Review: Hamzah Khan Overview Report*. http://www.bradford-scb.org.uk/scr/hamzah_khan_scr/Serious%20Case%20 Reveiw%20Overview%20Report%20November%202013.pdf (accessed on 23 March 2014).

Brandon M, Thoburn J. (2008) Safeguarding children in the UK: A longitudinal study of services to children suffering or likely to suffer significant harm. *Child and Family Social Work* 13: 365–377.

Brandon M, Beldersone P, Warren C, et al. (2008) *Analysing Child Deaths and Serious Injury Through Abuse and Neglect: What Can We Learn? A Biennial Analysis of Serious Case Reviews 2003–2005*. London: DCSF Research Review DCSF-RR023.

Brandon M, Bailey S, Beldersone P, et al. (2009) *Understanding Serious Case Reviews and Their Impact: A Biennial Analysis of Serious Case Reviews 2005–2007*. London: DCSF Research Review DCSF-RB129.

Children's Workforce Development Council. (2000) *The Assessment Framework*. Leeds, UK: CWDC.

Cleaver H, Freeman P. (1995) *Parental Perspectives in Cases of Suspected Child Abuse*. London: HMSO.

Davies C, Ward H. (2013) *Safeguarding Children across Services: Messages from Research*. London: Jessica Kingsley.

Department for Education. (2011) *Munro Review of Child Protection Final Report – A Child-Centred System*. London: DfE.

Department for Education. (2013a) *Working Together to Safeguard Children*. London: DfE.

Department for Education. (2013b) *Characteristics of Children in Need in England 2012–2013*. London: DfE and National Statistics.

Department for Education. (2013c) *Children Looked After in England Year Ending 31 March 2013*. London: DfE and National Statistics.

Department of Health. (1995) *Child Protection: Messages from Research*. London: HMSO.

Department of Health. (2014) *Child Protection Information Sharing Project*. https://www. gov. uk/government/news/child-protection-information-sharing-project. Accessed 24 March 2013.

Department of Health and Social Security. (1974a) *Report of the Committee of Inquiry into the Care and Supervision Provided in Relation to Maria Colwell*. London: HMSO.

Department of Health and Social Security. (1974b) *Non-Accidental Injury to Children*. London: HMSO.

Dickens J, Howell D, Thoburn J, Schofield G. (2005) Children starting to be looked after by local authorities in England: An analysis of inter-authority variation and case-centred decision-making. *British Journal of Social Work* 37: 597–617.

Farmer E, Lutman E. (2012) *Effective Working with Neglected Children and Their Families: Linking Interventions to Long-Term Outcomes*. London: Jessica Kingsley.

Featherstone B, White S, Morris K. (2014) *Reimagining Child Protection: Towards Humane Social Work with Families*. Bristol: Policy Press.

Ghate D, Hazel N. (2002) *Parenting in Poor Environments: Stress, Support and Coping*. London: Jessica Kingsley.

Gibbons J, Conroy S, Bell C. (1995) *Operating the Child Protection System*. London: HMSO.

Gilbert R, Kemp A, Thoburn J, et al. (2009) Recognising and responding to child maltreatment. *The Lancet* 373(9658): 167–180.

Gill O, Jack G. (2007) *Child and Family in Context: Developing Ecological Practice in Disadvantaged Communities*. Lyme Regis: Russell House.

Griffiths D, Moynahan FJ. (1963) Multiple epiphysial injuries in babies ('battered baby' syndrome) *British Medical Journal* 2(5372): 1558–1561.

Hallett C. (1995) *Interagency Coordination in Child Protection*. London: HMSO.

Her Majesty's Government. (2004) *Every Child Matters*. London: The Stationery Office.

Her Majesty's Government. (2006) *Working Together to Safeguard Children*. London: The Stationery Office.

Her Majesty's Government. (2008) *Information Sharing: Guidance for Practitioners and Managers*. London: The Stationery Office.

Her Majesty's Government. (2013) *Working Together to Safeguard Children*. London: The Stationery Office.

Home Office, Department of Health, Department of Education and Science, Welsh Office. (1991) *Working Together Under the Children Act 1989*. London: The Stationery Office.

House of Commons Health Committee. (2003) *The Victoria Climbié Inquiry Report (The Laming Report)*. London: The Stationery Office.

Jack G. (2011) Using local areas data to improve the lives of disadvantaged children and families. *Child and Family Social Work* 16(1): 61–70.

Jones R. (2014) *The Story of Baby P: Setting the Record Straight*. Bristol, UK: Policy Press.

Kempe CH, Silverman FN, Steele BF, et al. (1962) The battered child syndrome. *Journal of American Medical Association* 181: 17–24.

Lindsay G, Davies H, Band S, et al. (2008) *Parenting Early Intervention Pathfinder Evaluation: Research Brief*. London: Department for Children, Schools and Families.

Morris K, Hughes N, Clarke H, et al. (2008) *Families at Risk: Literature Review*. Birmingham, UK: University of Birmingham.

Neil E, Beek M, Ward E. (2013) *Contact After Adoption: A Follow-Up Study in Late Adolescence*. Norwich, UK: UEA Centre for Research on Children and Families. http://www.uea.ac.uk/documents/3437903/0/Contact+report+NEIL+dec+20+v2+2013.pdf/f2d766c7-39eb-49a3-93b7-1f1368a071a1 (accessed on 23 March 2014).

Parton N, O'Byrne P. (2000) *Constructive Social Work: Towards a New Practice*. London: MacMillan.

Quinton D. (2004) *Supporting Families*. London: HMSO.

Reading R, Bissell S, Goldhagen J, et al. (2009) Promotion of children's rights and prevention of child maltreatment. *The Lancet Child Maltreatment Series* 373: 332-342.

Sidebotham P. (2001) An ecological approach to child abuse: Creative use of scientific models in research and practice. *Child Abuse Review* 10: 97–112.

Sidebotham P, Heron J, Golding J. (2006) Child maltreatment in the 'Children of the Nineties: Deprivation, class and social networks in a UK sample'. *Child Abuse and Neglect* 26: 1243–1259.

Sinclair I, Baker C, Lee J, Gibbs I. (2007) *The Pursuit of Permanence: A Study of English Child Care Systems*. London: Jessica Kingsley.

Social Exclusion Task Force. (2007) *Reaching Out, Think Family: Analysis and Themes from the Government's Families at Risk Review*. London: Cabinet Office.

Stein M. (2009) *Quality Matters in Children's Services: Messages from Research*. London: Jessica Kingsley.

Stein M, Rees G, Hicks L, Gorin S. (2009) *Neglected Adolescents: Literature Review. Research Brief; DCSF-RBX-09-04*. London: Department of Children, Schools and Families.

Stevenson O. (2013) *Reflections on a Life in Social Work – A Personal and Professional Memoir*. Buckingham, UK: Hinton House.

The Lancet. (2008) *Child Maltreatment Series*. London: *The Lancet*.

Thoburn J. (2010) Towards knowledge-based practice in complex child protection cases: A research-based experts' briefing. *Journal of Children's Services* 5(1): 9–24.

Thoburn J. (2013) Services for vulnerable and maltreated children'. In Wolfe I, McKee M, eds. *European Child Health Services and Systems: Lessons without Borders*. Maidenhead, UK: Open University Press/McGraw-Hill.

Thoburn J, Cooper N, Brandon M, Connolly S. (2013) The place of "Think Family" approaches in child and family social work: Messages from a process evaluation of an English pathfinder service. *Children and Youth Services Review* 35(2): 228–236.

Turnell A, Edwards S. (1997) Aspiring to partnership: The signs of safety approach to child protection. *Child Abuse Review* 6: 179–190.

Tunstill J, Aldgate J, Allnock D. (2007) *Understanding the Contribution of Sure Start Local Programmes to the Task of Safeguarding Children's Welfare*. London: DfES.

United Nations. (1989) *United Nations Convention on the Rights of the Child*. New York: United Nations.

Webster-Stratton C, Herbert M. (1999) Researching the impact of parent training programmes on child conduct problems. In Lloyd E, ed. *Parenting Matters: What Works in Parenting Education?* Barkingside, UK: Barnardos.

PART 2

THE CHILD IN THE FAMILY

Foundation years: The foundations of health

5

SARAH COWLEY

Early child development is an indeterminate period, but is generally considered to comprise the period between conception and 7 years of age (Irwin et al. 2007). This important life stage is described as a *social determinant of health*, because it exerts such a critical influence on the infant's later health and development, to the extent that it affects inequalities across the population. This gave rise to the title of one report: 'Early child development – a powerful equalizer' (Irwin et al. 1997). Other reports have suggested the foundation years (Field 2010) are the most important period within that, referring to the first '1001 critical days' from conception to aged 2, because of the extent of robust evidence showing the later effect of this very early period of life (Wave Trust 2012; All Party Parliamentary Group for Conception to Age 2 – The First 1001 Days 2015). This chapter focuses mainly on this very early period of life, but wherever the emphasis is placed, there is a clear consensus in the evidence that early childhood matters, not only to individual children and their families, but to the whole of society.

This chapter is in three sections. First it will explain why the connection between early life and health inequalities is such an important public health phenomenon. Second, it will consider some of the most recent and emerging science of the early years. Finally, it will look in more detail at some of the key *foundations of health* that can be influenced to set children on a positive and healthy life course or that may, conversely, set lifelong barriers in their way.

CASE STUDIES

Before reading on, consider what it is like to be an infant in Britain today. There is no single reality, but the brief case studies set out two very different scenarios. Which baby do you think is likely to have the biggest hurdles to overcome in future? In what way?

Case study 5.1: Daisy

Daisy was determined to be more organized today. It was 11 AM and she had just finished putting the breakfast dishes into the dishwasher, so she would go and get dressed now. She became aware of a baby crying, then a butterfly caught her eye through the window, landing on the rose in her back garden. She had planted that rose bush herself and recalled the pleasure she had last summer, when it first came into bloom. Her mind wandered back to the day when her mother had helped her to choose it and everything had seemed so right, unlike now. She felt so strange these days – as if she was watching a world that was separate from herself, somehow. Everything was heavy, like wading through mud. Tears came into her eyes, along with that familiar sense of loss and grief; her beloved mother had died without even knowing that she was pregnant, would never see her grandson who was now 5 weeks old. Daisy thought she had learned to cope with her loss as it had happened so long ago – why was it on her mind now, nearly 2 years later? She sat down in the living room, looking at the small carriage clock that had been her mother's favourite. Why did she feel so hopeless, as though she couldn't cope now? The tears came again as the clock chimed two o'clock – she still wasn't dressed. Where did the morning go? Daisy became aware of a baby crying again.

Case study 5.2: Kayleigh

Kayleigh turned as she heard the first signs that Dwayne was stirring, stubbing out her cigarette on the outside window left before lifting her baby out of the cot. She only ever smoked out of an open window these days, to make sure her baby wouldn't have to breathe in bad air. 'Come on, little pickle', she said, blowing an enormous raspberry on his neck as he squirmed and nestled into her ample bosom, fixing his wide eyes on her face. She loved the way he smiled and cooed back at her chatter and enjoyed cuddling him so much – but how was she going to manage, as he got bigger? Their bedsit was damp and cluttered, she had to share a kitchen and bathroom. At 6 weeks, he was already showing signs of needing more space to stretch out, but there was hardly any room on the floor, unless his buggy and her sofa-bed were both folded away, which was a fiddle. She'd make an effort today, though, because her ex was supposed to come round this afternoon. Not that he always turned up, of course, but he said he would. She needed to talk to him about giving her some money every week, because even though they broke up before Dwayne was born and he isn't in work, he is still his dad and her benefits didn't go nearly as far as she needed them to. 'Things will work out somehow', she said to Dwayne, stroking his face as he gazed at her. 'Let's just get you changed now, then you will be ready for your bottle'.

UNDERSTANDING HEALTH INEQUALITIES

The Commission for the Social Determinants of Health (CSDH) was set up by the World Health Organisation to look at what can be done to improve health equity through an international focus on the social determinants of health. Their report began with a fierce reminder of the importance of health inequalities and of their social nature, stating baldly that: 'Social justice is a matter of life and death' (CSDH 2008, p. iii). This is explained further in their introduction, which is reproduced in Box 5.1.

The CSDH report (2008, p. iii) emphasizes the fact that *avoidable health inequalities* are social in nature, linked to questions of justice. The term *inequity* is used to show the fundamental lack of fairness and political choice involved in the way opportunities and resources are distributed in society. The directness in this report drew surprised comments from some who preferred to downplay the social and political basis of health inequalities, perhaps by describing them only

---

BOX 5.1: Introduction to Commission on Social Determinants of Health 2008 piii

- Social justice is a matter of life and death. It affects the way people live, their consequent chance of illness and their risk of premature death. We watch in wonder as life expectancy and good health continue to increase in parts of the world and in alarm as they fail to improve in others. A girl born today can expect to live for more than 80 years if she is born in some countries – but less than 45 years if she is born in others. Within countries there are dramatic differences in health that are closely linked with degrees of social disadvantage. Differences of this magnitude, within and between countries, simply should never happen.

- These inequities in health, avoidable health inequalities, arise because of the circumstances in which people grow, live, work and age, and the systems put in place to deal with illness. The conditions in which people live and die are, in turn, shaped by political, social and economic forces.

- Social and economic policies have a determining impact on whether a child can grow and develop to its full potential and live a flourishing life, or whether its life will be blighted. Increasingly the nature of the health problems rich and poor countries have to solve are converging. The development of a society, rich or poor, can be judged by the quality of its population's health, how fairly health is distributed across the social spectrum, and the degree of protection provided from disadvantage as a result of ill-health.

---

as *disparities* or *variations*. However, Sir Michael Marmot (who chaired the CSDH) went on to chair a strategic review of health inequalities in England, where he responded to a critic who had labelled the CSDH *ideology with evidence*, writing: 'We do have an ideological position: health inequalities that could be avoided by reasonable means are unfair. Putting them right is a matter of social justice. But the evidence matters. Good intentions are not enough' (Marmot 2010, p. 3).

This chapter takes its cue from these seminal reports, by drawing attention to the evidence of avoidable inequalities that affect babies and young children, before going on to explore the expanding knowledge base that shows that a focus on those early years is also the key to reducing inequity. The United Kingdom (UK) is one of the most unequal countries in which to be born (UNICEF 2010). It is the sixth richest country in the world, yet above one in three (39%) households with children have less than the Minimum Income Standard required to meet a 'standard of living in the UK today (that) includes, but is more than, just food, clothes and shelter. It is about having what you need in order to have the opportunities and choices necessary to participate in society' (Padley et al. 2015, p. 8). Among the Organisation of Economically Advanced Countries (OECD) the UK was ranked 13th of 24 countries for education, 11th for health and 19th for material well-being (UNICEF 2010). Inevitably, limiting these opportunities will affect how well parents are able to provide for their growing children.

At its most extreme, health inequity is manifest as a greater likelihood of death in the early weeks or months. Childbirth and the early months have become far safer for infants in the UK, as in the rest of the developed world, with steadily declining rates of child mortality over the last 30 years. Even so, infants are more likely to die before reaching their first birthday than at any other time in childhood. Wolfe et al. (2014) compiled the figures in Table 5.1 from national data, and examined why some children are more at risk of dying than others. They suggest that something could have been done to prevent these early deaths in around 21% of cases, clearly pointing to the social, economic and environmental factors that influence the progress of pregnancy, birth and even maternity care, which all influence a child's chances of survival. These infant mortality rates tend to be in the mid-range for European countries, and are associated with low birth weight, maternal smoking and maternal age (being either over 35 years

Table 5.1 Infant and childhood mortality rates by age and sex, UK, 2012

Age, years	Male	Female	Total	Numbers of deaths
Infant deaths per 1,000 live births				
	4.4	3.5	4.0	3,219
Deaths per 100,000 population in age group				
1–4	18	15	16	523
5–9	9	8	9	325
10–14	11	8	10	340
15–19	33	15	24	959

Source: Wolfe I et al. *Why Children Die: Death in Infants, Children and Young People in the UK*, London: Royal College of Paediatrics and Child Health, 2014.

or under 20 years old is a risk for pregnancy outcomes). In the UK, both stillbirths and Sudden Unexplained Deaths in Infancy are higher than elsewhere in Europe (Euro-Peristat 2013).

Fortunately, the vast majority of children survive to adulthood, but their life expectancy and life chances are dramatically affected by social factors. Not only are those from poor backgrounds more likely to die in infancy, they are also more likely to experience difficulties as they develop. Waldfogel and Washbrook (2008) recorded a clear social gradient in measures of school readiness for children aged 3 years, with those living in worse off areas being far less likely to be ready than their better off counterparts. They showed similar inequalities in children's vocabulary and conduct at aged 5 years.

In another example, the Social Exclusion Task Force (2007) examined the distribution of *family disadvantage indicators*, which are listed in Box 5.2. These indicators were derived from the *families at risk review* and examined the life chances of children born in 2000, who participated in the Millenium Cohort Study.

Where even one or two of these disadvantage indicators were present, children experienced worse outcomes – and the indicators were increasingly more likely to arise where there was more deprivation. The Social Exclusion Task Force (2007) mapped the percentage of children under 5 years old living with these *family disadvantage indicators* to areas of deprivation, as measured by the Index of Multiple Deprivation (IMD), which is compiled by government every few years to show where social and economic difficulties occur in different geographical areas. The results can be seen in Figure 5.1.

The graph shows a clear gradient, which is to say that at each step, from the 10% best off to the 10% worst off areas, the likelihood of children experiencing these disadvantage indicators grew, as did the likelihood of experiencing a higher number of them. This is known as

---

BOX 5.2: Family Disadvantage Indicators, from *Families at risk* review

- No parent is in work
- Family lives in poor quality or overcrowded housing
- No parent has qualifications
- Mother has mental health problems
- At least one parent has longstanding, limiting illness, disability or infirmity
- Family has a low income below 60% of the median
- Family cannot afford a number of food or clothing items.

Source: Social Exclusion Task Force, *Think Family: Analysis from 'Families At Risk' Review*, London: Cabinet Office, 2007.

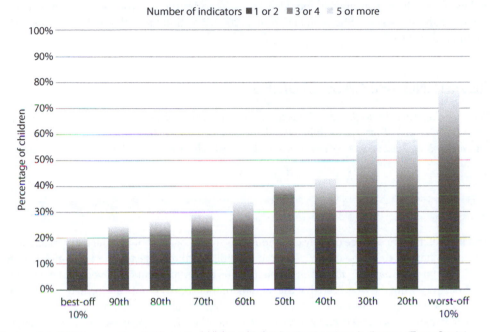

% of children with disadvantage indicators

Number of indicators ■ 1 or 2 ■ 3 or 4 ▪ 5 or more

Figure 5.1 Children aged under 5 years old living with *family disadvantage indicators*. (From Social Exclusion Task Force, *Think Family: Analysis from 'Families At Risk' Review*, London: Cabinet Office, 2007.)

the *social gradient* – poverty and deprivation matter a great deal, but it is not a simple matter of having enough money. Instead, social determinants are graded across the population, with each step up or down the social scale making it more or less likely that children will be able to flourish. At each stepped increase in markers of disadvantage, proportionately more children would be likely to experience poorer outcomes in the long term. The report (Social Exclusion Task Force 2007) goes on to explain that starting with multiple disadvantages exposes children to a greater likelihood of being rated by their parents as well below average in English and mathematics; more likely to have been suspended or excluded from school; more likely to have poor social networks; and more likely to have been in trouble with the police by the time they leave school. As they grow up, their early disadvantage translates into greater likelihood that they will, like their parents, be more likely to be without work, without qualifications and possibly in trouble with the police, so perpetuating the inequalities.

The Millenium Cohort Study, from which these data originated, is one of many longitudinal studies, some of which have followed infants from birth through childhood and into adulthood since the middle of the last century. Internationally, the studies show that children born in disadvantaged areas or in difficult circumstances then go on to lead lives of similar disadvantage. In the early days of such research, it seemed that these children were effectively 'born to fail' (Wedge and Prosser 1973), or trapped in 'cycles of deprivation' (Rutter and Madge 1976).

More recently, research attention has focused in two directions – first, exploring not only what these studies can tell us about predicting future problems, but also examining what helps to protect children and enables them to develop resilience in the face of the difficulties (Werner 2006). Second, which is where this chapter turns next, is a modern version of what was once called the 'nature versus nurture' debate. It is realized now that, even during pregnancy, and certainly from birth onwards, each infant has a unique biological and genetic endowment, which is intimately moulded and shaped by the environment and interactions that he or she encounters (Shonkoff and Phillips 2000; Ben-Shlomo and Koh 2002; Rutter 2006; Shonkoff et al. 2012).

REVISITING THE CASE STUDIES

Consider Daisy and Kayleigh again. Do you think either of their babies was born into a disadvantaged situation? Can you identify some difficulties that may arise for their future life and well-being? See if you can list issues that might be of concern, or which might help protect the baby in each of the two cases.

UNDERSTANDING EARLY CHILD DEVELOPMENT

At one level, the importance of early childhood has always been known – the early Jesuits were reputed to have lived by the motto, 'Give me the child until he is seven and I will give you the man'. Yet, far from being a *tabula rasa*, or blank slate, as our forebears believed, much development occurs within the womb, so that the human infant is born completely formed, yet still able to adapt. New-born babies (*neonates*), are both amazingly adaptable and uniquely vulnerable to what they can see, feel, hear and experience. Chamberlain (2003) proposes 12 senses that are already formed before birth (which Chamberlain calls *prenates*). These are summarized in Box 5.3. So much awareness at birth seems amazing, but modern scanning technology has made it possible to demonstrate them in utero and to show how rapidly these same senses develop after birth.

The African saying that 'it takes a village to raise a child' appears equally applicable wherever children live, speaking to another long-held awareness of the impact of the environment on the child. Parents and the family setting provide the most intimate environment, but that is only part of the story. Bronfenbrenner (1986) described the 'nested systems' that demonstrate the way that children live with their parents, who are part of a family, within a particular neighbourhood, which is part of a wider community (see Figure 5.2). Within each community and the wider society, it is necessary for an infant to be able to grow up with the particular knowledge required to survive in that milieu. It is only within the last 20–30 years that science has advanced to the point of understanding the incredible processes through which the human infant adapts from birth to meet such a complex challenge. (See chapter *'Approaches to Parenting'* below.)

THE DEVELOPING BRAIN

The basic architecture, or blueprint, for the developing infant is present at birth, in that brain and genes are present, but the wiring, connections and patterns that join them all together and prioritize the way they function in the infant, toddler and eventually adult have yet to be developed (Gerhardt 2004). The brain increases in size fourfold between birth and the age of 6 years, when it is 90% of its adult size (Stiles and Jernigan 2010), as those new connections are first made, extended, then pruned and reshaped according to the infants' experience. After birth, there is an 'unparalleled burst of synaptogenesis, neuronal growth and differentiation' (Courchesne

---

BOX 5.3: Twelve Proposed Foetal Senses

- Touch (both receiving and reaching out to touch) is the first sense to develop.
- Thermal sensing of hot and cold is real.
- Pain sensing (nociception) involves crushing and nerve damage, which needs to be borne in mind when creating protocols for obstetrics and neonatology.
- Hearing begins as early as 14 weeks after conception, improving steadily with the arrival of cochlear resources and full growth of the external ear.
- Balance and orientation in space develops from weeks 7 to 12 of pregnancy.
- The chemosensors of smell, which operate in close association with (7).
- The chemosensors of taste. Both (6) and (7) are bathed by amniotic fluids passing through the nasal area.
- *Mouthing* is used to explore texture, hardness and contours of objects; this sense is not about eating and nutrition.
- Sucking and licking in the womb are mouth-related pleasure senses. The sucking of fingers and toes is not nutritive. Ultrasound reveals prenates licking the placenta and twins licking each other, suggesting pleasure in bodily contact.
- Eyelids are fused shut for about 6 months, yet vision seems functional in being able to hit targets like needles during amniocentesis at 14–16 weeks of age. Some form of vision seems to facilitate twins boxing, kicking, kissing and playing together in the womb.
- Prenates demonstrate attunement with parents whether they are near or far from each other; they discern emotional disposition and character of those around them.
- Finally, prenates also demonstrate transcendent sensing as they report out-of-body and near-death experiences. In transcendent states, even immature senses function well and events are stored in memory – as can be demonstrated years later.

Source: The Association for Prenatal and Perinatal Psychology and Health, https://birthpsychology.com/free-article/fetal-senses-twelve-not-five-new-proposal#.VOHse_OsXVU, accessed June 7, 2015.

---

and Pierce 2005, p. 153), which is to say the infant's neurons grow and join at newly developed synapses (which connect the neurones to each other) in different patterns, depending upon the individual's experiences. This growth not only occurs at an astronomical rate, as illustrated in Figure 5.3, but also follows a strict order and timetable, so that, for example, the basic functions of vision and hearing develop earlier than areas of the brain governing higher-order functions, like speech, language comprehension, social communication and self-awareness (Courchesne and Pierce 2005).

The rate of change during this early development is phenomenal. Synapses, where the newly developed neurones connect, are generated at the rate of 1–200,000 per second during the first months of life, as the brain expands and matures. Simultaneously, in response to environmental interactions, familiar and often used neural pathways become more established, while others are pruned back and refashioned. There is an established order for this neuro-development, but this process rapidly ensures that each infant's brain rapidly becomes unique to that individual, reflecting her or his life experience from the very start. Although the brain remains plastic and malleable throughout childhood, this very early period of exponential growth and neurological development provides the best and easiest opportunity to provide the kinds of experiences that will positively shape the infant's future physiology, including their mental, emotional and cognitive capacity (Wave Trust 2012).

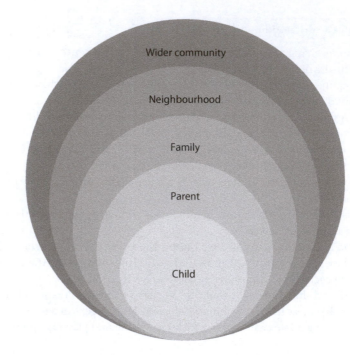

Figure 5.2 Bronfenbrenner's (1986) concept of nested systems.

GENE-ENVIRONMENT INTERACTION

Gerhardt (2004, p. 18) suggests that 'Babies are like raw material for a self. Each one comes with a genetic blueprint and a unique range of possibilities'. Changes in this genetic blueprint are intimately connected with the rapidly developing brain in these early weeks and months. Scientists have now discarded the old idea that the genes an infant is born with are 'set in stone'. Instead, the National Scientific Council on the Developing Child (2010) use the analogy of computer hardware and software to explain how infant development proceeds after birth. A neonate has a *structural genome*, made up of around 23,000 genes, inherited from her or his parents, which (like a computer) cannot function without some form of operating system, the equivalent of software, to activate the genes within it. Multiple environmental factors cause chemicals to be released in the infant's body, which serve this purpose. These environmental triggers are what the baby experiences, which results in certain gene sequences or variations cause chemicals and proteins to be produced in the brain. In turn, these affect the response to adversity or stress (National Scientific Council on the Developing Child 2015), or to sensory experiences, which are particularly important at specific critical periods (Ben-Shlomo and Kuh 2002; Faglioni et al. 2009). The genes will be switched on or off, either temporarily or permanently, so that the features governed by that particular gene or group of genes can be given expression. The chemical triggers may come from the external environment (physical, built or chemical) or from the environment of relationships within which the baby lives (National Scientific Council on the Developing Child 2010).

The science of epigenetics is, itself, still very young, so understanding how interactions between the environment and the developing infant lead to the lifelong outcomes is developing rapidly as new knowledge comes on stream. However, the effect of genetics on the developing brain is sufficiently well studied to say with some certainty that biological *imprints* are

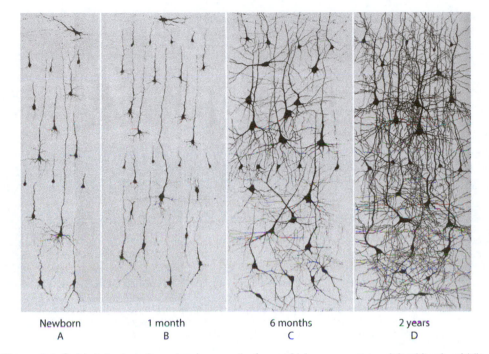

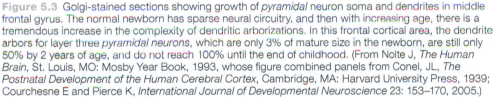

Newborn	1 month	6 months	2 years
A	B	C	D

Figure 5.3 Golgi-stained sections showing growth of *pyramidal* neuron soma and dendrites in middle frontal gyrus. The normal newborn has sparse neural circuitry, and then with increasing age, there is a tremendous increase in the complexity of dendritic arborizations. In this frontal cortical area, the dendrite arbors for layer three *pyramidal neurons*, which are only 3% of mature size in the newborn, are still only 50% by 2 years of age, and do not reach 100% until the end of childhood. (From Nolte J, *The Human Brain*, St. Louis, MO: Mosby Year Book, 1993, whose figure combined panels from Conel, JL, *The Postnatal Development of the Human Cerebral Cortex*, Cambridge, MA: Harvard University Press, 1939; Courchesne E and Pierce K, *International Journal of Developmental Neuroscience* 23: 153–170, 2005.)

created through the interaction of a child's genes and experiences in these early years of life. Figure 5.4 from the Harvard Centre on the Developing Child (2014) shows how the biological mechanism known as *epigenetic adaptation* shapes the way that infants' brains and bodies develop, leading to different (healthy or not) adaptations throughout their lives.

This new knowledge has added to earlier observations made by the late epidemiologist, David Barker, who formulated what became known as the 'Barker hypothesis of the foetal and infant origins of disease' (Barker 1990). His research team had identified a detailed cache of health visitors' records for 16,000 babies born between 1911 and 1930 in Hertfordshire, which recorded birth weight and feeding patterns for the first year of life. Barker's team followed up these infants 60 years later and found that those who had weighed more at birth, particularly if they were breast-fed, had significantly lower death rates from ischaemic heart disease and stroke. The research teams hypothesized a genetic link as the basis for these observations, proposing that some genes were *primed* or *triggered* by intra-uterine and early life nutrition. Since then, there has been a mass of research largely supporting the hypothesis and extending it to encompass a range of chronic conditions (such as diabetes) that arise in later life (Hill 2015). There have also been some critiques on grounds of incomplete knowledge, some methodological flaws and lack of information to confirm a direct and independent link between foetal and early life and later disease (Hill 2015; Skogen and Øverland 2012). However, it remains a hugely influential part of the spectrum of research about how and why health and illness develops across the life course (Ben-Shlomo and Kuh 2002).

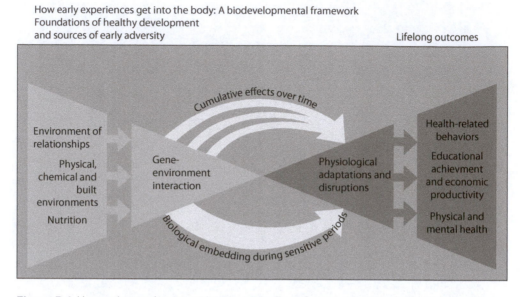

How early experiences get into the body: A biodevelopmental framework
Foundations of healthy development
and sources of early adversity

Lifelong outcomes

Cumulative effects over time

Environment of
relationships

Physical,
chemical and
built
environments

Nutrition

Gene-
environment
interaction

Physiological
adaptations and
disruptions

Biological embedding during sensitive periods

Health-related
behaviors

Educational
achievment
and economic
productivity

Physical and
mental health

Figure 5.4 How early experiences get into the body. (From Center on the Developing Child at Harvard University, *Building the Brain's 'Air Traffic Control' System: How Early Experiences Shape the Development of Executive Function*. Working Paper No.11, 2011. http://www.developingchild. harvard.edu)

THE MICROBIOME

An even newer area of scientific development concerns the human microbiome, which may eventually complete the picture that Barker started to paint about the early origins of later disease. Once the human genome had been mapped, it became clear that much of the genetic material actually belongs to the trillions of micro-organisms that form part of the human body. The human microbiome project set out to map these micro-organisms (Turnbaugh et al. 2007) and to understand the part they play in human development and health. The interplay between the core human microbiome within the *host organism*, that is, the human being, is shown in red in Figure 5.5, with pertinent features of the environment with which it interacts shown in blue.

Ursell et al. (2012) indicate that there is not yet agreement about whether it is more help-ful to speak of an individual's microbiome as a single organ or entity, or if it is more accurate to describe several, such as the microbiome of the skin, or that of the gut. Terminology aside, this developing science is beginning to clarify the basis for some of the rapid changes that occur within minutes and weeks of birth and to provide further clues to the mechanisms involved in early life influences on later health. As an example of the kinds of variations that have been shown, the foetal gut is sterile, but within 20 minutes of a vaginal birth, the microbes found in the infant's gut resemble that of the mother's vagina, while infants delivered by caesarean section show microbes typical of the human skin (Ursell et al. 2012). It is not yet certain how long this difference lasts, since there are many naturally occurring periods of rapid change and stability in the microbiome in the subsequent weeks of life, as the infants interact with the environment. These naturally occurring changes may help to explain features of long-term development, including predisposition to certain diseases

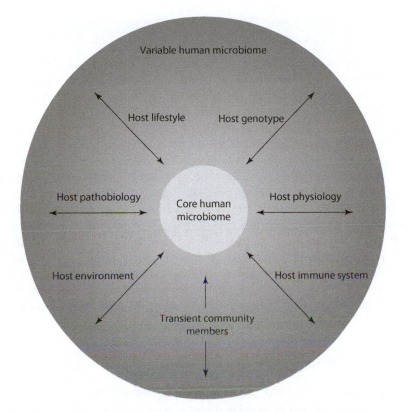

Figure 5.5 The concept of the core human microbiome. (From Turnbaugh PJ et al., *Nature*, 449, 804–810, 2007.)

or developmental traits like weight gain or sensitive skin (including tendency to infantile eczema).

These new areas of developmental science are expanding rapidly, with some exciting results, which also point to opportunities for changing what, at one time, appeared to be inevitable outcomes – that infants born into poverty and deprivation were somehow destined to live unequal lives, with poorer health, educational attainments and consequent low-paid employment. We know now that these depressing predictions do not have to be realized, because future health and social well-being are not inevitably pre-determined at birth. However, studies across the life course have shown equally conclusively that the early life period is immensely influential in setting the foundations for an infant's future health and development. Further, now the mechanisms involved are better understood, it has been possible to identify key areas of influence that can help to protect and enable positive development. These are considered next.

REVISITING THE CASE STUDIES

Look back at the list of issues you identified that might help or hinder the case study babies' development. Can you think of any more now? Which baby has the best chances and in which way?

FOUNDATIONS OF HEALTH

Studies of early development all emphasize the importance of the environment, which enables or hinders positive development in the infant. Babies do not live alone, so the environment for most consists of their birth family – mother, father, possibly siblings and other family members, like grandparents. The amount of support a family receives, whether from other family members or the wider community, directly affects any infants in that family. The Centre for the Developing Child (2010) set out a framework for policies that would strengthen lifelong health, explaining that parents and other carers need support from the wider society to facilitate them having the time, commitment, skills and knowledge about how to care for a new infant. Financial, psychological and institutional resources all play their part in enabling the biological processes described above to happen, including the political will to enable good, supportive physical and community environments for families to live in. If those supports are in place, it is easier for the parents and other caregivers to support three central concepts described as the *foundations of health*, detailed below. These are stable responsive relationships; safe, secure environments and appropriate nutrition, which collectively influence the physiological adaptations (or disruptions) that accumulate over time and become embedded at particular sensitive periods (Centre for the Developing Child 2010).

STABLE, RESPONSIVE RELATIONSHIPS

This is the most widely studied and, some would argue, essential of the three foundations of health. Young children develop in an environment of relationships, which make up the *active ingredients* (National Scientific Council on the Developing Child 2009) of the multiple biological changes that happen at this time. Through relationships, infants experience everything they need for their development. These experiences become embedded and imprinted into their physiology, influencing the way they feel, think, react, speak, see, hear and learn as they grow up; in short, 'affecting virtually all aspects of their development – intellectual, social, emotional, physical, behavioural and moral' (National Scientific Council on the Developing Child 2009, p. 1). Furthermore, if a child is loved unconditionally and passionately, by at least one person – usually the mother, or both birth parents – that main caregiver will strive, even against extreme odds, to ensure that everything else the child needs is provided.

At birth, the new infant experiences a burst of sensations, as all the foetal senses (Chamberlain 2003) suddenly come into play. The parturient mother, likewise, experiences a flood of emotions and responds through her senses – reaching for the infant, touching, nuzzling and smelling, gazing into the baby's eyes, examining her minutely all over, licking, nuzzling and stroking. Even at birth, babies can respond, turning towards the mother's voice or smell, reaching out a tiny tongue to copy a father's tongue reaching out to him – amazing, incredible, everyday events captured on film and photo in so many birthing rooms now that portable photography is everywhere, and interpreted skilfully by Murray and Andrews (2005) in their picture documentary of a baby's earliest moments.

Over the next hours and weeks, parents learn to interpret and respond to their baby's smallest sound or changing expressions, telling him what he is experiencing – 'oh, you are hungry now', or why she is feeling it – 'you are all wet and need changing, soon have you dry again'. These murmurings and comforting actions help to soothe the baby, which encourages the carer to continue and reinforces the growing bonds of attachment with the baby. This responsiveness is described as *serve and play* – as each cue requires and receives a response, by carer and baby. Simultaneously, the infant's neurones are growing, multiplying, making new connections, responding by logging the events and building the framework that the brain needs to make sense of the world. Each new pathway becomes an embedded experience, providing a scaffolding into which the baby's developing brain can grow as she or he begins to make sense of the world – not just learning new words (although that is important) but understanding how it operates, how to interpret bodily sensations and what to expect from caregivers, who are usually parents.

Mothers seem, almost automatically, to raise the pitch of their voice to a timbre that is more easily heard by infants, perhaps humming or singing, repeating words and phrases, which helps this embedding and understanding. Fathers are important, of course (and babies learn to turn to their fathers voice as readily as to their mothers), but the higher tone of a female voice is more easily heard at first, and this manner of *baby-talk* is known as *mother-ese*. During the critical periods of early development, babies learn the sound of their own language (their *mother tongue*) and dialect, with all its unique pronunciations and sounds. They become familiar with the key sights and order of house and home, embedding expectations about smells, colours, feelings and those all-important relationships, all the time being completely dependent upon their caregiver for interpreting and explaining, both in words and deeds, as they learn about the world and their place in it. Infants' abilities to understand and manage their emotions and to organize their basic thinking skills – cognitive function – stem from these very early interactions, which provide the basic capabilities required for later behaviour and intellectual capacity. Mastery of these *executive functions* allows a child to focus attention, remember how things are ordered and understand the basic rules to operate in society (like, waiting your turn; knowing when to use a spoon or fork at mealtimes; understanding that books mean stories, which are made up; enjoying music). Cognitive ability (*thinking concepts*) and vocabulary, essential as a basis for later school success among other things, stem from these early interactions and attendant neurological developments (Center on the Developing Child at Harvard University 2011).

Also, these early expressions of caring and nurturing provide the building blocks for the infant's emotional development and attachment between child and primary carer, usually the mother. The style of care has a direct impact. If a crying infant is soothed, comforted, fed and nurtured, those responses will wire the brain in the way that primes the baby to assume the world is a safe and predictable place, enabling them to learn how to regulate their own emotions. This provides the solid basis needed to develop later decision-making ability and self-management of behaviour – the executive functions of the brain.

On the other hand, if a baby is left to cry unattended for long periods, or when evident discomfort provokes no caring response, the developing brain is unable to settle to a clear orientation, resulting in stress. Minor stressful episodes, termed 'positive stress' (for example, if a baby is left to cry for a few minutes while his mother finishes eating her meal or deals with a phone call), can be beneficial in enabling the baby to experience and learn to manage variations in emotion, particularly in the context of knowing that relief will soon be forthcoming. Even higher levels or more frequent stress can be tolerable and, as long as a baby is supported in due course, has no permanent adverse effects (National Scientific Council on the Developing Child 2014). This is important, as parents can sometimes feel overwhelmed by the responsibility and all-consuming neediness of a small child, leading to feelings of guilt and unrealistic expectations to avoid stress for a baby at all costs.

Prolonged or severe stress is different, and can be potentially toxic to the developing brain (National Scientific Council on the Developing Child 2014). The hormones adrenaline and cortisol, released in the brain during periods of acute stress, are designed to help the organism deal with threats by providing a surge in energy, memory and immune response, among other beneficial functions. However, when stress is prolonged and unrelieved, particularly during this sensitive period of early neuro-development, these hormones become highly toxic and damaging to the actual fabric of the brain. Positive, caring relationships can act as a buffer against this stress, even in conditions of extreme hardship, such as family poverty, homelessness or strife. Conversely, unmoderated stress in early infancy has a profoundly adverse impact on the developing brain, making later conduct disorder, mental health problems and learning difficulties far more likely.

There are many barriers and stressors on new parents that potentially impede the development of nurturing, responsive relationships (Sanger et al. 2015), with mental health issues being one of the most significant areas of concern, not least because of their ubiquity, as shown in Box 5.4. Mental illness impedes parents' (particularly mothers) ability to respond to their infant's cues, potentially leading to impaired attachment and a range of adverse outcomes as the baby's brain develops without the predictable and regular responses and experiences needed. Even stress hormones circulating in the mothers' blood during pregnancy can have an adverse effect on the baby's brain, leading to calls for policy action to moderate the commonest causes of perinatal distress (Hogg 2013; All Party Parliamentary Group for Conception to Age 2 – The First 1001 Days 2015).

Indeed, there is a strong economic case for more attention to be paid to maternal (and paternal) mental health, with one group estimating the total cost to British society at £8.1 billion (Bauer et al. 2014). Almost three-quarters (72%) of these costs stem from the adverse impact of maternal mental illness on the developing child. The extent and seriousness of these outcomes varies, depending upon many other factors, such as responses from other family members, the extent of their ability to support both mother and baby, and the seriousness of the mental illness. Infant death is the most extreme adverse outcome, with infanticide being a rare but potential danger, in the case of the 2%–3% of puerperal women who develop psychosis. More frequently, infants of mentally ill mothers are at risk of growing up to experience special educational needs, lower than anticipated school achievement, anxiety and conduct problems and later depression or other mental illness themselves. All of these adverse outcomes are potentially preventable by timely identification and treatment of the mothers' mental health problems, so that secure, responsive relationships can be established or re-established and the infant's early development can proceed unimpeded.

SAFE, SUPPORTIVE ENVIRONMENTS

One of the key aims of parenthood is to ensure the safety and survival of offspring and every parent will work hard to see that this aim is achieved. Political will to legislate for the safety and protection of a nation's youngest citizens is of particular interest for this basic foundation of health (Center on the Developing Child at Harvard University 2010), since so much depends upon public funding and national culture. The system in which policymakers operate is part of the wider society in which the family is situated, as described by Bronfenbrenner (1995) and shown in Figure 5.1.

Policies to overcome infectious diseases are a good example. Once the greatest fear of new parents, deaths and disability from this cause are increasingly unusual in the developed world,

BOX 5.4: Mental Health Issues

THE ANTENATAL PERIOD

- Depression and anxiety affect 10%–15% of pregnant women.
- Post-traumatic stress disorder (PTSD) occurs in about 8% of pregnant women.
- 1 million children in the UK suffer from the type of problems (including Attention deficit hyperactivity disorder [ADHD], conduct disorder, emotional problems and vulnerabilities to chronic illness) that are increased by antenatal depression, anxiety and stress.

THE PERINATAL PERIOD

- Mental health problems affect up to 20% of women during the perinatal period.
- About 11% of pregnant women experience some form of depression, with 3% suffering from a major depressive disorder.
- Anxiety and panic disorders affect 2%–4% of pregnant women.

INFANT MENTAL HEALTH

- 122,000 babies under one are living with a parent who has a mental health problem.
- Infant regulatory disturbances such as excessive crying, feeding or sleeping difficulties and bonding/attachment problems are the main reasons for referrals to child health clinics.
- Around one-fifth of children aged 18 months have regulatory problems.
- About 15% of children have Disorganized Attachment behaviour, which is associated with high levels of entry into care, poor relationship skills through life, high levels of disruptive behaviour in school and pre-school, school exclusion, poor physical and mental health, aggression and entry into the criminal justice system.
- Around half (49.9%) of infants and toddlers (12–40 months) still have emotional and behavioural problems 1 year after initial presentation.

Source: All Party Parliamentary Group for Conception to Age 2 – The First 1001 Days, *Building Great Britons*, London: Wave Trust, 2015.

thanks largely to the success of immunisation programmes, which are considered to be among the most successful public health interventions of all time. Even so, some parents need convincing that these immunisations are still required, when such infections have become locally rare. Resistance stems from unfounded worries about the possibility that side-effects of the immunisation may outweigh the benefits from reduced risk of infection. Parents who have never seen a baby with a serious disease like measles or polio might have only a hazy idea of the devastating potential of the disease, which leads to misunderstandings and insufficient knowledge to make properly informed decisions. Explanation or reassurance in such circumstances can help improve take-up of immunisations (Leask et al. 2012). Lower take-up can reduce what is called *herd immunity* (that is the total number of infants in the community who are protected), so that individual incidents of infection occur and risk reintroducing epidemics again. Immunisation is compulsory in some countries, such as Australia and parts of the United States (Salmon et al. 2006), but the UK relies upon persuasion, free availability of a government-backed and a strongly evidence-based schedule of immunisations, as listed in Table 5.2 (Public Health England 2015).

Safety from non-infectious hazards is somewhat easier for parents to achieve in developed countries, where laws are in place to protect their youngest citizens, for example by specifying

Table 5.2 Routine childhood immunisations from July 2014

2 months old	Diphtheria, tetanus, pertussis, polio and *Haemophilus influenzae* type b (Hib)
	Pneumococcal disease
	Rotavirus
3 months old	Diphtheria, tetanus, pertussis, polio and Hib
	Meningococcal group C disease (MenC)
	Rotavirus
4 months old	Diphtheria, tetanus, pertussis, polio and Hib
	Pneumococcal disease
Between 12 and 13 months old	Hib/MenC
	Pneumococcal disease
	Measles, mumps and rubella (German measles)
2, 3 and 4 years old	Influenza
3-years 4-months old or soon after	Diphtheria, tetanus, pertussis and polio
	Measles, mumps and rubella

Source: Public Health England, Routine Childhood Immunisations from July 2014. Poster, 2014. https://www.gov.uk/government/publications/routine-childhood-immunisations-from-july-2014.

standards for the width of bars in a cot to avoid an infant's head being caught, outlawing lead in household paint and plumbing and requiring toys to be manufactured in ways that avoid risks of inhaling or trapping. Infants born in the developing world are less fortunate, where health protection laws are less well established, or where toxic environmental substances are prevalent – heavy metals (lead, mercury, manganese) and organophosphates (used in agriculture, fertilizers etc.) are particularly injurious to early development (National Scientific Council on the Developing Child 2006). Infants absorb these through breast milk, food, water, house dust or soil (Walker et al. 2011). Such environmental risks and toxins remain a concern in developed countries, like the UK, as industrialization brings new and different ways of spreading the substances.

Given the wide health inequalities that exist in the UK, it is to be expected that some population groups will face greater difficulties than others in protecting their infants from environmental harm. Families that have no secure home are particularly likely to face difficulties in keeping their child safe. Substandard accommodation can be hard to keep clean and free from hazards that may be dangerous as a small infant begins exploring her or his environment. Hogg et al. (2015) have drawn attention to the *unstable start* faced by many English babies – the figures they compiled are summarized in Box 5.5.

These data refer only to families that local authorities have accepted a responsibility for – known as *statutorily homeless* – and there are many other families, such as asylum seekers or those who have been classified as *intentionally homeless,* who are not counted. Hogg et al. (2015) point out that homeless families often have a history of adversity, so the baby is exposed to multiple issues of concern. The accommodation they live in might be small, damp, cold, noisy and unsafe, which adds to the pressure on parents who are often vulnerable themselves. Although not actually living on the streets, many vulnerable families live in non-decent or over-crowded housing, which may fall outside the legal requirements for home safety in the UK, with likely risks from unsafe electric sockets, unguarded fires, dampness and ingrained dirt, poor heating and ventilation. The figures for families recognized by authorities as homeless may be regarded as only the 'tip of the iceberg', with many more families living in overcrowded, temporary and

> ### BOX 5.5: Homeless Babies in England, 2015
>
> - Around 15,700 babies under the age of 2 years old are classed as statutorily homeless in England.
> - Of these, about 710 live in bed-and-breakfast (B & B) accommodation, many without access to a kitchen and with shared bathrooms.
> - Of these, up to 170 have been in B & B accommodation for longer than 6 weeks.
> - Highly mobile families or those living in poor conditions featured in 45% of Serious Case Reviews.
>
> *Source:*   Hogg S et al. *An Unstable Start — All Babies Count: Spotlight on Homelessness.* London: NSPCC, 2015.

inadequate housing conditions, with no national data to reflect the extent of the difficulties. Vulnerable families are particularly at risk of exploitation from unscrupulous landlords and the spectre of slum housing (such as the so-called 'sheds with beds', which lack basic requirements like safe power supply, clean running water and ventilation) is rising in England again. Such poor living conditions are highly risky for the health, development and even survival of young infants.

Families living with stress are more likely to turn to external supports, such as smoking, alcohol or drugs, either from prescription or obtained through other means. Such substances, used legally or not, may damage the infant's developing brain, particularly where they are used antenatally and cross the placenta into the baby's bloodstream (National Scientific Council on the Developing Child 2006). Damage from illegal drugs like cocaine or methampthetamine ('speed') may not have immediately noticeable effects on a new baby or toddler, but can lead to attention disorders and mood difficulties as the child reaches adolescence. Both nicotine and alcohol are potentially harmful, with alcohol being one of the most dangerous neurotoxins in its effects on the developing foetus. However, after birth, the impact from drugs and alcohol is most marked by the way it impairs the ability of parents to successfully care for their child. Evidence for this comes from the observation that parental substance misuse was noted in 25% of child protection plans and 42% of Serious Case Reviews (Rayns et al. 2013). The same authors drew on evidence from national surveys to show the high number of babies living in families where drugs or alcohol misuse are present (see Box 5.6). The risk of child maltreatment, with all the attendant harms that sets in train, is particularly high in this group of children. More information about this is included in Chapter 5.

NUTRITION

The last of the three *foundations of health* is as essential as the other two – babies must be fed and a sound, balanced diet through childhood is fundamental to ensuring infants reach their full potential. Malnutrition for mothers and babies remains a problem worldwide, with up to 34% of children affected by stunting or growth retardation as a result (Walker et al. 2011). The obesity epidemic is a global problem, as well, being often cited as one of the biggest threats to future public health. There are concerns about the effect on children in school, with increased risk of bullying, poor self-esteem and social isolation. However, the major public health concerns stem from evidence that overweight children are more likely to become overweight adults (Singh et al. 2008), which significantly increases their risk of earlier death, disability and chronic illness. Being overweight is likely to reduce life expectancy by up to 3 years, while obesity may

> **BOX 5.6: Babies Living with Parents who Misuse Drugs or Alcohol**
>
> - Around 79,000 babies under 1 are living with a parent who is classified as a *hazardous or harmful* drinker – this equates to 93,500 babies in the UK.
> - Around 26,000 babies under 1 are living with a parent who would be classified as a *dependent* drinker – this equates to 31,000 babies in the UK.
> - Around 43,000 babies under 1 are living with a parent who has used an illegal drug in the past year. This is equivalent to 51,000 across the UK.
> - Around 16,500 babies under 1 are living with a parent who has used Class A drugs in the past year. This is equivalent to 19,500 across the UK.
>
> *Source:*   Rayns G et al., *All Babies Count: Spotlight on Drugs and Alcohol*, London: National Society for the Prevention of Cruelty to Children, 2013.

take off as many as 8 years, as it leads to a higher risk of diabetes, cardiovascular disease and many types of cancer (World Health Organisation 2012). Overweight and obesity are key markers for poor nutrition, since they are often reflective of a diet that is high in fats, sugars, snacks and sweetened drinks, rather than including the preferred range of vegetables, fruit and regular balanced meals (Rudolf 2009; Willis et al. 2014; All Party Parliamentary Group on a Fit and Healthy Childhood 2015).

The *social gradient* applies in obesity, as with so many other concerns, so its adverse impacts affect those who already have the most difficulties to face; on the other hand, reducing obesity could have a significant impact on health inequalities. In 2013/2014, more than one in five (22.5%) English children measured on school entry (Reception Year) for the National Child Measurement Programme were either overweight or obese, with 9.5% being obese (Health and Social Care Information Centre 2014). Among these 4- to 5-year olds, 12% of children starting school in the most deprived of areas were obese, compared with 6.6% among those at school in the least deprived areas. One local survey of 300 children (cited by the All Party Parliamentary Group on a Fit and Healthy Childhood 2015) suggested that over 90% of excess weight gained by girls and over 70% gained by boys is acquired before they start school.

At its most basic, excess weight is easy enough to explain – it arises when the amount of energy consumed through eating exceeds that used, through daily activities. While that summarizes the immediate cause, the causes of that cause are far wider and more varied. Key risk factors associated with excess weight in the preschool period include the mother being obese before becoming pregnant and smoking during pregnancy, children's screen time – television and other media (Hawkins and Law 2006). McPhie et al. (2014) identify maternal controlling, parenting, general and eating psychopathology, socio-economic status (SES) and maternal child feeding practices. Data from a US (Wisconsin) longitudinal study makes specific links between lower SES and excess body weight (Pudrovska et al. 2014), with the authors helpfully identifying the key mechanisms that have been proposed to explain this phenomenon.

First, the critical (or sensitive) period model (Ben-Shlomo and Kuh 2002) reflects a biological imprinting mechanism and posits that early life experiences can have long-lasting effects on biological and behavioural systems, which are irreversible and permanent. This idea connects with developmental models outlined above, describing the way that chronically raised cortisol levels can cause long-term damage, by causing biochemical disruptions early in the postnatal period that are programmed into the infant's metabolism. In this case, the changes relate to the way the developing infant processes nutrients and, while these changes are imprinted early, they become evident many years – even decades – later, leading to obesity in middle or later life.

This observation would explain the one made by Singh et al. (2008), that many obese adults did not carry excess weight as children.

Pudrovska et al. (2014) identify other factors implicated in early life social origins of later overweight, which are also relevant to whether or not infants are offered appropriate nutrition. These include the accumulation of risks model, since disadvantage is also associated with risks and harms that accumulate through the life course. Also, the *pathway model* and health behaviours early in life are identified as possible mechanisms that can be influenced in childhood, and which have a long-term impact on the infant's life into adulthood. Hawkins and Law (2006) found community-level factors were less strongly supported in the research literature than immediate parenting (especially maternal) behaviours. However, where fast-food outlets exceed easy and cheap access to fruit and vegetables, particularly in a population that has limited access to their own means of transport, it is easy to see why parents might opt for the former.

Food habits and behaviours are strongly ingrained, and parents act as influential role models. There is evidence that children's diets and eating behaviours closely match those adopted in the family, particularly by mothers. Family activity levels are also copied, although there are suggestions that fathers are somewhat more influential than mothers in this (Rudolf 2009). Infants are able to regulate their intake from birth, but all too often parents over-ride this by pushing the baby to feed for a little longer, just to finish the bottle or take some more, or earlier, solid foods. Controlling parenting styles are associated with overweight (Rudolf 2009; McPhie et al. 2014), for example if food is used as a reward (sweets, chocolate) or withheld as a punishment ('no dessert unless you finish your mains'). Rudolf suggests working to the motto of '*parent provides and child decides*', which is to say that the parent should decide which food to offer and when, but if the child shows signs of satiety by pushing food away or of hunger by seeking more, this should be respected.

There is limited research about how best to promote good food habits in pre-school children, but there is general agreement about the key issues. In one of the few studies, Willis et al. (2014) focused on the main family lifestyle and parenting factors needed for healthy weight management, listed in Box 5.7.

One key protective factor that is mentioned often, is breastfeeding (Arenz et al. 2004; Cathal and Layte 2012; UNICEF 2013). The World Health Organization (2011) recommends that all babies are exclusively breast-fed until they are 6 months old. It not only provides the infant with exactly the right amount of nutrients, but allows the infant to control the amount of food taken and introduces different flavours, which stem from the mother's food passing through into the breast milk (Rudolf 2009). This helps to increase acceptability of the range of flavours familiar in the household, so reduces fussiness as well as likelihood of overweight. The benefits from breastfeeding far exceed those of protection against obesity reduction alone, as summarized in Box 5.8.

Even so, breastfeeding rates remain relatively low in England, despite recent improvements. Breastfeeding initiation rates rose to 81% in 2010, but by the time their infant is 3 months old, only 17% of mothers still exclusively breastfed their babies, falling to 1% by 6 months (McAndrew et al. 2012). In 2010, 35% of mothers still gave their infants some breast milk at 6 months, but there were large social variations, with the more affluent mothers tending to breastfeed for longer (McAndrew et al. 2012).

While modern formula milks are extremely sophisticated and modified to match breast milk as far as possible, there are key aspects that can never be replicated. In particular, recent evidence points to the important role of breast milk as one of the key mechanisms involved in facilitating beneficial microflora in the neonatal gut, with lifelong implications for health (Schwiertz et al.

BOX 5.7: Key Lifestyle and Parenting Factors for a Healthy Weight

PARENTING

- Parental self-efficacy
- Authoritative style of parenting
- Modelling of a healthy lifestyle

EATING PATTERNS

- Regular family mealtimes
- Limited grazing behaviour (snacking)

HEALTHY EATING

- Appropriate child-sized portions
- Less energy dense foods and sugar-sweetened beverages
- More fruit and vegetables

PHYSICAL ACTIVITY

- More active play
- Less sedentary behaviour, especially television viewing
- Emotional well-being
- Emotional well-being of the child and all family members

Source: Willis TA et al. *Pediatric Obesity* 9(5): 339–350, 2014.

BOX 5.8: Summary of Key Benefits from Breastfeeding

- Fewer hospital admissions (Department of Health 2013; UNICEF 2013) from
  - Lower respiratory tract infections
  - Infant feeding difficulties, wheezing
  - Gastroenteritis, rd
  - Non-infective gastroenteritis
  - Eczema
  - Otitis media
  - Infant feed intolerance
  - Lactose intolerance
  - Asthma
- Lower risk of Sudden and Unexplained Deaths in infancy (Wolfe et al. 2014)
- Reduced risk of obesity (Arenz et al. 2004; Cathal and Layte 2012; UNICEF 2013)
- Enhanced opportunities for mother-infant attachment, with fewer reports of maternal neglect (Strathearn et al. 2009)
- Some evidence of (infant) having higher cognitive ability (Kramer et al. 2008)

2003; Madan et al. 2012). The foetal gut is sterile, but is rapidly colonized by bacteria from the mother after birth. Fully breast-fed infants tend to have higher concentrations of protective bacteria, with a lower level of potentially harmful ones. These are not established through a single movement, but by a series of dynamic changes influenced by diet and exposure to a range of other environmental factors. These influence the way the neonatal microbiome develops, with lifelong implications for the immune system, affecting both infections and allergies, and future carbohydrate metabolism, which helps explain why some people are more prone to weight gain than others. Indeed, Madan et al. (2012, p. 753) suggest that *'establishment of the microbiome in the critical neonatal period is potentially foundational for lifelong health and disease susceptibility'*. This new science has the potential to explain some of the intricate mechanisms behind the well-known fact that breastfeeding provides a good nutritional start to life.

REVISITING THE CASE STUDIES

If you met Kayleigh or Daisy, what would you tell them about the foundations of health for their babies? How much do you think the mothers could change themselves and how much depends upon their families or the wider society?

CONCLUSION

Mothers and babies have always been of primary interest to the public health community, not only for their own sake, but because their well-being shines a light into what is happening to the health of the wider society. As infant and child mortality has decreased so dramatically over the last half century, some might have felt this marker had lost its potency, whereas this period attracts as much interest as ever, or more. This chapter began by explaining the reason for the continuing relevance of these early, foundational months and years of life. Health inequalities, both between countries and within them, remain stark. An infant's life chances remain intimately linked to the social status of their parents or the part of the country they were born in, even in resource-rich, highly-developed countries like the UK. Now, there is sufficient evidence to understand the mechanisms that create these destructive inequalities. That same science can be used to help ameliorate the early disadvantage and help promote good health and well-being for our youngest citizens.

Throughout, this chapter has drawn attention to the way that much of the new science confirms knowledge that has been long-held in society – such as that early childhood is important for future health, that loving relationships between mother (or other primary caregiver) and baby matter and that good nutrition is foundational. The new science also draws attention to long-held beliefs that have been shown to be untrue. It is not inevitable that poor babies will become poor adults. Furthermore, many of the changes needed to protect and enable positive developments in infants are simple to implement – cuddling and talking to babies, reading to them, breastfeeding and ensuring they are provided with safe space in which to play. All of these actions sound reasonable and will be straightforward for many parents.

However, the chapter has also pointed to the underlying difficulties faced by so many parents in achieving these apparently simple measures. In the end, political will is needed to support new babies and their parents. The need is to ensure safe conditions for families to live and play in, affordable nutritious food and speedy access to care for mental as well as physical health problems for parents who are struggling. Life has become increasingly difficult for many young families since the global downturn in 2008. We find evidence of this in the increasing health inequalities and worrying statistics about babies whose life chances are still being blighted by an unsatisfactory start to life. We have grounds for optimism in the number of official reports and in the extent of political interest in the phenomenon of the first 1001 critical days, and foundation years. Perhaps this interest will soon turn to action soon for the benefit of all new babies and the wider society.

REFERENCES

All Party Parliamentary Group for Conception to Age 2—The First 1001 Days. (2015) *Building Great Britons*. London: Wave Trust.

All Party Parliamentary Group on a Fit and Healthy Childhood. (2015) *Healthy Patterns for Healthy Families: Removing the Hurdles to a Healthy Family*. London: All Party Parliamentary Group on a Fit and Healthy Childhood.

Arenz S, Rucket R, Koletzko B, von Kreis R. (2004) Breastfeeding and childhood obesity—a systematic review. *International Journal of Obesity* 28: 1247–1256.

Barker DJ. (1990) The fetal and infant origins of adult disease. *BMJ* 301(6761): 1111.

Bauer A, Parsonage M, Knapp M, et al. (2014) *The Costs of Perinatal Mental Health Problems*. London: Centre for Mental Health and London School of Economics, for Maternal Mental health Alliance.

Ben-Shlomo Y, Kuh D. (2002) A life course approach to chronic disease epidemiology: Conceptual models, empirical challenges and interdisciplinary perspectives. *International Journal of Epidemiology* 31: 285–293.

Bronfenbrenner U. (1986) Ecology of the family as a context for human development: Research perspectives. *Developmental Psychology* 22(6): 723–742.

Cathal MC, Layte DR. (2012) Breastfeeding and risk of overweight and obesity at nine years of age. *Social Science & Medicine* Jul;75(2):323-30.

Center on the Developing Child at Harvard University (2011) *Building the Brain's 'Air Traffic Control' System: How Early Experiences Shape the Development of Executive Function*. Working Paper No.11. http://www.developingchild.harvard.edu.

Chamberlain D. (2003) Communicating with the mind of a prenate. *JOPPPAH* 18(2): 99–100.

Commission on Social Determinants of Health (CSDH). (2008) *Closing the Gap in a Generation. Health Equity through Action on the Social Determinants of Health*. Geneva: World Health Organization.

Courchesne E, Pierce K, Schumann CM, et al. (2007) Mapping early brain development in autism. *Neuron* 56(2): 399–413.

Courchesne E, Pierce K. (2005) Brain overgrowth in autism during a critical time in development: Implications for frontal pyramidal neutron and interneuron development and connectivity. *International Journal of Developmental Neuroscience* 23: 153–170.

Euro-Peristat Project with SCPE and EUROCAT. (2013) *European Perinatal Health Report. The Health and Care of Pregnant Women and Babies in Europe 2010*. 2. www.europeristat.com.

Faglioni M, Jensen CL, Champagne FA. (2009) Epigenetic influences on brain development and plasticity. *Current Opinion in Neurobiology* 19: 207–212.

Field F. (2010) *The Foundation Years: Preventing Poor Children Becoming Poor Adults*. London: The Stationery Office.

Gerhardt S. (2004) *Why Love Matters: How Affection Shapes a Baby's Brain*. Hove, UK: Routledge.

Hawkins SS, Law C. (2006) A review of risk factors for overweight in preschool children: A policy perspective. *International Journal of Pediatric Obesity* 1(4): 195–209.

Hill MA. (2015) *Embryology Abnormal Development – Developmental Origins of Health and Disease*. Retrieved March 7, 2015 https://embryology.med.unsw.edu.au/embryology/index.php/Abnormal_Development-Developmental_Origins_of_Health_and_Disease.

Hogg S. (2013) *Prevention in Mind. All Babies Count: Spotlight on Perinatal Mental Health*. London: NSPCC.

Hogg S, Haynes A, Cuthbert C, Baradon T. (2015) *An Unstable Start – All Babies Count: Spotlight on Homelessness*. London: NSPCC.

Irwin LG, Siddiqi A, Hertzman C. (2007) *Early Child Development: A Powerful Equalizer, A Report for the WHO Commission on Social Determinants of Health*. Geneva: WHO.

Kramer MS, Aboud F, Mauchand E, et al. (2008) Promotion of breastfeeding intervention trial (PROBIT) study group. Breastfeeding and child cognitive development: New evidence from a large randomized trial. *Archives of General Psychiatry* 65(5): 578–584.

Leask J, Kinnersley P, Jackson C, et al. (2012) Communicating with parents about vaccination: A framework for health professionals. *BMC Pediatrics* 12: 154.

Madan JC, Farzan SF, Hibberd PL, Karagas MR. (2012) Normal neonatal microbiome variation in relation to environmental factors, infection and allergy *Current Opinion in Pediatrics* 24(6): 753–759.

McPhie S, Skouteris H, Daniels L, Jansen E. (2014) Maternal correlates of maternal child feeding practices: A systematic review. *Maternal and Child Nutrition* 10: 18–43.

Marmot M. (2010) *Strategic Review of Heath Inequalities in England post-2010: Fair Society, Healthy Lives*. London: Institute of Health Equity, University College London.

Murray L, Andrews L. (2005) *The Social Baby: Understanding Babies' Communication from Birth*. Richmond, UK: CP Publishing.

National Scientific Council on the Developing Child. (2006) *Early Exposure to Toxic Substances Damages Brain Architecture*. Working Paper No. 4. Retrieved from http://www.developing-child.net.

National Scientific Council on the Developing Child. (2009) *Young Children Develop in an Environment of Relationships*. Working Paper No. 1. Updated edition, Retrieved from http://www.developingchild.net.

National Scientific Council on the Developing Child. (2010) *Early Experiences Can Alter Gene Expression and Affect Long-Term Development*. Working Paper No. 10. http://www.developingchild.net.

National Scientific Council on the Developing Child. (2005/2014) *Excessive Stress Disrupts the Architecture of the Developing Brain*. Working Paper 3. Updated Edition. http://www.developingchild.harvard.edu.

Nolte J. (1993) *The Human Brain*, St. Louis, MO: Mosby Year Book, 1993.

Padley M, Valadez L, Hirsch D. (2015) *Households below a Minimum Income Standard*. York: Joseph Rowntree Foundation.

Public Health England. (2014) Routine Childhood Immunisations from July 2014. poster. https://www.gov.uk/government/publications/routine-childhood-immunisations-from-july-2014.

Pudrovska T, Logan ES, Richman A. (2014) Early-life social origins of later-life body weight: The role of socioeconomic status and health behaviors over the life course. *Social Science Research* 46: 59–71.

Rayns G, Dawe S, Cuthbert C. (2013) *All Babies Count: Spotlight on Drugs and Alcohol*. London: National Society for the Prevention of Cruelty to Children.

Rudolf M. (2009) *Tackling Obesity through the Healthy Child Programme – A Framework for Action*. Leeds, UK: Leeds Community Healthcare, University of Leeds.

Rutter M, Madge N. (1976) *Cycles of Disadvantage: A Review of Research*. London: Heinemann.

Rutter, M. (2006) *Genes and Behaviour: Nature–Nurture Interplay Explained*. Malden, MA: Blackwell Publishing.

Salmon DA, Terret SP, MacIntyre CR, et al. (2006) Compulsory vaccination and conscientious or philosophical exemptions: Past, present, and future. *The Lancet* 367(9508): 436–442.

Sanger C, Haynes A, Rayns G, et al. (2015) All babies count: Reducing the pressure on new families. *Midwifery* 31: 345–348.

Schwiertz A, Gruhl B, Löbnitz M, et al. (2003) Development of the Intestinal bacterial composition in hospitalized preterm infants in comparison with breast-fed, full-term infants. *Pediatric Research* 54(3): 393–399.

Shonkoff JD, Phillips D. (2000) *From Neurons to Neighborhoods: The Science of Early Childhood Development.* Washington, DC: National Academy Press.

Shonkoff JP, Akil H, Chang HI, et al. (2012) *From Neurons to Neighborhoods: An Update.* National Research Council and Institute of Medicine. Washington, DC: National Academy Press.

Singh S, Mulder C, Twisk JWR, et al. (2008) Tracking of childhood overweight into adulthood: A systematic review of the literature. *Obesity Reviews* 9: 474–488.

Skogen JC, Øverland S. (2012) The fetal origins of adult disease: A narrative review of the epidemiological literature. *JRSM Short Reports* 3(8): 59.

Social Exclusion Task Force. (2007) *Think Family: Analysis from 'Families At Risk' Review.* London: Cabinet Office.

Stiles J, Jernigan TL. (2010) The basics of brain development. *Neuropsychology Review* 20: 327–348.

Strathearn L, Mamun AA, Najman JM, O'Callaghan MJ. (2009) Does breastfeeding protect against substantiated child abuse and neglect? A 15-year cohort study. *Pediatrics* 123(2): 483–493.

The Health and Social Care Information Centre. (2014) *National Child Measurement Programme: England, 2013/14 School Year.* London: Health and Social Care Information Centre.

Turnbaugh PJ, Ley RE, Hamady M, et al. (2007) The human microbiome project. *Nature* 449: 804–810.

UNICEF. (2010) *Innocenti Report Card 9: The Children Left Behind.* A league table of inequality in child well-being in the world's rich countries. Florence, Italy: UNICEF.

UNICEF. (2013) *The Evidence and Rationale for the UNICEF UK Baby Friendly Standards.* London: UNICEF.

Waldfogel J, Washbrook E. (2008) *Early Years Policy.* London: Sutton Trust.

Walker SP, Wachs TD, Grantham-McGregor S, et al. (2011) Inequality in early childhood: Risk and protective factors for early child development. *The Lancet* 378: 1325–1338.

Wave Trust. (2012) *Conception to Age 2: The Age of Opportunity.* London: Wave Trust.

Wedge P, Prosser H. (1973) *Born to Fail.* London: Arrow Books for National Children's Bureau.

Werner E. (2006) What can we learn about resilience from large-scale longitudinal studies? In: Goldstein S, Brooks RB, eds. *Handbook of Resilience in Children.* New York: Springer Science, 91–105.

WHO. (2011) *Exclusive breastfeeding for six months best for babies everywhere.* http://www.who.int/mediacentre/news/statements/2011/breastfeeding_20110115/en/.

Willis TA, George J, Hunt C, et al. (2014) Combating child obesity: Impact of HENRY on parenting and family lifestyle. *Pediatric Obesity* 9(5): 339–350.

Wolfe I, Macfarlane A, Donin M, Viner R. (2014) *Why Children Die: Death in Infants, Children and Young People in the UK.* London: Royal College of Paediatrics and Child Health.

World Health Organization (2012) Population-based approaches to childhood obesity prevention. Geneva: World Health Organization.

Approaches to parenting

MAGGIE FISHER AND DIANE DeBELL

6

INTRODUCTION

The most important and probably the most influential setting for childhood is the home environment, whether that setting is with the child's natural or adoptive parent(s), reconstituted families, carers, extended family members, foster parents or within the supervision of the state (children in care). But what do we mean when we refer to the parenting role and why is there such a burgeoning contemporary interest in parenting within government policy, the media and the general public?

Bornstein (2002) defined parenting in the following way:

> Parents create people. It is the entrusted and abiding task of parents to prepare their offspring for the physical, psychosocial and economic conditions in which they will eventually fare, and it is hoped flourish... parents are the 'final common pathway' to children's development and stature, adjustment and success.
>
> **(Bornstein 2002, p. ix)**

> Parenting is something that parents do, not something they have.
>
> **(Quinton 2004, p. 27)**

Parenting involves tasks such as physical care, boundary setting and the teaching of social behaviour. Optimal child and adolescent behaviours such as responsiveness, affection and positive regard are, of course, the ideal outcome of parenting. In theory, those relationship qualities that indicate emotional security and secure attachment are the aspiration *for* parenting.

However, parental ability to achieve this ambitious agenda is influenced by many factors, including genetics; childhood experiences of the parenting role; socio-economic circumstances such as relative poverty; housing; culture; the community/neighbourhood environment and the health or ill-health of the child or the parent(s). And these factors rarely remain stable throughout the school-age years. The child, furthermore, is a purposive actor in this relationship and we find that individual children respond in different ways to the parenting they experience.

Some children are more resilient than others and the parenting role can, intentionally or not, support that resilience or it can introduce risks that the child or adolescent is unable to negotiate. The factors that produce risk for children are poverty, mental illness, struggling schools, violence (in the community or in the home) and disabilities. We still know little about the factors that produce resilience in individual children (Ghate and Haxel 2002; Bartley 2006). However, the Harvard Center on the Developing Child is currently investing serious research into understanding the science of resilience, *giving children a sense of mastery over difficult experiences* (2015).

Every Child Matters (2003) specified the importance of the parental relationship in a child's growth and development in the United Kingdom,

> The bond between the child and their parents is the most critical influence on a child's life. Parenting has a strong impact on a child's educational development, behaviour and health.

(Chief Secretary to the Treasury 2003, p. 39)

Government policy in all four countries of the United Kingdom during the twenty-first century has been moving rapidly to a position of concern about the parenting role; about what the state's responsibility for assisting parents to carry out this role should be and the design of legislation that can support parenting (e.g. the *Carers and Disabled Children Act 2000*; the *Children Act 2004*; the *Children and Families Act 2014*). It is a policy position we find repeated by the Department of Health, Department for Education and Skills (DfES), the Treasury, the Social Exclusion Unit, the Home Office Family Policy Unit, the Children and Young Persons Unit, the Children and Families Directorate within the Department for Education, and other governmental agencies and departments, including the integrating role now assigned to the four Ministers for Children – one in each of the four countries of the United Kingdom.

In January 2007, the Treasury and the DfES published an evidence-based discussion paper, *Policy Review of Children and Young People* (HM Treasury and DfES 2007) in preparation for the 2007 Comprehensive Spending Review. The intention was to plan family support investment for the years 2008–2009, 2009–2010 and 2010–2011.

This work marked an important recognition of the need for sound evidence about *how best* to assist parents in their work with children and young people. Also see Quinton's valuable overview of research in 2004. Writing in 1999, DeBell found little evidence of agreement about either the value base or the relative effectiveness of work by professional and voluntary or community agencies in delivering parenting support initiatives.

What is also needed, in addition to shared definitions of what parental support means, is greater clarity about the specific objectives of individual programmes or interventions. The currently poor research knowledge about the relative effectiveness of different approaches is directly linked to poor articulation of the desired outcomes of both individual and joint services.

The evidence also suggests that there is no agreed philosophy or shared vision of parenting. In other words, for partnership working to succeed, a shared understanding of the value base of parenting programmes is needed.

(DeBell 1999, p. 4)

Much work has been conducted since the turn of the century in an effort to probe these questions. But, writing specifically about the critical issue of child abuse and neglect in *The Lancet* in 2005, Barlow and Stewart-Brown repeated this discouraging picture:

Whilst there is some evidence emerging about the potential effectiveness of preventive initiatives, there is considerably less consensus about what works when abuse has already occurred.

(Barlow and Stewart-Brown 2005, p. 1750)

This chapter explores the child and young person in the context of 'the family'; the many influences that impact on the family; how *parenting* affects the child's health and well-being and the role of the public health practitioner in the broad field known as parenting support.

THEORIES OF PARENTING AND OF CHILDHOOD

Parenting is a complex matter that generates extensive debate. It is an activity in which parents engage almost unconsciously. Historically and, indeed in contemporary Britain, parenting skills and knowledge are passed on through families from generation to generation.

It was with the emergence of psychology and psychoanalysis in the latter part of the nineteenth century that parenting practices began to be studied as a factor that affects a child's health and development. The very concept of childhood itself did not emerge as a focus for philosophical debate in western nation-states until the eighteenth century with writers such as Adam Smith, Rousseau, Blake, Boswell and Hume. These earlier philosophical enquiries were largely concerned with the relationship between child development and educational philosophy but, together, they early theorized childhood as a separate sphere from the adult world and one that is shaped by adult actions.

Blake's *Songs of Innocence and Experience* (1788 and 1794) broke important ground when he posed the sentimental view of childhood unworldliness against the reality of what he saw of childhood in the streets of London.

I wander thro' each charter'd street,
Near where the charter'd Thames does flow
And mark in every face I meet
Marks of weakness, marks of woe.
In every cry of every Man,
In every Infant's cry of fear,
In every voice; in every ban,
The mind-forg'd manacles I hear …

(Blake 1794, in Keynes 1970)

To put it very simply, the child in Blake is conceived and made manifest as a consequence of how the adult organizes the world.

It was not until the 1970s that a new sociology of childhood emerged, which broke free of the concept of the child as a consequence, primarily, of adult imagination and control – in other words, the child as actor in his or her own life placed the child's voice and the child's active volition at the centre of attention (MacKay 1973; Speier 1976; James and Prout 1997; Qvotrup et al. 1994; Christiansen and James 2000; Alderson 2001; Mayall 2002). This is to oversimplify complex arguments but it is an important concept when we talk about parenting. The child's physical, emotional and psychological vulnerabilities are set within a context of both the parental function and the child's own strategies for negotiation of, and response to, parental actions. In other words, parenting is a dynamic between the child and the adult.

Following three centuries of theorization in western cultures about the child in relation to the parental figure, we have recently become accustomed in Britain to thinking about the child–parent relationship from a mainly behaviourist approach in classical learning theory. In other words, the thinking here is that parents who behave towards their children in unhelpful ways, either through ignorance or intention, are generally believed to produce behaviours in their children that are counterproductive to the child's health and well-being. It is fair to say that this is the starting point for contemporary government policy in Britain and for public health interventions that seek to 'support parents'. In fact, from the softer world of how to manage emotional and behavioural problems in young children and adolescents to the harsher world of antisocial behaviour orders (ASBOs) as well as the realities of child abuse and neglect, the behaviourist approach is dominant in contemporary thinking about how to support parenting.

In this approach to parental support, reward is encouraged, such that it should bring about desired behaviour and ignore undesirable behaviour. It is based on the principle that what you pay attention to is what you get more of. Supporters of this approach believe that teaching parents behaviour management techniques is the most effective way of changing unhelpful parenting practices (Utting et al. 1993; Webster-Stratton 1999). Such thinking goes back to Skinner in the 1950s and 1960s, and it is a powerful voice in contemporary government policy. It is also a fairly rapid approach that can be 'taught' quickly and can be 'taught' to parents as a group. It is thereby a cost-effective approach for statutory services in providing parenting support interventions.

The psychotherapeutic approach, on the other hand, attributes unhelpful parental behaviours to parental distress. Here, the argument is that effective parenting is, in contemporary popular language, *emotionally literate*. Attending to the emotional relationship between the parent and the child is argued to be the key to supporting parents. Holistic qualities such as empathy, respect and genuineness are here emphasized, and parents are encouraged to understand the *feelings* that cause their children's behaviour. In this way, parents are encouraged to respond in helpful ways to children (Gordon 1975; Bavolek 1990; Gottman and Declaire 1997). The argument is that adult self-reflection and analysis can enable parents to help their children manage their own feelings in emotionally positive ways, and can thus improve children's and young people's relationships with others. Praising desirable behaviour and ignoring unhelpful behaviour, as in the behaviourist approach, is also advocated as a strategy and is designed to help foster positive parent–child relationships that can lead to emotional well-being.

A further school of thought suggests that difficulties begin with the baby and the 'goodness of fit' (Thomas and Chess 1977) between parent and infant. Temperamental or genetically determined neuropsychological differences can here make parenting more or less challenging and can be the cause of unhelpful parenting practices.

Parents' perceptions of their child are known to be important factors in influencing parenting behaviours.

(Ghate and Hazel 2002, p. 15)

All the proponents of the different approaches agree that changing parental behaviour can have a critical impact on children's behaviour, and that low self-esteem, feelings of guilt and inadequacy in parents and in children can be substantial barriers to positive behavioural change in the child. The varying schools of thought, however, begin from different theories of childhood, and thereby describe different approaches to the most expedient way of changing parental behaviour and thus child or adolescent behaviour where that would benefit the child. There are various studies that provide evidence to support each model.

What is common to these different approaches is that parenting can be defined as the feelings, attitudes, behaviours and beliefs that parents have with regard to their children, including rejection of the child. Researchers examining parenting and parenting programmes have identified a number of adult attributes that arguably are necessary for successful parenting and healthy parent–child relationships. But, there is also much that is in common between parent–child relationships and social well-being within communities and societies (Wilkinson 1996) and within schools (Weare 2000). In other words, articulations of the determinants of healthy adult relationships are identical between those needed for healthy parenting and those needed for effective teaching and for healthy communities. The argument is that the critical skill needed for creating emotional well-being in the home, at school and in the community is reciprocity in human relationships.

APPROACHES TO PARENTING STYLES

Diverse research programmes have theorized parenting styles (e.g. the statistical classification generated by Stevenson et al. 2004). In 1973, Diana Baumrind identified three parenting styles that are frequently used as a point of reference by public health practitioners. She argues that parenting styles derive from parental behaviours along the four dimensions as follows:

* Warmth and responsiveness or nurturance – often reflected in the emotional tone of a family
* Parental expectations of a child ('is this a realistic expectation for a child of this age?')
* Clarity and consistency of rules
* Style and level of communication between parent and child

Using the above four dimensions, Baumrind described three specific combinations of these features and referred to them as 'parenting styles':

* The permissive style, which is high in nurturance, but low in parental expectation, control and communication
* The authoritarian style characterized as high in control and parental expectation, but low in nurturance and communication
* The authoritative style, which is high in all four dimensions

In 1983, Maccoby and Martin took Baumrind's (1973) model a step further and identified a fourth category: the neglecting style. This insight has been widely accepted and underpinned by research findings (Steinberg et al. 1989, 1991, 1992, 1994, 1995; Dornbusch et al. 1987; Lamborn et al. 1991; Glasgow et al. 1997). Maccoby and Martin (1983) adjusted Baumrind's dimensions to propose a two-dimensional model along a continuum from level of control/demand to acceptance/rejection or responsiveness as depicted in Figure 6.1. Where these two dimensions intersect they create four distinctive parenting styles, which are similar to Baumrind's (1973) original three styles described above.

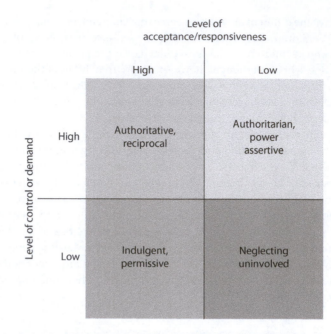

Figure 6.1 Parenting styles. (From Bee H, *The Developing Child*. 9th edition. Boston: Allyn & Bacon, p. 385, 2000. With permission.)

It is frequently argued that parenting *styles* can be highly predictive of particular outcomes for children but these assertions, significantly, focus attention on family systems rather than on individual parental behaviours. And, of course, parents do not fall neatly into these categories. Parenting styles vary and change in response to the child's age, behaviours, temperament, and health profiles (e.g. child or parental ill-health or disability). Indeed, individual children within the same family act, respond and see their worlds differently from each other. Nevertheless, the following styles provide us with a way of organizing and thus describing diverse parental behaviours in relation to the child.

- *Authoritarian parenting* can be characterized by an insistence on unquestioning obedience, order and respect for authority. Authoritarian parents make high demands on their children and can be emotionally unresponsive. This style of parenting is associated with children who perform less well in school, have less social competence with peers and have lower self-esteem (Maccoby and Martin 1983; Baumrind 1991). Children of authoritarian parents may appear subdued or, conversely, may display high aggression or appear to be out of control.
- *Permissive parenting* may also be associated with some poor outcomes for children such as underperformance at school during adolescence or tendencies towards aggression if the parents are very lax about aggressive behaviour. Children of permissive parents are more likely to be immature, to evade responsibility and to be dependent on others for help (Maccoby and Martin 1983).
- *Parents who neglect their children* can trigger disruptive child behaviours and there is a high association between neglect and delinquent behaviours (Patterson 1992). These children often display disturbance in their relationships with peers and adults. Children of uninvolved, emotionally abusive, or neglecting parents can be impulsive and/or antisocial and tend to be less motivated at school (Block 1971; Pulkkinen 1982; Lamborn et al. 1991). Parents who neglect their children are often themselves overwhelmed

by their own complex problems; may be suffering from mental health problems; may be repeating family patterns of parenting and can be psychologically or emotionally unavailable to the child. In other words, the parent who neglects a child is likely to have little emotional connection to the child. These children are often described as 'insecurely attached' (Ainsworth et al. 1978). Steele (2002) argued the importance of fathers in the attachment role, while Utting and Pugh (2003) extended this to include friends and communities. Sanders (2004) also investigated the ways in which sibling relationships can compensate for or can become congruent with parental relationships.

- *Authoritative parenting* is consistently associated with the most positive outcomes for children (Dornbusch et al. 1987; Steinberg et al. 1989, 1991, 1992, 1994, 1995; Lamborn et al. 1991; Glasgow et al. 1997). Authoritative parents are warm and nurturing. They set clear limits and boundaries and positively reinforce desirable behaviour. These parents are characterized as highly responsive to their child's individual needs, and are less likely to use physical punishment. High demands are placed on the child to achieve realistic social and academic goals. Children experiencing this type of parenting tend to show higher self-esteem, greater independence and self-confidence and more altruistic behaviour. Academically they perform better (Steinberg et al. 1992).

One disadvantage in using this model is that it cannot capture important patterns of family interaction in diverse cultural or ethnic groups. For example, in some Asian cultures, expectations about strict obedience are often understood by the child to be aspects of parental caring and concern, and may not be perceived to be demonstrating lack of warmth.

NEGATIVE CONSEQUENCES OF PARENTING STYLES

Nevertheless, parenting style is repeatedly associated with outcomes that can affect child health and well-being. Desforges and Aboiuchaar (2003) identified parenting as one of the most important determinants of educational achievement:

> The most important finding … is that parental involvement in the form of 'at-home good parenting' has a significant positive effect on children's achievement and adjustment, even after all factors shaping attainment have been taken out of the equation.

(Desforges and Aboiuchaar 2003, p. 4).

Parental involvement in a child's schooling between the ages of 7 and 16 years is a more powerful predictor of attainment than family background, family size and level of parental education (Feinstein and Symons 1999). In particular, a father's interest in a child's schooling is strongly linked to good educational outcomes for the child (Hobcraft 1998; Flouri and Buchanan 2001; Goldman 2005).

Neglectful, permissive and authoritarian parenting are linked with antisocial behaviour (Sanders and Dadds 1996); low self-esteem (McClun and Merrell 1998) and drug and alcohol abuse (Cohen et al. 1994). Conversely, authoritative parenting is predictive of good peer relationships and educational achievement (Baumrind 1978; Steinberg et al. 1992).

Research by Patterson et al. (1989) indicates that a combination of coercive parenting, poor supervision, and lack of parental warmth or affection could account for 30%–40% of antisocial behaviour and criminality, delinquency and violence in adolescence. Child abuse (Egeland 1997) and family conflict/domestic violence, even if children are not directly involved, have been found to be contributory causes of mental health and social problems in later life (Amato et al. 1995).

Furthermore, studies by Wilkinson (1996) and Brummer (1997) indicate that emotional distress can cause physical illness by affecting the immune response. Smoking, drinking in excess and the consumption of high-fat foods were also found to be valued by young people and adults for their ability to relieve emotional distress (Cameron and Jones 1985). Stress caused by school examinations has indicated susceptibility to viral infections (Cohen et al. 1994), while Marmot et al. (1991 and again in 2005) early argued that lack of control over life events (also see Rosengren et al. 1933) can create long-term vulnerability to cardiovascular disease. The collective picture indicates a link between emotional distress and physical illness and disease, both in children and long into adulthood.

Research has also repeatedly found greater vulnerability to physical and mental ill-health in boys than in girls. Boys are at greater risk of developing seizure disorders; autism and related problems; dyslexia; and hyperactivity; and are more susceptible to maternal mental health problems (Murray and Cooper 1997). Boys have been found to be more likely to develop conduct disorders, to be involved in criminality and to be more likely to attempt suicide (Lewis and Slogget 1998).

Hodgson et al. (1996) suggest that social and psychological factors are linked in the aetiology of mental health and illness. How individuals respond to stressful events is dependent on their individual strengths or vulnerabilities, which in turn will determine their coping styles and resilience. This is influenced by individual personality profiles that have a genetic component, but is also powerfully shaped by the social and emotional environment in which children grow and develop.

The child is not, however, a passive actor in these profiles. We have called attention to the dynamic that develops between child and adult carer, and we have also referred to the resilience versus risk factors that operate to help or hinder the child in his/her negotiation of the familial, social and psychosocial environment. See Chapter 8 for discussion of these factors in the context of child and adolescent mental health. Figure 6.2 is a visualization of that dynamic in terms of the child's environment and its potential for impact on the child.

THE INTERACTING ECOLOGICAL FRAMEWORK – THE CHILD WITHIN THE FAMILY SYSTEM

Bronfenbrenner's model (1979) of the ecology of human development takes these arguments further by producing a useful framework for considering the child in its real-world setting, because it helps us to understand how interrelated and complex systems outside the family connect in ways that affect the child and the family. Bronfenbrenner argued that the ecology of human development consists of four distinct but interrelated systems or types of settings (see Figure 6.3). The child is at the centre of the model and the child affects and is affected by the settings in which that child spends time. The family is, arguably, the most important setting for the child because this is, quite simply, where the child spends the most time and has strong emotional ties.

- The *microsystem* consists of the child in the family but also includes the immediate settings with which the child has direct personal experience such as the family, the school, after-school activities and the neighbourhood/community setting. The family, however, it is articulated, is the major microsystem for child development in Britain and in many parts of the world.

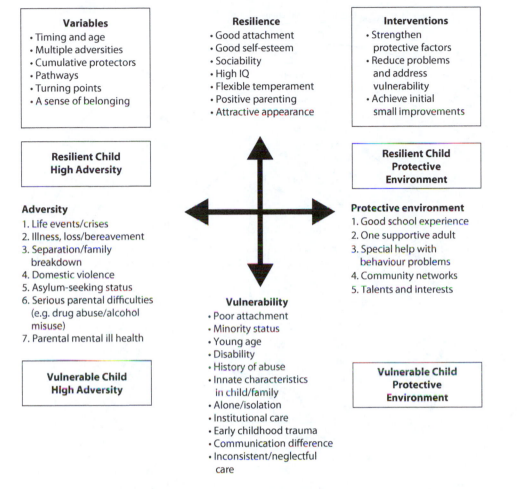

Variables
- Timing and age
- Multiple adversities
- Cumulative protectors
- Pathways
- Turning points
- A sense of belonging

Resilience
- Good attachment
- Good self-esteem
- Sociability
- High IQ
- Flexible temperament
- Positive parenting
- Attractive appearance

Interventions
- Strengthen protective factors
- Reduce problems and address vulnerability
- Achieve initial small improvements

Resilient Child High Adversity

Resilient Child Protective Environment

Adversity
1. Life events/crises
2. Illness, loss/bereavement
3. Separation/family breakdown
4. Domestic violence
5. Asylum-seeking status
6. Serious parental difficulties (e.g. drug abuse/alcohol misuse)
7. Parental mental ill health

Protective environment
1. Good school experience
2. One supportive adult
3. Special help with behaviour problems
4. Community networks
5. Talents and interests

Vulnerability
- Poor attachment
- Minority status
- Young age
- Disability
- History of abuse
- Innate characteristics in child/family
- Alone/isolation
- Institutional care
- Early childhood trauma
- Communication difference
- Inconsistent/neglectful care

Vulnerable Child High Adversity

Vulnerable Child Protective Environment

Figure 6.2 Resilience and vulnerability in children. (From Lifelong Learning Directorate of Somerset County Council, *Somerset Behaviour Support Service Guidance Notes*. Taunton, UK: Somerset County Council, p. 19, 2004. With permission.)

- The *mesosystem* was described by Bronfenbenner as

  … the interrelations among major settings containing the developing person at a particular point in his or her life.

  (Bronfenbrenner 1977, p. 515)

For example, an interaction between a parent and a child can be influenced by what has happened to the parent at work that day. Or a change in family organization or circumstances, including bereavement or parental divorce can disrupt the child's understanding of his or her world.

- The *exosystem* is an extension of the mesosystem and refers to all the outside influences that the child does not experience directly but which affect one of the microsystems of which the child is part, particularly the family. We can think here of housing, financial resources, adult employment, education and family history.

111

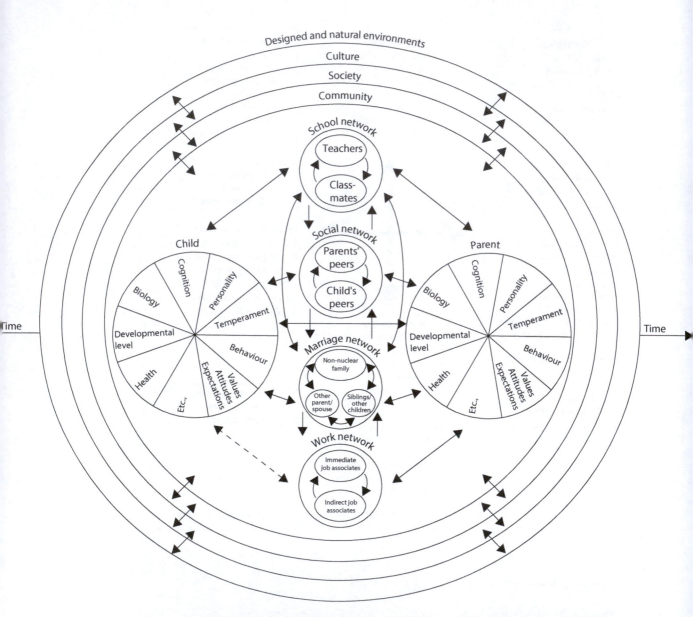

Figure 6.3 Ecology of human development. (From Lerner RM, Castellino DR, Patterson AT, et al., Developmental contextual perspective on parenting. In: Bornstein M, ed. *Handbook of Parenting*. Vol. 2. Mahwah, NJ: Lawrence Erlbaum Associates, pp. 287–297, 1995. With permission.)

- The *macrosystem* is the larger cultural setting in which all the other systems are embedded. It includes the neighbourhood in which the family lives; the family's social circumstances; the family's ethnic identity, cultural values, beliefs, political philosophies; the family's economic circumstances and the larger cultural/historical events such as war, civil strife, famine, floods or environmental catastrophe that may affect the other ecological systems.

Bronfenbrenner's model allows us to represent the reality that bidirectional socialization (the child and the family) is embedded in a more complex system of social networks, and societal, cultural and historic influences.

THE FAMILY IN THE UNITED KINGDOM

The family in the United Kingdom is understood to be the basic social formation responsible for the growth and development of children and young people. Such is generally the case across all developed countries. The family is a biological reality for most children, and children are generally cared for in a social context, in which their survival depends on a family formation. In fact, children in the care of the state are theoretically placed in a context that is designed to replicate the biological family. However, there are alternatives to the conventional family, which presume a collectivist approach to child rearing such as Kibbutzim, The Nayar of Malabar, collective communities in North America, and the continued existence of large-scale residential care in many of the post-soviet countries of Eastern Europe and in China.

The family takes many forms within the four countries of multicultural Britain, but it is a vital influence on a child's well-being and health. Nevertheless, socio-biologists suggest that the *mother–child* relationship represents the basic family unit and that it is predetermined by nature. This gender bias is reflected in much government parenting policy. The weight of parental responsibilities, apart from financial responsibility, generally appears to fall upon women. For example, parenting orders have been described as *mothering orders*, simply because they are mainly made against mothers. Some professionals have expressed concern that parenting orders can be seen as discriminatory in practice because they criminalize mothers (Coleman et al. 1999; Ghate and Ramella 2002). In reality, of course, many of these mothers are the sole carers of these children and the fathers may be non-resident or absent.

Changing social expectations and values, attitudes to gender, marital and relationship breakdown have all had an impact on the family as a unit in Britain and on contemporary government policy. In the United Kingdom, roughly 40% of first marriages end in divorce, and the number of lone parents has been on the increase for the last three decades at least. Parents may be divorced, single, same-sex, or adoptive. Many children live in reconstituted families with step-parents and step-siblings. Many children live between different homes, with parents who do not live together, and do so without apparent distress. Nevertheless, family breakdown and marital discord have been associated with an increase in disorders such as child depression and anxiety (Wallace et al. 1997; Harold et al. 2001).

The traditional two-parent nuclear family is often argued in developed countries to be the ideal arrangement for raising children. This view is supported by evidence suggesting that there are better outcomes for children raised in these circumstances (Morgan 1999; Wells and Rankin 1991). Government policy across the United Kingdom, however, also acknowledges the private domain of the family by recognizing the rights of individuals to be self-determining within a landscape of changing social mores. This is reflected, for example, in government policy that argues its support for lone parents and for families in relationships other than marriage.

As Bronfenbrenner's model (1979) demonstrates, however, the child is embedded in the family in a context in which there are many interacting pressures, including socio-economic and psychosocial factors that arise from the surrounding culture and the implicit values of the political system of the day – all exerting influences on the family system itself.

The whole premise of the 'ecological' framework – in terms of the way people experience everday life – is that children and parents inhabit ecological systems where these levels flow into, and interact with, one another to produce complex nested relationships and layered or overlapping effects.

(Ghate and Hazel 2002, p. 100)

GOVERNMENT POLICY AND PRACTICE: PARENTAL EMPOWERMENT OR SOCIAL CONTROL?

The Beveridge Report (1942) recommended that the government of the time should find ways of fighting the five 'giant evils' of want, disease, ignorance, squalor and idleness (Timmins 1996). The outcome was the British welfare state and the establishment of the National Health Service (NHS) in 1948, providing free medical care for all at the point of access. The NHS was part of Beveridge's crusade to tackle disease. Squalor and idleness were tackled by a massive post-war building programme to improve housing, schools, the roads and the nation's infrastructure at a time when the country was near bankruptcy. National Service was also introduced with a view to reducing idleness and unemployment as well as ensuring a standing army. The 1944 *Education Act* introduced by Rab Butler sought to tackle ignorance and to reduce unemployment. The school-leaving age was raised to 15 in 1944, and universal free schooling was provided in grammar, secondary modern and technical schools. The school-leaving age was raised to 16 in 1972. In 1952, the last workhouse was closed.

Since the Second World War, government interest in parenting has sharply increased. It has been fuelled more recently by concerns about social exclusion, social cohesion, the criminal justice agenda, and the potential links between the quality of parenting and the potential for better outcomes for children.

> Parenting is probably the most important public health issue facing our society. It is the single largest variable implicated in childhood illness and accidents, teenage pregnancy and substance misuse, truancy, school disruption and under achievement, child abuse, unemployability, juvenile crime and mental illness. These are serious in themselves but are even more important as precursors of problems in adulthood and the next generation.

(Hoghughi 1998, p. 1545)

The concerns reflected here have provided impetus for government policy intervention in the parenting role in the United Kingdom and internationally. Since *Supporting Parents* (1998) there has been a steep rise in the range and scale of parenting support interventions. In 2005, the Treasury with the DfES published *Support for Parents: The Best Start for Children*, and in 2007 a *Policy Review of Children and Young People: A Discussion Paper* (HM Treasury and DfES 2005, 2007).

These publications are linked, and they contextualize children's and young people's ability or not to thrive within four factors: family prosperity; parenting; the wider community and services. It is fair to say, however, that greatest attention is focused on parenting rights and responsibilities, with concomitant government investment in parent education, usually time limited.

Some observers have suggested that parent education is a form of social control, and it is important to consider who benefits (Smith 1997). There have been contradictions and tensions in government policy and legislation since the late twentieth century. Policy makers are faced with the need to juggle contradictory pressures about adult employment (e.g. women's employment and methods to improve men's involvement in the care of their children); a liberal approach to ensuring parental autonomy and, at the same time, rationales for government interventions in the private sphere of parenting and the family.

For example, the *Crime and Disorder Act 1998*; the *Anti-Social Behaviour Act 2003*; the *Criminal Justice Act 2003*; the *Respect Action Plan 2006* and the *Social Exclusion Action Plan 2006* early indicated a move towards direct intervention in parenting work. There is serious need for government investment in evaluations to determine the impact of these measures on children and families (see National Children's Bureau 2007).

Furthermore, concerns about child protection have increased since 1989 when the UK Government became a signatory to the UN Convention on the Rights of the Child (UNCRC 1989). The Laming Report (Department of Health and Home Office 2003) marked a turning point in recognition that statutory services have a responsibility to protect children from harm by carers (see Chapters 4 and 9). Yet, the current government has not provided children with the same protection from assault as adults, including assault by a parent.

By failing to give children equal protection under the law, the United Kingdom breaches obligations under the UNCRC, the European Social Charter, the International Covenant on Economic, Social and Cultural Rights and other human rights treaties. In 1995, the UN Committee on the Rights of the Child, the Human Rights Treaty Body for the UNCRC, made a formal recommendation to the UK Government to prohibit corporal punishment, and raised the following concerns over the use of reasonable chastisement:

> The committee is worried about the national legal provisions dealing with reasonable chastisement in the family. The imprecise nature of the expression of reasonable chastisement as contained in these legal provisions may pave the way for it to be interpreted in a subjective and arbitrary manner. This committee is concerned that the legislative and other measures relating to the physical integrity of children do not appear to be compatible with the provision and principles of the convention, including those of articles 3, 19, and 37.

> **(Henricson 2003, p. 48)**

Other contradictions in government policy can still be found in the targeting of parents to provide sex and relationship education in the home, whilst simultaneously bypassing the family when providing confidential sexual health services to children. However, control of children continues to be an issue for which the UK Government has attributed primary responsibility to parents who are then expected to be supported by schools and the youth justice system in a secondary manner.

> Families are the core of our society. They should teach right from wrong. They should be the first defence against antisocial behaviour.

> **(Labour Party Manifesto 1997, p. 19)**

Parenting orders were introduced by the *Crime and Disorder Act 1998*. Magistrates could then direct a parent to attend some form of counselling or guidance if their child has committed an offence or has frequently truanted from school. However, the parent cannot be compelled to receive help until help has been offered and rejected by the parent. Many observers have expressed concern about holding parents responsible for their children in this way. Henricson (2003, pp. 46–48) first summarized these concerns:

> A critical element of parent education programmes is that they should engage parents in the process; this is unlikely to be achieved if parents are having to attend under compulsion and in the context of a humiliating court order.

> There is the possibility that the parenting order could be challenged from a legal and human rights perspective because it attributes blame for the conduct of one person to another, and in effect criminalizes a parent without their having committed a crime.

The approach rests on an assumption that the primary responsible relationship in bringing up children rests with parents. This undermines the role of the wider community. It also undermines children's agency.

(Morrow 1999)

The burden of responsibility in the execution of the legislation tends to fall on the mother with the majority of parenting orders being made against mothers rather than fathers. This has adverse implications for equal opportunities and equality under the law.

(Ghate and Ramella 2002; Morrow 1999)

This is another stick with which to beat disadvantaged parents where supportive carrots are to be preferred. It continues a regrettable trend of intervening in the family life of the least well-off in society.

(Henricson 2003, p. 41)

Despite these protestations over compulsion, the evaluations from parenting orders have found that parents who have been required to attend a programme have, nevertheless, reported a benefit from them (Ghate and Ramella 2002). The Scottish Government has not adopted parenting orders because of its reservations about the efficacy of coercing parents.

Parliament struggles to tighten definitions of parental responsibility on child safety, such as the age at which a child may be left alone at home. In the absence of government guidelines, the National Society for the Prevention of Cruelty to Children (NSPCC) has produced a code recommending that babies and very young children should not be left unattended, while children under 13 years should not be left at home alone for long periods. The code suggests that children under 16 years should not be left alone overnight or in charge of younger children (Papworth 2002). Parental rights and responsibilities are, effectively, ill-defined. It has been suggested that Parliament should conduct a policy review to reconcile 'disparate strands of policy', and should produce a parental code to define parental rights and responsibilities, thereby enhancing relations between government and parents (Henricson 2003).

FAMILY RELATIONSHIPS AND CHANGE DURING CHILDHOOD: THE ROLE OF PARENTING SUPPORT

As children grow and develop from dependent infant to independent adult, the relationship between child and adult inevitably changes. This requires an adjustment in parenting skills for each stage of a child's life. During the cycle of child growth and development, parents themselves also develop and change as they cope with their own life-cycle stages, and the changes that occur in their circumstances. This profile can have a significant impact on how parents actually parent their children and how they manage their children's lives and their children's changing relationships to the world in which they are growing up and the world they are learning to negotiate.

The concept of parenting support at a whole-population level is relatively new as a feature of government policy. It is also, as we have already noted, a difficult concept to define. What we can do is describe diverse approaches to intervention.

Quinton (2004) argued that parenting support tends to fall into three categories: formal, informal and semi-formal. In this profile, it is the work of professionals that constitutes formal support (e.g. mainly delivered by health, social care and education practitioners but also by the youth justice system). Informal support is that help and assistance that comes from family, friends and neighbours. Semi-formal support is generally provided by voluntary, charitable or faith-based organizations. There is, however, little systematic co-ordination between these sources of assistance for parents. And there is little systematic and co-ordinated training for parenting support, even for professional services. The exceptions tend to be health visiting, and child and adolescent mental health services (CAMHS). And, in some cases, school nurses are trained in parenting support skills. Telephone and Internet links are a further form of growing assistance to parents.

There is also repeated evidence that parents who have access to one form of support tend also to use multiple forms of assistance – formal, informal, and semi-formal. In other words, 'relationships lie at the heart of support' (Quinton 2004, p. 130), and those parents who are more socially effective are also more likely to receive help. This implies that the most severe parenting problems are often closely linked to isolation of the adult parent(s)/carer(s) from family and/or community networks (see Section 'Thinking about Risk in Approaches to Parenting').

In 2004, Whittaker designed a model of both formal and informal approaches to parenting education and support (Bidmead and Whittaker 2004; see Figure 6.4). 'Informal' here subsumes Quinton's (2004) concepts of *informal* and *semi-formal* approaches, by collapsing these into one category. Whittaker's model reflects a birth-to-adolescence perspective, and is useful as a starting point for visualizing the structure of parenting support in Britain. What it cannot do is fully reflect the internal system of support that accrues from family members, friends and neighbours, who are integral to any analysis of parenting support. What Figure 6.4 also disguises is the accidental nature of support systems across the country. In other words, where a family lives will largely determine the scope, scale and accessibility of services, including family and community assistance.

Furthermore, gender bias towards support for mothers has been repeatedly identified in research evidence. On the whole, professionals and community groups tend to focus their work on mothers, and do so at the expense of fathers. Williams (1999) early identified the process of exclusion of fathers that tended to occur in home visiting. This *father-blind* approach by public services has been identified by Ferri and Smith (1996); Barclay and Lupton (1997); Burghes et al. (1997); Grimshaw and McGuire (1998); Warin et al. (1999); Williams and Robertson (1999) and Ghate et al. (2000).

Professionals who work with families wrestle with many complex issues, and need to become adept at managing that complexity (see Section 'The concept of need in parenting children and young people').

Hall and Elliman (2003, p. 34) suggest that success in providing parental support is determined not only by what potential helpers do but by the characteristics of the person/people providing the service. The relationships they develop with the parents are critical to the success or failure of the intervention and to the parent's ability to implement effective strategies for parenting. For example, the style of relationship that professionals establish with parents will influence how the professionals are perceived, and will influence parental expectations of their role. This is repeated throughout much of the evidence (e.g. Ghate and Hazel 2002; Quinton 2004; Bartley 2006).

Cunningham and Davis (1985) identified three parent–professional relationships:

1. The *expert model* in which the professional feels he/she has all the expertise; takes control of the situation and makes the decisions. Mutual respect, sharing of information, negotiation and parental views are given low priority. This approach can undermine parental confidence and/or create dependency. It may also lead to important information and problems being missed. It is not a holistic view and pays little attention to the environmental context in which the family lives.

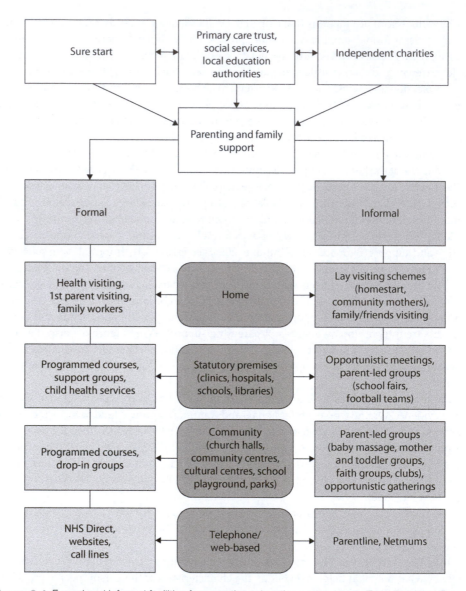

Figure 6.4 Formal and informal facilities for parenting education and support. (From Bidmead C, Whittaker K. *Postitve Parenting: A Public Health Priority*. London: CPHVA, p. 30, 2004. With permission.)

2. The *transplant model* sees the parent as having useful skills to augment the professional's skills. Here, the professionals see themselves as *transplanting* skills to the parent in their absence (e.g. carrying out treatments for technology-dependent children). In such cases, professionals understand themselves to be managers of family situations. In this profile, the professional retains overall control and identifies objectives, treatments and teaching methods. The parents may not share these aims and objectives, yet the professional may expect the client to comply with the instructions and to become competent. Furthermore, the family may not have the necessary physical, practical or emotional resources to comply. If excessive demands are made on the family, the outcome can be hostility and a breakdown in the professional–parental relationship.

3. The *consumer model*, which evolved to become the *parent advisor model* (Davis et al. 2002), and subsequently developed further to become the *family partnership model*. This approach is based on a shared partnership between professional and parent. Control remains with the parent, and the professional's role is to share information with the parent and to explore options. In this model, the professional acknowledges the parent's expertise, skills and depth knowledge of the family/child situation. The professional acts as a *skilled helper*, with an emphasis on understanding the needs of the family/parent, and negotiates a way forward, a form of counselling. To establish this partnership approach, the professional must have appropriate personal qualities such as respect, empathy, personal integrity and excellent communication skills. In such cases, the parent selects the parenting options that most suit the family's needs. The professional's skills lie in establishing the negotiating process and helping to find solutions. In this model, aims and expectations are openly stated and explored, and this forms the basis of a contract. The professional also needs to have an understanding of the helping process, the skills and qualities necessary to enable families to change their practices.

These relationship skills are important for professionals working with parents either on an individual basis or in groups. Parenting UK, for example, (formerly the Parent Education Support Forum) advocates specific training for all those who offer parent support and who facilitate parent groups. Parenting UK has developed National Occupational Standards (NOS) for Working with Parents (www.parentinguk.org). Training includes provision of adequate supervision for the practitioner and encourages reflective practice and professional development.

Research rarely concentrates on the process of help itself and the parent–helper interaction, elements that can determine success or failure. In such cases, the context of the relationship will determine the outcome. Fonagy et al. (2001), for example, argued that positive outcomes in specialist treatments are dependent on the style of treatment rather than the choice of treatment. The core skills he identified were listening to and respecting children and parents, and valuing their views and experience. Quinton (2004) also argued that how professionals work with parents is as important as what they do.

Crowley (Parenting UK) suggests that parenting education and support is like performing heart surgery, where professionals are delving into the most intimate relationships between parent and child. Everyone feels vulnerable. She compares this to a surgeon performing open-heart surgery. The expectation from the public is that the surgeon will be suitably qualified to perform such operations. So, it is with providers of parent education and support. Practitioners need to have the skills and personal attributes appropriate to working with parents. The NOS for Working with Parents supports this contention.

Similarly, Miller (2002) in an important presentation to the Parent Child Conference reported research carried out in Newcastle and commissioned by the Healthy Action Zone in the North East (2000). From the findings, she identified three types of approaches to parental perceptions of parent education. This qualitative study interviewed parents from four target groups comprising teenage parents, school children, pre-school children and parents of children with special educational needs. The following models were developed:

- *The dispensing model*: Parents ask 'what can I do to change my child?'. Parent educators focus on the child as a problem. Surface learning only takes place at this level, and this type of learning is viewed as instruction by an expert.
- *The relating model*: Parents ask 'how do I feel about this situation?'. Parent educators focus on the parent as a problem. This stimulates a different type of learning.

- *The reflecting model*: Parents ask 'why is this happening?'. Parent educators focus on the relationships in the family as a legitimate area for exploration. A deep level of learning can take place. This type of learning is associated with skilled facilitation and an ongoing supportive relationship.

One repeated criticism of research studies (Hall and Elliman 2003) is that the interventions under study often use highly skilled facilitators, who are well trained, have regular quality supervision and support, and are often from a mental health background. When such programmes are replicated, they are often facilitated by less well-qualified staff who have infrequent supervision and operate in less well-organized work environments. As a consequence, the outcomes can be disappointing because replication is not possible. The skill and ability of the facilitator is one of the most critical ingredients in successful outcomes (e.g. the ability to recruit and retain parents from the outset, notably when trying to work with families most in need).

THINKING ABOUT RISK IN APPROACHES TO PARENTING

Despite the generic and the public health definitions of risk, thinking about approaches to parenting actually involves thinking about factors that can cause risk to the parenting function. By this we do not refer to risk in terms of child protection only. Rather, we are concerned with those families who are most in need, whether as a consequence of material or emotional need. What we mean by this is to indicate those factors that complicate the difficult work that parenting involves for all parents.

> Parenting in a modern industrial society includes a formidable range of tasks and responsibilities. For parents to pull these off requires sufficient resources and social supports, that can be drawn on to help them.

> (Quinton 2004, p. 180)

Quinton's work is a useful starting point because it is an overview of 14 studies (in addition to Ghate and Hazel's work 2002) of diverse challenges that parents encounter. Its purpose is to try to identify the kinds of support that parents themselves want and might use, including how such support is or should be organized. The determination in Quinton's work was to provide an analytical addition to systematic literature reviews, which tend to foreground analyses of interventions themselves (e.g. Barlow and Stewart-Brown 2001; Patterson et al. 2002; Moran et al. 2004; Sanders and Morawska 2006). In other words, Quinton and his team were asking broader questions about the parenting experience, and they did this by commissioning individual studies from expert teams (on behalf of the DfES).

> Research on the effects of supportive interventions – i.e. on 'what works' – needs more specific attempts to understand the direction of effects through well-evaluated trials of different approaches.

> (Quinton 2004, p. 181)

Much of the work discussed in Quinton (2004) indicated severe problems with public services. Perhaps one of the most striking studies involved South Asian parents' experiences of living with a child with severe disabilities. The incidence of disabilities amongst South Asian families is three times the national average. This is a public health matter. The findings of Hatton et al. (2004) are alarming. They found that these families are not provided with the diagnostic information from healthcare professionals that they need from the outset of diagnosis, nor do they receive information about services that might help them. Many in the study did not speak

English and, contrary to popular perceptions, most did not have extended families to assist them. The emotional support that parental partners provided for each other was a key feature of these parents' ability to parent their disabled children in severely adverse circumstances.

Of the commissioned studies, imprisoned fathers were the least likely group to be assisted in their parenting role (Boswell and Wedge 2004). This confirms work by DeBell (2003) that studied the effect on adolescents of having a close family member in custody. Approximately 125,000 children each year will have a parent in prison (Brown 2003, p. 4). But, this figure increases when close family members are included (e.g. siblings, mothers, uncles, grandfathers). The stigma attached to imprisonment means that most children at school who have a close family member in custody, do not reveal this fact to the school. Yet, the distress caused by imprisonment of a close family member can lead to poor health, poor educational attainment because of exam disruption, and either social isolation or truancy, anxiety, distress or inability to manage anger. Considerable recent work is focusing on the potential relationship between sibling custody and child and adolescent delinquency (Murray and Farrington 2006), and between parental imprisonment and children's own eventual criminal behaviour (Murray et al. 2007).

What interventions would be appropriate in each of these cases? Little work has focused on these kinds of difficulty that are encountered by parents attempting to manage their parenting role effectively. The reason is largely linked to the isolation caused by the way these problems are handled by public agencies such as the criminal justice system and the healthcare system. From a public health practice perspective, these examples are neither intractable nor insolvable. But, they do tend to be invisible.

Quinton speaks of parental support as a process, and this fits with our earlier argument that the parenting role is itself a process over time, affected by the ecology of the family system itself and the changes experienced by all members of a family as children grow and develop, as family circumstances change and mutate.

Families coping with disabilities (in the child or in the parent/carer) are a stark example of the long-term issues implied by a process approach to parenting development (see Chapter 9). The findings suggest little inter-agency co-ordination and poor information to assist children and their parents/carers. For example, the tendency to medicalize such experiences fails to understand the social context in which these families lead their lives.

THE CONCEPT OF NEED IN PARENTING CHILDREN AND YOUNG PEOPLE

The following is a real case study in the United Kingdom, but rendered anonymous.

The Jones family is Mum (Marie) age 29 and Dad (Tom) age 31. Marie has two sons (Daniel, age 12 and Mark, age 10) fathered in an earlier relationship that was characterized by domestic violence. The boys no longer have contact with their birth father. Together, Marie and Tom have a daughter (Kylie, age 4). Marie's first child was born when she was 17. Her own mother is remote and Marie was sexually abused by her step-father. Marie and Tom are heavy smokers and Marie suffers from depression. Husband Tom drinks in excess and is an occasional drug user. He has spent time in prison for theft and drug dealing.

The family lives in a three-bedroom house rented from the local authority, located in what is characterized as a deprived estate. They are in rent arrears and are threatened with eviction. Debt is a serious problem. The house is in poor structural condition, is uncared for, and is unsafe. The family has a number of pets living in the house with them.

> Daniel's behaviour is difficult for his Mum to manage. He has been excluded from school in the past and he often clashes with his brother. Daniel at age 12 is enuretic and has been in trouble with the police for stealing from local shops and fighting with other boys.
>
> Mark has been diagnosed with attention deficit hyperactivity disorder (ADHD) and is currently prescribed with Ritalin. His mother says that she cannot 'handle him', and her husband Tom shows little interest in either of the boys. Mark is a poor sleeper and frequently wanders the house at night.
>
> Kylie is her father's favourite. She is about to start school but is a fussy eater, goes to bed late and wakes frequently in the night.
>
> Marie is six months pregnant and has had a difficult pregnancy. There have been medical concerns about the baby's growth, and Marie often forgets to attend antenatal appointments.

The complexity of this family's situation and their children's needs will have attracted attention from a range of service providers, including school, health, social care, and community services as well as housing and police officers. The challenge is twofold. On the one hand, the parents and their children can only be assisted in so far as they seek assistance. On the other hand, without assistance, they could potentially be subject to legal interventions – from local authority housing offices, debt agencies and/or the police.

This one family's situation has virtually all the elements that public health practitioners highlight in their work. School nurses, health visitors, CAMHS teams, midwives, children's services, education welfare officers (EWOs), and crisis support teams are all orientated towards assisting with one or more of the presenting problems. The difficulty from a service provision perspective is that the over-riding need is co-ordination and interagency work. A lead professional could be helpful in such a profile of need, but local authority and integrated children's services, across the United Kingdom are stretched, under-funded, under-resourced, and they are continuing to experience change at the local level.

> Time and again, our research revealed that those welfare professionals who listened, who were not judgemental, gave their clients time, who were prepared to advocate for their clients and seek solutions which were appropriate to their needs, were highly valued and made a positive difference to their lives. These were the exception, however, and when interviewed it was often the case that state welfare workers felt that their approach was despite their employing agency, rather than positively endorsed by the agency.

(Bartley 2006, p. 23)

The challenge is and, it remains, to determine

> The extent to which there is overlap between what parents want, what services provide and 'what works' … a more thorough understanding of all three should help considerably in our efforts to improve the way in which we deliver services in this field.

(Ghate and Hazel 2002, p. 10)

Having said that, we do not know what forms of help and assistance the Jones children have or do not have from relatives, from friends and from schools. Furthermore, the danger is that public policy tends to focus on the parental difficulties, without thinking about each child's individual perspective on the problems he/she is confronting, whether that method of confrontation is successful for the child or not. *Behavioural problems*, for example, are the presenting and public manifestation of the child's experience. And behavioural problems are the generic term with which children like those in our case study will find themselves generally labelled – for the simple reason that it is their behaviour that is public and observable.

Ghate and Hazel (2002) conducted some of the most extensive research we currently have about the experiences of families who live and parent their children in poor environments in twenty-first century Britain. Their findings reveal the stunning capacity that parents actually demonstrate in managing family life in the most adverse circumstances – situations that include seriously poor housing; very low income; parental and child ill-health; an absence of safe play areas outside the home; insufficient resources for food and clothing. These would be risk factors for successful parenting for any parent.

> The results of the study confirmed that parents living in poor environments are typically exposed to high levels of risk factors at all levels of the ecological model. Whether we explore stressors at the level of the individual, the level of the family and household or at the level of the community and environment, we find clear evidence of elevated levels of adversity for parents and their children relative to the wider population. Based on the data we gathered, there can be little doubt that parenting in a poor environment is a particularly difficult job.

(Ghate and Hazel 2002: 233)

There are two obvious approaches we can take to child poverty: invest in removing material poverty; invest in strengthening resilience and capability in the child and family. This is not an either/or agenda. There is emerging evidence of links between the two in some few deprived areas of the United Kingdom where communities, and thus families within them, are being strengthened by developing civil society strategies that start from co-ordinated service delivery (Stewart et al. 1999; Mitchell 2003; Mitchell and Backett-Millburn 2006).

In addition, considerable research is being undertaken in an effort to understand the factors that produce 'the enormous capabilities and resilience that people show in their everyday lives and under crisis conditions' (Bartley 2006, p. 3). Thus far, the evidence suggests two common factors that can make resilience in the child or young person more likely.

> Those mostly have to do with the quality of human relationships, and with the quality of public service responses to people with problems…. . Good public services enable and encourage people to maintain social relationships, but badly provided ones can create social isolation.

(Bartley 2006, p. 3)

CONCLUSION

We intentionally chose to title this chapter 'Approaches to parenting', and not to use the term *parenting support*. The latter, as Quinton (2004) argues, is a conceptually problematic term. Furthermore, we have argued that the issue is not merely a matter of parenting skills, important though they are. Children and young people thrive or fail to thrive as a consequence of multiple factors within the ecological framework in which the family finds itself. And child well-being in the family setting is rarely examined from the child's or young person's perspective.

Our purpose in this chapter has been to explore the public health practice issues that arise from the school-age child's home environment, whatever form that might take. In doing this, we sought to explore the factors within family life that can affect the health and well-being of children and young people of school age.

The public health practice perspective on the school-age child requires us to consider the three settings children and young people inhabit during their school-age years: the home; the school; the neighbourhood/community. Within the home setting, the features that matter are the approach to parenting that the child experiences and the social and material circumstances that constitute the family environment, including the services the family can draw upon within the local community. The child and his or her carer(s) live within an ecological framework that interacts with and has consequences for the family unit and thus for children and young people.

We have emphasized the dynamic between the child and the adult carer(s), and we have sought to explore the way in which the child as actor in the family setting has a consequence for the approach to parenting. There is, of course, an imbalance of power within the home, but it remains the case that how a child responds to the carer(s) can affect the approach to parenting, and practitioners need to be sensitive to that dynamic.

It is also widely recognized that individual children and young people have various degrees of resilience when confronting emotional and/or material risk in the family setting. Yet, we know little about the delicate balance between risk and resilience. For public health practitioners, the task is to build resilience in whatever way possible. It is this ingredient that public health practitioners need to nurture in children and young people whose home lives are difficult. To do that requires services that are not judgemental, that listen to the child and to the family, and that act as advocates for the family. This means reorienting much existing practice.

KEY POINTS

- It is the *quality of human relationships* that determines the health and well-being of the family. All child outcomes eventually flow from the nature of reciprocity that develops within the family, the community within which the family lives and with the public and voluntary services that seek to support families.

- The quality of public service responses to children, young people and their families, when they encounter problems, is determined by the nature of the relationship that develops between service providers and the individual members of the family. In contemporary Britain, public services are still far from integrated across government departments in most communities.

- Parenting is a process over time, and is affected by the ecology of the family system itself, the changes experienced by all members of the family as children grow and develop, as family circumstances change and mutate.

- Children and their parents/carers live family life as a dynamic between the child and the adult. Furthermore, sibling relationships can help or hinder the child's experience of family life. Having said that, children and young people are ultimately vulnerable to adult carer(s)' behaviours.

- We know little about how capability and resilience develop in individual children who are faced with risks from or within family life. Yet, it is resilience that helps to protect children and young people in circumstances where the family is potentially damaging.

- Public health practitioners need to start their work with families from the position of relationship building, and they need to help families to create environments that can build resilience in children and young people. This means listening to the child's perspective on family life and creating contexts of assistance that can start from the child's innate strengths (the child's capacity for resilience).

- Service delivery to assist children, young people and their families in the United Kingdom is not yet generally integrated or effectively focused.

REFERENCES

Ainsworth M, Blehar M, Waters E, Wall S. (1978) *Patterns of Attachment.* Mahwah, NJ: Lawrence Erlbaum Associates.

Alderson P. (2001) Research by children. *International Journal of Social Research Methodology* 4: 139–153.

Amato P, Loomis L, Booth A. (1995) Parental divorce, marital conflict and offspring wellbeing during early adulthood. *Social Forces* 73: 895–915.

Barclay L, Lupton D. (1997) *Constructing Fatherhood: Discourses and Experiences.* London: Sage.

Barlow J, Stewart-Brown S. (2001) Understanding parenting programmes: Parents' views. *Primary Health Care Research and Development* 2: 117–130.

Barlow J, Stewart-Brown S. (2005) Child abuse and neglect. *The Lancet* 365: 1750–1752.

Bartley M, ed. (2006) *Capability and Resilience: Beating the Odds.* London: UCL Department of Epidemiology and Public Health on behalf of the ESRC: Priority Network on Capability and Resilience (2003–2007). www.ucl.ac.uk/capabilityandresilience (accessed on 19 January 2007).

Baumrind D. (1973) The development of instrumental competence through socialization. In: Pick AD, ed. *Minnesota Symposium on Child Psychology.* Vol. 7. Minneapolis: University of Minnesota Press, 3–46.

Baumrind D. (1978) Parental disciplinary patterns and social competence in children. *Youth and Society* 9: 239–275.

Baumrind D. (1991) The influence of parenting style on adolescent competence and substance use. *Journal of Early Adolescence* 11: 56–95.

Bavolek S. (1990) Parenting: Theory, policy and practice. *Research and Validation Report of the Nurturing Programmes.* Eau Claire, WI: Family Development Resources Inc.

Bee H. (2000) *The Developing Child.* 9th edition. Boston: Allyn & Bacon.

Bidmead C, Whittaker K. (2004) *Positive Parenting: A Public Health Priority.* London: CPHVA.

Block J. (1971) *Lives through Time.* Berkeley, CA: Bancroft.

Bornstein MH. (2002) *Handbook of Parenting.* 2nd edition. Mahwah, NJ: Lawrence Erlbaum Associates.

Boswell G, Wedge P. (2004) The parenting role of imprisoned fathers. In: Quinton D, ed. *Supporting Parents: Messages from Research.* London: Jessica Kingsley Publishers, 247–251.

Bronfenbrenner U. (1977) Toward an experimental ecology of human development. *American Psychologist* 32: 513–531.

Bronfenbrenner U. (1979) *The Ecology of Human Development.* Cambridge, MA: Harvard University.

Brown K. (2003) Introduction. In: DeBell D, ed. *Starting Where They Are Project: Supporting Young People with a Prisoner in the Family.* London: Action for Prisoners' Families, 4–5.

Brummer E. (1997) Stress and the biology of inequality. *British Medical Journal* 314: 1472–1475.

Burghes L, Clarke L, Cronin N. (1997) *Fathers and Fatherhood in Britain.* London: Family Policy Studies Centre.

Cameron D, Jones ID. (1985) An epidemiological and sociological analysis of alcohol, tobacco, and other drugs of solace. *Community Medicine* 7: 18–29.

Center on the Developing Child. (2015) *The Science of Resilience.* www.developingchild.harvard.edu.

Chief Secretary to the Treasury. (2003) *Every Child Matters (Cm 5860).* London: Stationery Office. www.everychildmatters.gov.uk/_content/documents/EveryChildMatters.pdf (accessed on 17 January 2007).

Christiansen P, James A. (2000) *Research with Children. Perspectives and Practices*. London: Falmer Press.

Cohen D, Richardson J, Labree L. (1994) Parenting behaviours and the onset of smoking and alcohol use: A longitudinal study. *Paediatrics* 94: 368–375.

Coleman J, Henricson C, Roker D. (1999) *Parenting in the Youth Justice Context*. London: Youth Justice Board.

Cunningham C, Davis H. (1985) *Working with Parents: Frameworks for Collaboration*. Oxford: Oxford University Press.

Davis H, Day C, Bidmead C. (2002) *Working in Partnership with Parents: The Parent Advisor Model*. London: The Psychological Corporation.

DeBell D. (1999) *What Do We Know about the Effectiveness of Parenting Support Initiatives: A Review of Research in the Field*. Norwich, UK: Healthy Norfolk 2000.

DeBell D. (2003) *Starting Where They Are Project: Supporting Young People with a Prisoner in the Family*. London: Action for Prisoners' Families.

Department of Health and Home Office (2003) *The Victoria Climbié Inquiry. Report of an Inquiry by Lord Laming*. London: HMSO.

Desforges C, Aboiuchaar A. (2003) *The Impact of Parental Involvement, Parental Support and Family Education on Pupil Achievement and Adjustment: A Literature Review. Report No 433*. London: Department for Education and Skills.

Dornbusch S, Ritter P, Liederman P, et al. (1987) The relation of parenting style to adolescent school performance. *Child Development* 58: 1244–1257.

Egeland B. (1997) Mediation of the effects of child maltreatment on developmental adaptation in adolescence. In: Cicchetti D, Toth SL, eds. *Rochester Symposium on Developmental Psychopathology. Volume VII: The Effects of Trauma on the Developmental Process*. Rochester, NY: University Press, 403–434.

Feinstein L, Symons J. (1999) *Attainment in Secondary School. Discussion Paper 341*. London: Centre for Economic Performance, London School of Economics and Political Science.

Ferri E, Smith K. (1996) *Parenting in the 1990s. Family and Parenthood Series*. London: Family Policy Studies Centre.

Flouri E, Buchanan A. (2001) *Father Involvement and Outcomes in Adolescence and Adulthood*. Oxford, UK: Oxford University Press.

Fonagy P, Target M, Cottrell D, et al. (2001) *A Review of Outcomes of Psychiatric Disorder in Childhood. Final Report to the National Health Service Executive. Project ID MCH 17-33*. London: Department of Health. www.doh.gov.uk.

Ghate D, Hazel N. (2002) *Parenting in Poor Environments: Stress, Support and Coping*. London: Jessica Kingsley Publishers.

Ghate D, Ramella M. (2002) *Positive Parenting: The National Evaluation of the Youth Justice Board's Parenting Programme*. London: Youth Justice Board for England and Wales.

Ghate D, Shaw C, Hazel N. (2000) *Fathers and Family Centres: Engaging Fathers in Preventative Services*. York, UK: Joseph Rowntree Foundation.

Glasgow K, Dornbusch S, Troyer L, et al. (1997) Parenting styles, adolescents' attributions and educational outcome in nine heterogeneous high schools. *Child Development* 68: 507–529.

Goldman R. (2005) *Father's Involvement and Outcomes in Adolescence and Adulthood*. Oxford, UK: Oxford University Press.

Gordon T. (1975) *Parent Effectiveness Training*. New York: Peter Wyden.

Gottman J, Declaire J. (1997) *The Heart of Parenting; How to Raise an Emotionally Intelligent Child*. London: Bloomsbury.

Grimshaw R, McGuire C. (1998) *Evaluating Parenting Programmes*. London: National Children's Bureau.

Hall D, Elliman D. (2003) *Health for All Children*. 4th edition. Oxford, UK: Oxford University Press.

Harold G, Pryor J, Reynolds J. (2001) *Not in Front of the Children? How Conflict Between Parents Affects Children*. London: One Plus One.

Hatton C, Akram Y, Shah R, et al. (2004) Supporting South Asian families with a child with severe disabilities. In: Quinton D, ed. *Supporting Parents: Messages from Research*. London: Jessica Kingsley Publishers, 235–240.

Henricson C. (2003) *Government and Parenting: Is There a Case for a Policy Review and Parents' Code?* York, UK: Joseph Rowntree Foundation (for the National Family and Parenting Institute).

HM Treasury and Department for Education and Skills. (2005) *Support for Parents: The Best Start for Children*. London: HMSO.

HM Treasury and Department for Education and Skills. (2007) *Policy Review of Children and Young People: A Discussion Paper*. London: HMSO.

Hobcraft J. (1998) *Childhood Experience and the Risk of Social Exclusion in Adulthood. CASE Briefing. Centre for Analysis for Social Exclusion*. London: London School of Economics.

Hodgson R, Abbasi T, Clarkson J. (1996) Effective mental health promotion: A literature review. *Health Education Journal* 55: 55–74.

Hoghughi M. (1998) The importance of parenting in public health. *British Medical Journal* 316: 1545–1550.

James A, Prout A, eds. (1997) *Constructing and Deconstructing Childhood: Contemporary Issues in the Sociological Study of Childhood*. 2nd edition. London: Falmer Press.

Keynes G, ed. (1970) *Blake: Songs of Innocence and Experience*. Oxford: Oxford University Press.

Labour Party. (1997) *New Labour Because Britain Deserves Better. Labour Party Manifesto*. www.psr.keele.ac.uk/area/uk/man/lab97.htm (accessed on 19 January 2007).

Lamborn S, Mounts N, Steinberg L, Dornbusch S. (1991) Patterns of competence and adjustment among adolescents from authoritative, authoritarian, indulgent and neglectful families. *Child Development* 62: 1049–1065.

Lerner RM, Castellino DR, Patterson AT, et al. (1995) Developmental contextual perspective on parenting. In: Bornstein M, ed. *Handbook of Parenting*. Vol. 2. Mahwah, NJ: Lawrence Erlbaum Associates, 287–297.

Lewis G, Sloggett A. (1998) Suicide, deprivation and unemployment: Record linkage study. *British Medical Journal* 317: 1283–1286.

Lifelong Learning Directorate of Somerset County Council. (2004) *Somerset Behaviour Support Service Guidance Notes*. Taunton, UK: Somerset County Council.

Maccoby E, Martin J. (1983) Socialization in the context of the family: Parent–child interaction. In: Hetherington EM, ed. *Handbook of Child Psychology: Socialization, Personality and Social Development*. Vol. 4. New York: Wiley, 1–102.

MacKay. (1973) Conceptions of children and models of socialization. In: Dreitzel HP, ed. *Childhood and Socialisation*. New York: Macmillan, 22–43.

Marmot MG, Davey Smith G, et al. (1991) Health inequalities amongst British civil servants: The Whitehall Study II. *The Lancet* 337: 1387–1393.

Marmot M. (2005) Presentation to the Tackling Health Inequalities Governing for Health Summit. In: *Reaching Out: An Action Plan on Social Exclusion*. Vol. 46. London: The Cabinet Office.

Mayall B. (2002) *Towards a Sociology for Childhood. Thinking from Children's Lives*. Buckingham: Open University Press.

McClun L, Merrell K. (1998) Relationship of perceived parenting styles, locus of control orientation and self-concept among junior high age students. *Psychology in the Schools* 35: 381–390.

Miller S. (2002) *Parental Perceptions of Parenting Education*. Paper presented at: The National Family and Parenting Institute, The Parenting Education and Support Forum, One Parent Families, The Open University and the Trust for the Study of Adolescence Parent Child Conference, sponsored by The Children and Young People's Unit, HSBC Bank, The Teenage Pregnancy Unit and the Home Office, April 18–19, 2002, London.

Mitchell R. (2003) *Greater Expectations: The Parts of Britain Where People Live Longer Than They Should. RUHBC Findings Series 4*. Edinburgh: University of Edinburgh.

Mitchell R, Backett-Millburn K. (2006) *Health and Resilience: What Does a Resilience Approach Offer Health Research and Policy? RUHBC Findings Series 11*. Edinburgh: University of Edinburgh.

Moran P, Ghate D, Van der Merwe A. (2004) *What Works in Parenting Support? A Review of the International Evidence. Research Report 574*. London: Department of Education and Skills.

Morgan P. (1999) *Farewell to the Family? Public policy and breakdown in Britain and the USA*. London: London Institute of Economic Affairs.

Morrow V. (1999) Conceptualising social capital in relation to the well being of children and young people: A critical review. *The Sociological Review* 47: 745–765.

Murray J, Farrington DP. (2006) Evidence-based programs for children of prisoners. *Criminology and Public Policy* 5: 721–736.

Murray J, Janson CL, Farrington DP. (2007) Crime in adult offspring of prisoners. A cross-national comparison of two longitudinal samples. *Criminal Justice and Behaviour* 34: 133–149.

Murray L, Cooper P. (1997) Effect of postnatal depression on infant development. *Archives of Disease in Childhood* 77: 99–101.

National Children's Bureau. (2007) *NCB Response to the Comprehensive Spending Review 2007: Joint Policy Review on Children and Young People*. London: National Children's Bureau.

Papworth J. (2002) *When you are old enough? The Guardian 19 June 2002*. www.guardian.co.uk/parents/story/0,,739853,00.html (accessed on 19 January 2007).

Patterson G. (1992) *Antisocial Boys*. Eugene, OR: Castalia Press.

Patterson G, DeBaryshe B, Ramsey E. (1989) A developmental perspective on antisocial behaviour. *American Journal of Psychology* 44: 329–335.

Patterson J, Barlow J, Mockford C, et al. (2002) Improving mental health through parenting programmes: Block randomised controlled trial. *Archives of Disease in Childhood* 87: 472–477.

Pulkkinen L. (1982) Self-control and continuity from childhood to late adolescence. In: Baltes P, Brim G Jr, eds. *Lifespan Development and Behaviour*. Vol. 4. New York: Academic Press, 64–107.

Quinton D. (2004) *Supporting Parents: Messages from Research*. London: Jessica Kingsley Publishers.

Qvotrup J, Bardy M, Sgritta G, Wintersberger H, eds. (1994) *Childhood Matters. Social Theory, Practice and Politics*. Aldershot, UK: Avebury.

Rosengren A, Orth-Gomer K, Wedel H, Wilhelmsen L. (1933) Stressful life events, social support and mortality in men born in 1933. *British Medical Journal* 307: 1102–1105.

Sanders MR, Markie Dadds CL. (1996) Triple P. A multi-level family intervention programme for children with disruptive behaviour disorders. In: Cotton P, Jackson HE, eds. *Early Intervention and Prevention in Mental Health Application of Clinical Psychology*. Melbourne, Australia: Australian Psychological Society, 59–87.

Sanders R. (2004) *Sibling Relationships: Theory and Issues for Practice*. Hampshire, UK: Palgrave Macmillan.

Sanders RS, Morawska A. (2006) Towards a public health approach to parenting. *The Psychologist* 19: 476–479.

Smith R. (1997) Parent education: Empowerment or control? *Children and Society* 11: 108–116.

Speier M. (1976) The adult ideological viewpoint in studies of childhood. In: Skolnick A, ed. *Rethinking Childhood: Perspective on Development and Society*. New York: Little Brown, 168–186.

Steele H. (2002) State of the art: Attachment. *The Psychologist* 15: 518–522.

Steinberg L, Darling N, Fletcher A, et al. (1995) Authoritative parenting and adolescent adjustment: An ecological journey. In: Moen P, Elder GH Jr, Luscher K, eds. *Examining Lives in Context: Perspectives on the Ecology of Human Development*. Washington, DC: American Psychological Association, 423–66.

Steinberg L, Elmen J, Mounts N. (1989) Authoritative parenting, psychosocial maturity, and academic success among adolescents. *Child Development* 60: 1424–1436.

Steinberg L, Lamborn S, Darling N, et al. (1994) Overtime changes in adjustment and competence among adolescents from authoritative, authoritarian, indulgent and neglectful families. *Child Development* 65: 754–770.

Steinberg L, Lamborn S, Dornbusch S, Darling N. (1992) Impact of parenting practices on adolescent achievement: Authoritative parenting, school involvement and encouragement to succeed. *Child Development* 63: 1266–1281.

Steinberg L, Mounts N, Lamborn S, Dornbusch S. (1991) Authoritative parenting and adolescent adjustment across varied ecological niches. *Journal of Research on Adolescence* 1: 19–36.

Stevenson J, Sonuga-Barke E, Thompson M, et al. (2004) Effective strategies for parents with young children with behaviour problems. In: Quinton D, ed. *Supporting Parents*. London: Jessica Kingsley Publishers, 218–219.

Stewart M, Reid G, Buckles L, et al. (1999) *A Study of Resiliency in Communities*. Ottawa, Canada: Ottawa Office of Alcohol, Drug and Dependency Issues, Health Canada.

Thomas A, Chess S. (1977) *Temperament and Development*. New York: Brunner/Mazel.

Timmins N. (1996) *The Five Giants: A Biography of the Welfare State*. London: Fontana Press.

United Nations. (1989) *United Nations Convention on the Rights of the Child*. Geneva: UN. www.unhchr.ch/html/menu3/b/k2crc.htm (accessed on 19 January 2007).

Utting D, Bright J, Henricson C. (1993) *Crime and the Family: Improving Child Rearing and Preventing Delinquency. Occasional Paper 16*. London: Family Policy Studies Centre.

Utting D, Pugh G. (2003) The social context of parenting. In: Hoghughi M, Long N, eds. *The Handbook of Parenting*. London: Sage, 19–37.

Warin J, Solomon Y, Lewis C, Langford W. (1999) *Fathers' Work and Family Life*. London: Family Policy Studies Centre.

Wallace SA, Crown JM, Cox AD, Berger M. (1997) *Child and Adolescent Mental Health*. Abingdon: Radcliffe Medical Press.

Weare K. (2000) *Promoting Mental, Emotional and Social Health: A Whole School Approach*. London: Routledge.

Webster-Stratton C. (1999) Researching the impact of parent training programmes on child conduct disorder. In: Lloyd E, ed. *What Works in Parenting Education?* Barkingside, UK: Barnaodo's Basildon Essex, 85–114.

Wells L, Rankin J. (1991) Families and delinquency: A meta-analysis of the impact of broken homes. *Social Problems* 38: 71–89.

Wilkinson RG. (1996) *Unhealthy Societies: The Afflictions of Inequality.* London and New York: Routledge.

Williams R. (1999) *Going the Distance: Fathers and Health Visiting.* Reading, UK: The University of Reading in association with the Queen's Nursing Institute.

Williams R, Robertson S. (1999) Fathers and health visitors: 'It's a secret agent thing'. *Community Practitioner* 72: 56–58.

ACTS OF PARLIAMENT

All these Acts are published by HMSO in London, and all can be accessed from the UK Parliament website (www.publications.partliament.uk).

Education Act 1944
Crime and Disorder Act 1998
Carers and Disabled Children Act 2000
Anti-Social Behaviour Act 2003
Criminal Justice Act 2003
Children Act 2004
Children and Families Act 2014

PART 3

THE CHILD IN
SCHOOL

The school as location for health promotion

7

DIANE DeBELL AND MARGARET BUTTIGIEG

INTRODUCTION

The school as location for health promotion prompts a number of questions. Why the school? What is health promotion? What do we mean by health? In England, the policy context for child health in the school years and in the school environment has become the focus of significant attention during the twenty-first century. This is echoed in Scotland, Northern Ireland and Wales. Furthermore, cross-government departmental and joint ministerial approaches have become a prominent feature of upstream thinking.

Every Child Matters: Change for Children (HM Government 2004) originally specified national and local priorities for children's services by articulating five target outcomes for children and young people, and these were given a legal platform in the *Children Act 2004*, which remains applicable across the United Kingdom and is the enabling legislation for many of the current developments around services for children and young people. Services include local authority (LA) education (state maintained schools) and academies as well as health, social care, youth justice, Connexions, youth workers, and support from the voluntary/charitable sector. The five target outcomes of *Every Child Matters* are a description of what we might think of as a definition for health and well-being amongst children and young people from birth to age 19.

- Being healthy
- Staying safe
- Enjoying and achieving
- Making a positive contribution
- Achieving economic well-being

The *Every Child Matters* framework draws on the work of Hall and Elliman (2003). It dovetails with the Standards set by the *National Service Framework for Children, Young People and Maternity Services* (Department of Health and DfES 2004) and is elaborated by the *Children and Families Act 2014.*

Every Child Matters triggered a positive social policy programme in the United Kingdom. It required whole system change and a re-evaluation of service delivery across the four countries and it focused the need for a simple, bold, aspirational statement of policy for children and young people's health and well-being.

THE SCHOOL AS THE CHILD'S WORKPLACE

One of the determinants of health that has historically made a positive difference to adult health can be found in the developing legislation to improve health and safety in the workplace – safer working conditions; shorter working hours/working week; and legislation to improve the way people treat each other. For children, the school is their workplace, but legislation does not transfer to the school environment for children – only for teachers and staff.

Schools in the United Kingdom have historically been the site of endemic child bullying; toilet facilities are often unhygienic and younger children report menacing behaviours from older children in school toilets as well as on playgrounds and via cyber bullying. Food steadily declined in nutritional value during the latter part of the twentieth century and is only now beginning to improve; fresh drinking water has not been freely available but recently has been the subject of legislation; physical activity has declined as a proportion of the time spent at school; while achievement targets for all children's work at school have been steadily increasing throughout the period since the Second World War. In other words, children's health has not been consistently at the core of school planning yet expectations about children's achievement at school have steadily risen. Mayall et al. in 1996 first documented the damaging split between health and education in English schools.

> … education also takes place at home, and health care at school. Children themselves challenge the division of lived life into private and public sectors; they take their bodies and emotions as well as their minds, into school each day. For them the maintenance of health there is a key concern.

(Mayall et al. 1996, p. 1)

Yet we also know that some individual schools across the United Kingdom have created very successful communities of learning that simultaneously work to improve child health. The reality is that there has been inconsistency of approach, largely because of the executive power of the head teacher within Britain's schools. The values, ethos and leadership direction of the head teacher have historically had considerable effect on the culture of school life, for example on the question of how the school does or does not relate to its local community and whether or not the school integrates local community resources into school life. It is in this understanding of the school as part of a large community that we can begin to understand the public health orientation that makes health promotion, its prevention and health-improvement agenda, a part of school life.

Considerable research has begun to focus on establishing evidence of the link between educational attainment and positive emotional and physical health (see, for example, Flynn and Knight 1998; Prashar 2003). The current Extended Schools Program (Department of Education 2012) began from this perspective in May 2006.

Furthermore, secondary school league tables have been used to bring pressure on schools to engage in public health practice by indicating a link between schools' levels of success as a correlation with the levels of their work that reflect a public health framework (Department for Education and Skills [DfES] and the Department of Health 2003). And in July 2005, the Office for Standards in Education (Ofsted) published its *Framework for the Inspection of Children's Services* (Ofsted 2005b), with specifications based on the *Children Act 2004* and with principles that align precisely with *Every Child Matters: Change for Children* (HM Government 2004) thereby incorporating child health as a basic premise for the inspection of schools. Further strengthening should occur with implementation of the *Children and Families Act 2014*.

In other words, the upstream policy pressures to link health and education have been steadily increasing since the turn of the century (e.g. from the National Healthy Schools Programme (NHSP) in 1999 to the *Children and Families Act* 2014). And it is in the arena of public health practice that we need to look for evidence of downstream implementation of these national policy directives for the promotion of child health (e.g. see below in 'Health promotion as targeted interventions').

Yet, despite considerable pressure to eradicate the historic profile of separation between the child's learning environment and the child's health needs, child health promotion as an explicit curriculum requirement in schools has historically been driven by legislation apart from the school inclusion agenda, which secures education provision for children with special education and/or health needs. In other words, the promotion of the child's health in the school environment has become a matter of legislation in the United Kingdom and the 2014 Act provides comprehensive direction for schools and for families and for all other associated children's services. Interpretation of the Act and its implementation will focus attention for a further 5–10 years.

Thus, thinking about the school as a child's place of work helps us to be clearer about how to conceptualize the school as a location for health promotion because it enables us to think about the determinants of health that lie within the social and the physical/emotional context of school life itself as well as the determinants of health that lie within the local community outside the school environment. Attendance at school constitutes the second most important social and physical environment children inhabit outside the family or carer home. It is possible, furthermore, to argue that the school and the home interact with each other as determinants of child health (see previous chapter).

To think about the school environment in terms of its contribution to, or its potential for harm to child health necessarily precedes our ability to think of school as a location for health promotion. Whether and how to think about child health at school is a considerable challenge for head teachers and their staff, whose primary function is to deliver teaching that satisfies the requirements of the National Curriculum. It is also a challenge for public health practitioners who work with school-age children: 'Simply going into curriculum-led school lessons is not enough' (DfES and Department of Health 2006).

THINKING ABOUT HEALTH PROMOTION AND SCHOOL LIFE

Public health practitioners have argued that the school is a key location for health promotion since at least the beginning of the twentieth century. For example, a school nurse in New York during 1908 reported that she had identified the four schools in the city with the highest rates of school exclusions. From that specification (a public health assessment), she targeted her subsequent work on the family and school environments of these children in these schools for the purposes of identifying health-improvement strategies that could be conducted by nurses with assistance from schools.

> After a month's experimental work, made by one nurse as a demonstration, the results were considered so satisfactory that twelve nurses were appointed, and following the report of this month's work with twelve nurses in forty-eight schools (four schools for each nurse), the Board of Health considered that the work … had fully demonstrated its practical value as a supplement to the health inspectors. It was seen that the work of the nurses connected the efforts of the Department of Health with the homes of the children, thus supplying the link needed to complete the chain.

(Rogers 1908, p. 966)

This attention to the child's combined school and home environment as a key to health improvement was again repeated in New York in 1941.

> We called our enterprise 'public health nursing' … Our purpose was in no sense to establish an isolated undertaking. We planned to utilize, as well as to be implemented by, all agencies and groups of whatever creed which were working for social betterment, private as well as municipal. Our scheme was to be motivated by a vital sense of the interrelation of all these forces. For this reason we consider ourselves best described by the term 'public health nurses'.

(Wales 1941, p. xi)

These two early examples contain the principles of the health-promotion concept that would come to be theorized in the late twentieth century – interdepartmental work; a social and environmental understanding of child health; and the use of public health-measurement and risk-assessment tools. In both of these pre-war reports, we see the constituent elements of a social model of medicine – the perception that health involves more than a medical model of care, 'All medicine is inescapably social' (Eisenberg 1999, p. 164).

The history of modern medicine and particularly of public health as a medical discipline dates from mid-nineteenth century research and practice. The common thread throughout the public health movement has always been its attention to population health, and the public health pioneers have all been concerned with the social and economic determinants of health alongside questions of infectious and communicable disease control. This has not, however, been uncontested territory. For example, the post–World War II approach to health improvement in industrialized countries primarily focused on individual medicine, individualized health care and individualized health risk.

Even in 2004, *Choosing Health* (Department of Health 2004a) in England shifted the public health focus away from Acheson's (1998) social model to a medical model reminiscent of the approach that came to dominance after World War II in both the United States and Britain – a model that gave rise to what we now understand as *lifestyle medicine*, which focuses attention on a model of prevention that primarily seeks to change individual behaviour rather than address the social, economic and structural determinants of health and disease. The power of individualized health responsibility remains and can be problematic for schools.

The creation of population-based public health, however, has undergone a swift conceptual and practical boost in the twenty-first century. The most radical lead has come from Harvard University in the United States. And the most recent picture in the United Kingdom indicates a similar conceptual shift, notably via the creation of Public Health England, a national body within the Department of Health. In 2006, the English DfES, working with the Department of Health, wrote:

> Schools are particularly important to Every Child Matters because they are the universal service that has the most contact with school-age children and, increasingly, those children accessing the early education offer, as well as frequent and close contact with their families [sic].

(DfES and Department of Health 2006)

This quote from the 2006 Extended Schools Initiative suggests a policy position that seeks to locate the school in a local community context that is designed to integrate LA and health services 'in close contact with families' in such a way as to maximize ability to improve child health by changing the very culture of schools and by enlarging their functions. The Extended Schools Initiative itself did not wholly survive the change in government in 2010 but the close alignment of health, social care, and population focused health planning has become embedded in Public Health England's approach to health promotion for children and young people.

Analysis of the school health services in the United Kingdom makes plain the uncertainty that remains about who is and should be responsible for children's and young people's health improvement. The services have steadily reduced numbers employed for this task. Yet neither schools nor local authorities are required to provide the service.

> The school health service should be of such educational value that children learn how to protect their health, to secure medical care when it is needed, and to accept reasonable responsibility for their own health and that of others. Moreover, the parents should be taught how to give their children the care necessary to promote health and maintain efficiency and happiness.

(Department of Health 2004a)

In this approach, the school health services were tasked with the goal of improving individual child and individual parental behaviours that affect child health. *Choosing Health* is, in fact, an example of policy shift that moves away from the interpretation of health improvement as a social issue (Acheson 1998) to a prevention agenda based on increasing individual responsibility for health.

The tension between focusing on individual responsibility for individual health behaviours, on the one hand, and focusing on the social and economic determinants of health on the other hand, is a repeated theme in contemporary government policy on child health (see 'Thinking about health inequalities agenda'). Public health practitioners tend to respond to these messages by developing practical interventions that focus expertise either on single health issues (e.g. childhood obesity, drug and alcohol abuse, sexual health) or on individual groups of children and young people (e.g. adolescents, children with long-term conditions and/or disabilities, children excluded from school, looked-after children).

In other words, when we think about the school as location for health promotion, we immediately confront a range of questions about the meaning and practice of health promotion itself. In this context, it is helpful to conceptualize our understanding of both the school setting and of what we mean by health promotion, in order to ask ourselves whether and how the school can function as a setting for improving the health of children and young people. *Choosing Health* (Department of Health 2004a) signalled a focus on individual behaviour, *lifestyle medicine,* rather than on community responsibility, whereas *Extended Schools and Health Services* (DfES and Department of Health, 2006) articulated health improvement as a joint community, family and school responsibility.

The struggle to maintain a working school nurse service in all schools across the four countries of the United Kingdom has been an indicator of the difficulty there continues to be in ensuring child health is positioned as an integrated part of the child's schooling experience. The school nurse, a qualified nurse with specialist training (NMC recorded), is an integral feature of the public health workforce. For example, public health nurses who are specifically trained to guide families and teachers as they navigate the health and care of children at school during the ages 5–19 are a core part of the workforce in England (Nicholson 2014). Nevertheless, their numbers have been allowed to dwindle since the early part of the century.

This profile may or may not continue. The strength of the workforce's growth will depend on the commissioning process and the internal leadership of the nursing profession. At present, child and adolescent health is becoming increasingly sophisticated in its requirements and the workforce needs are for more staff.

In October 2015, school nurses (and health visitors) will move to LA management and they will use the Joint Strategic Needs Assessments (JSNAs) in order to plan services that match population needs. In addition, the Royal College of Paediatrics and Child Health (RCPCH) has published major training materials in its e-Learning investment. This is a major indication of the centrality of importance that Public Health England is signalling for child health.

At best, we can say that there are apparent oscillations in policy approach in the United Kingdom as we proceed with the *Children and Families Act 2014* but we can also see that the practice of health promotion itself is not a simple matter of single interventions despite their importance as a platform for practice.

WHAT DO WE MEAN BY HEALTH PROMOTION?

The concept of health promotion first developed out of the discipline of public health in the 1970s. The seminal moment occurred at the Alma Ata, Kazakhstan, International Conference on Primary Health Care in 1978, with commitment to an 'acceptable level of health for all the people of the world by the year 2000' (World Health Organization [WHO] 1978). What lay behind this decision was a conceptual shift away from a primary dependence on vertical healthcare systems (hospital-based and specialist-orientated medicine) to a vision of integrated family and community-based health care as the lead organizing principle for healthcare systems across the world. In other words, this was a social model of medicine aspiring to the principles of participation, inter-sectoral collaboration and equity – effectively, an empowerment agenda based within a primary healthcare system.

What made the Alma Ata declaration so radical in 1978 was the shift of focus away from a hospital/medicine-led concept of health and health care, to a vision of services delivered at community level – where people live and work. But Donald Court, in the United Kingdom, had already argued for the preventive community agenda by 1976 when he chaired the UK Commission of Enquiry into the Child Health Service.

The connection between health and education is one of the most important aspects of paediatrics. In general our understanding of disorders of learning is still rudimentary, and the problems of intellectual limitation, defective speech, inadequate reading ability, excessive clumsiness, disturbed behaviour, truancy, school phobia and delinquency create a formidable array of disability. These problems will yield only to the combined efforts of doctors, teachers, psychologists, social workers, and others. Yet we have found a good deal of evidence that as yet services were not disposed to co-operate in the interests of the child.

(Court 1976, p. 3)

In November 1986, the Alma Ata targets were re-invoked with the signing of the Ottawa Charter for Health Promotion in Canada at the First International Conference on Health Promotion (WHO 1986). This initial programme was more a checklist than a strategy. Yet the outcome has been the development of what we now refer to as health promotion, a sophisticated way of thinking about the improvement of health across whole populations. In effect, the primary healthcare movement and the health-promotion movement grew up alongside each other.

At the same time, health promotion, as a concept, has been fraught with debate and confusion. And where child health is concerned, health promotion is a concept that is often used when we actually mean health education, which is best described as a subset activity of work within health promotion.

For example, it is helpful to separate formal teaching programmes about health subjects (e.g. dental hygiene, puberty, and the subjects within the personal, social, and health education [PSHE] curriculum) from health-promotion work per se. Only when we have made this discrimination can we begin to talk about the vectors of activities, interventions and responsibilities that make up the work of health promotion in the school environment.

There is inevitably a pressure to define health promotion as a product in terms of interventions and activities (see below) when, in fact, it is part of an emerging pressure towards citizen participation and empowerment. Health promotion might best be thought of in terms of a political communication strategy, and it arises from arguments based in social medicine. And even here it is not without its critics, who argue that health promotion over-emphasizes interventions designed to modify individual behaviour, and neglects the social and economic contexts that determine behaviour (Sidell et al. 1997).

In other words, there is a basic uncertainty about the parameters of health promotion. How, for example, do you build strategies for health improvement if the social, economic or political environment is toxic?

The underpinnings of debate about the meaning of health promotion in the United Kingdom also arise from shifts and changes in government policy over the last three decades. For example, the Black Report in 1980 identified the correlation between poor health and low income in modern Britain, but the findings were suppressed by the Conservative government of the time (Black 1980). Public health practitioners and managers have reported to us that, until 1997, they were instructed by central government not to use the term *inequalities* in their analyses.

The Acheson Report (1998) signalled a re-focus of attention on the link between socio-economic and health inequalities as explanations for population health profiles (see 'Thinking about the health inequalities agenda'). Yet, by 2004 the policy agenda had shifted attention back again to individual responsibility for health (Department of Health 2004a). This kind of policy oscillation would return the United Kingdom (notably England) to roughly the position that preceded election of the Labour government in 1997. In the twenty-first century, there is now considerable pressure on both sides of the Atlantic to broaden the analysis of health

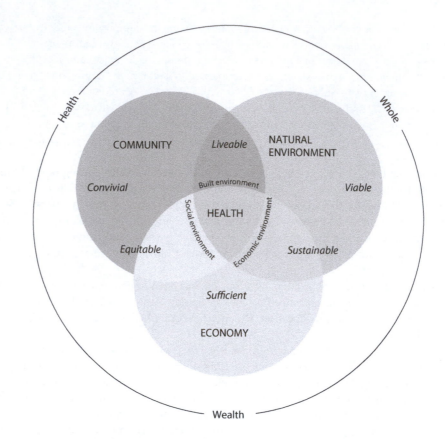

Figure 7.1 Labonte's 1993 holosphere of healthy and sustainable communities. (From Butler CD, Friel S, *PLoS Medicine* 3, 1693, 2006. Under Creative Commons Attribution License; Derived from Labonte, *Australian and New Zealand Journal of Public Health* 17, 4–12, 1993.)

determinants and to do so by means of a public health concept. Health promotion is thereby a view that encompasses the social, economic and structural factors that influence population-level differences in patterns of health and illness (Figure 7.1). The health inequalities arguments that are proving to have significant effect on both sides of the Atlantic focus on two of Labonte's spheres – the community and the economy. They do not, in fact, attend closely to the natural environment though they invoke the social environment (e.g. roads, housing, safe play areas). The natural environment is a contentious arena for health promotion, but at an international level, it is evident that Labonte's full model is important. Chernobyl (Ukraine) and Bhopal (India), for example, are only two of many longstanding examples of environmental damage that continue to compromise child health. War and civil strife are further examples of twenty-first century toxic environments.

LOOKING MORE CLOSELY AT HEALTH PROMOTION

At base, health promotion tends towards two areas of activity:

* Modifying people's behaviour
* Protecting the public through regulatory measures in law

These two directions often lead to debate about the trajectory and the purpose of health-promotion work. Which focus should take the lead – behavioural change or regulatory legislation? Government policy continuously oscillates between these two pressures. Reducing smoking and improving nutrition are two useful examples. One could argue that both behaviour change and legislation are necessary to achieve child health improvement in these areas, but they are by no means easy to reconcile.

The questions that arise are about how intrusive the state should be in seeking to improve the health of the public. For example, we are familiar with charges about 'the nanny state' in Britain. Yet, if we stay with examples of nutrition and tobacco use alone, we find both legislative and resource questions at play. Whether or not to ban tobacco smoking in public areas is only one example of difficult legislation. Regulating the food industry is even more complex and yet it can be equally damaging to child health, notably because food additives can be a contributor to obesity.

There are also linked resource questions. Taxes on cigarettes are a benefit to the Treasury; tension between industry regulation and the taxes accrued from the food and drinks industries are always problematic; costs to the Exchequer of providing subsidized school meals raise questions about whether or not to prioritize nutrition within the budget for state education. The list can be long and these are not new arguments.

Contemporary debates about school dinners are a useful example to use when we are thinking about child public health and the role of health promotion in the school in this way. For example, it is rather pointless to promote the 'five a day' fruit and vegetable programme, and then send the child into a lunch that has neither. But the school nutrition landscape began to change significantly from September 2006, including legislation to control food industry advertising directed at children from January 2007.

In 2007, Nutritional Standards and Requirements for School Food (England) were put in place and then revised in 2008, 2011 and 2014. From 1 January 2015, new revised standards came into force and these include the requirement to provide drinking water on all school premises and without charge. The regulations apply to all state funded schools, including academies and free schools.

To take the nutrition question one step further as an example for exploring what health promotion means, it is useful to note that, at base, these are arguments that link into the twenty-first century public health concern about childhood obesity. In other words, we find an intersection of mixed responsibility when thinking about nutrition, health, the school environment, financial costs to the government of healthy food, and individual child and eating behaviours (the family context and the food industry effect).

Nutrition has nevertheless become regulated in schools since the revised *School Food in England* (Department for Education [DfE] 2008, 2009, 2015a, 2015b). For example, drinking water must now be provided free of charge at all times on school premises. And from 1 January 2015, new revised standards have come into force that apply to all state maintained schools including academies and free schools. This is an extension of legislation passed in 2007 and then revised in 2008 and in 2011 (*Education [Nutritional Standards and Requirements for School Food] [England] Regulations* 2007).

Historically, successes in improving health have primarily derived from better housing, improved water supplies and sanitation; safer conditions in the workplace; education; the alleviation of poverty; and the general provision of health and social care services. These agenda items do not remain stable and they require continuous revisiting. For example, Pearson reported findings in 2002 from a health visitor and district nurse seconded to a Newcastle housing department,

> Housing officers often made their decisions about housing in the virtual absence of health information.
>
> (Pearson 2002, p. 59)

Second, the larger social and economic context in which children live their lives impacts on their health, regardless of individual health behaviours. Furthermore, Benzeval et al. were arguing, prior to the change of government in the United Kingdom in 1997,

> … since much health-related behaviour itself is socially determined, it is people's circumstances that are the most important determinant of health.
>
> (Benzeval et al. 1997, p. 17)

In 1991, Dahlgren and Whitehead conceptualized health promotion in a model that quickly became the dominant visual representation of the determinants of health (see Figure 7.2). Their purpose was to seek a way of identifying the factors that affect population health, in order to identify both the policy maker's and the practitioner's place in developing a preventive model of health care that could challenge the dominant curative or medical model. Dahlgren and Whitehead (1991) drew explicit attention to the complexity of social, political, economic and structural factors that determine health.This model has been an influential method for conceptualizing the vectors of health-promotion work in the United Kingdom for more than two decades and it remains relevant today. The outer circle refers to the upstream activities of governments at national and international levels, whereas the inner circle draws attention to the personal and the individual. It is at the inner two circles that health-promotion interventions tend to be found. Yet

> Effective action to improve people's health co-ordinates activities at all levels. There is a complex relationship between the worlds in which people live, how they collectively and individually make sense of what happens around them throughout their lives, and how those happenings affect their mental and physical health.
>
> (Heer and Woodhead 2002, p. 4)

It is this co-ordinating activity that is at the heart of repeated calls for cross-departmental and inter-professional collaboration that we find in recent UK policy. It is perhaps the most difficult agenda of all activities for health-promotion work to operationalize, and it is the task of public health practice to do just that.

Furthermore, when we think about child public health, we don't have a tradition of asking children themselves what their views are of their health and of their health needs. However, this is changing (See Moules and O'Brien in Chapter 11). The Department of Health (England) made consultation with children and young people a priority in *Action on School Nursing* (2012) and in *Getting it right for children, young people and families* (2014).

How, then, do we choose the health issues that we believe we should 'promote'? In other words, what do we know about children's wishes and desires about their own health? And if we did routinely seek the views of children and young people, would we be better able to promote their health?

There exist rarely mentioned and often forgotten human rights protections in Articles 23–27 of the 1948 Universal Declaration of Human Rights. Article 25 is stated as follows:

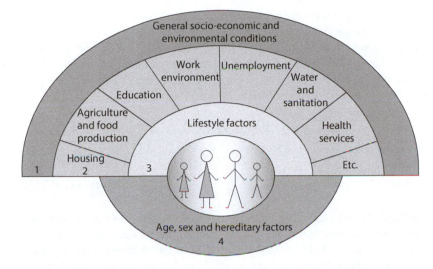

Figure 7.2 Determinants of health. (From Dahlgren G, Whitehead M, *Policies and Strategies to Promote Social Equity in Health*, Institute for Future Studies, Stockholm, 1991. With permission.)

Everyone has the right to a standard of living adequate for the health and well-being of himself and of his family, including food, clothing, housing and medical care and necessary social services, and the right to security in the event of unemployment, sickness, disability, widowhood, old age or other lack of livelihood in circumstances beyond his control.

(Universal Declaration of Human Rights 1948, Article 25)

In discussions of children's health within the context of children's rights, we generally refer to Article 12 of the United Nations Convention on the Rights of the Child 1989 (see Chapter 11), but Article 25 of the 1948 agreement provides us with a context for thinking about the rights of the child by specifying our responsibility to the total social context in which the child lives. This is perhaps as good a place as any to position our thinking when we seek to reflect on the meaning of health promotion for children and young people.

THINKING ABOUT THE HEALTH INEQUALITIES AGENDA

How far can people have responsibility for their health if the means to health are outside their control?

(Sidell et al. 1997, p. 2)

By the end of the twentieth century, the international evidence of the effect of socio-economic inequalities on health had become compelling. Findings from the United Kingdom 1991 Census, the 2001 and the 2011 Census all found that families with children were over-represented at the lower end of the income distribution scales, with research providing evidence of a strong association between low income and poor health. Yet in the 1960s, theorists had been convinced that social progress would effectively succeed in eliminating the socio-economic gap within the populations of industrialized countries. That has not happened. In fact, we see a widening gap.

Much of the recent evidence linking poor health and low income has derived from research initiated in the United Kingdom and in the United States. It is not an evidence base without argument and dissent but it is an evidence base that has influenced government policy in the United Kingdom since 1997 and continues to do so.

> People who live in disadvantaged circumstances have more illnesses, greater disability and shorter lives than those who are more affluent. Such injustice could be prevented, but this requires political will. The question is: can British policy makers rise to the challenge?
>
> **(Benzeval et al. 1997, p. 16)**

These insights are not new. They were documented in Britain as early as the 1860s. These insights did, however, immediately become the source of the new government's policy on public health in 1997. It was the first explicit public health position based in economic analysis by an incoming government. These are also the underlying factors that have directed public health practice since the turn of the twenty-first century.

Investment in research in the area known as *health inequalities* has also intensified with a view to proving in repeated studies that the link between socio-economic inequalities and poor health is without question (Wilkinson 1996; Kawachi et al. 1999; Bartley 2003; Marmot 2004; and others). Political economists have been seeking to refine this argument (Hofrichter 2003) but poverty is at the core of international debates about the determinants of health, notably child health. The WHO focus considerable work on the social determinants of health.

The question that thereby follows is about how health-promotion activities in the school setting can grapple with the effects of poverty on child health. Commenting on poor health in Scotland, Macintyre and Hart observed:

> There has been a lot of research describing, and attempting to explain, inequalities in health; but much less on effective ways of reducing them.
>
> **(Macintyre and Hart 2000, p. 2)**

Turn of the century policy in the United Kingdom, and differentially in other developed countries, has largely argued the health inequalities premise as the primary determinant of child health. Yet the resource costs to governments of seeking to eradicate socio-economic differences remain increasingly problematic and ideologically uncomfortable, and rather than diminishing, the gap between rich and poor has continued to widen. By 2004, the publication of *Choosing Health* (Department of Health 2004a) signalled a change in policy direction in England designed to shift responsibility back to the individual and away from the state as the primary vehicle for improving health.

In effect, this suggests a return to the earlier *lifestyle behaviours* approach that emerged, though in different forms, in both the United Kingdom and the United States after World War II, and it is located within a medical and individual self-care paradigm. It is also at the core of the debate about personal versus state responsibility for the cost of health, education and social care services.

Nevertheless, this shift of investment emphasis has been noticeably uneven. Preschool children in deprived areas of the United Kingdom continue to be the focus for resource investment – mainly via Sure Start – but investment varies significantly with each change of government in the United Kingdom. By 2015, the original target of 10,000 children's centres had dropped to a mere 3,000 still operating despite 33% of children in England living in poverty.

The school-age child's health has likewise come in and out of focus with each change in government. The Children's Fund for school-age children was launched in 2000 with a generous profile of resources (extended to 2008). Children's trusts, virtual organizations of co-ordinated care and support were first put in position from 2003 (operational from April 2004), and the re-organization of social care and education budgets for children into co-ordinated leadership by single, LA-based children's services was formalized in England from April 2006. School-based health services for school-age children, however, remain differentially resourced across all four countries of the United Kingdom. And school health services have returned to an uncertain future as primary healthcare services in the United Kingdom adjust simultaneously to structural change and demand for significant cost savings.

In other words, the overall policy picture is one that argues the health inequalities agenda while, at the same time, it often de-prioritizes services that meet the collective or community needs of school-age children compared with the size of resources for preschool children in deprived geographical areas. This is probably the case because of the resource implications and the complexity involved in restructuring public sector provision, the principle resource for child public health practice.

THE HEALTHY SCHOOLS PROGRAMME

A health promoting school is one in which all members of the school community work together to provide children and young people with integrated and positive experiences and structures, which promote and protect their health. This includes both the formal and the informal curriculum in health, the creation of a safe and healthy school environment, the provision of appropriate health services and the involvement of the family and wider community in efforts to promote health.

(Burgher et al. 1999, p. 4)

This vision is a fully holistic paradigm of health promotion for school-age children and was agreed by the WHO in 1995. However, from its outset, the United Kingdom's response to the WHO agenda, the NHSP, has always been a voluntary code of practice. Schools have not been obliged to participate in the NHSP. The target initially was to achieve 100% of state-maintained schools participating in England by the end of 2009 (75% had achieved recognized standards by that first date).

Scotland, Wales and Northern Ireland also set targets for participation. The programme was first announced in England in 1993 as a response to intended collaboration with the European Network of Health Promoting Schools. It is fair to say that little activity followed until the late 1990s when the NHSP was formally launched in October 1999. By 2005/2006, however, the profile of NHSP was demonstrating active cross-departmental collaboration because of its position as a dual responsibility of both the Department of Health and the DfES.

The pressure on schools to participate in the NHSP has waxed and waned since the turn of the century. At the outset, however, the programme was a teacher-led initiative and this, in itself, slowed initial progress simply because of the absence of the health sector on so many of the key decision-making bodies that led the NHSP in each LA in the early years.

The Healthy Schools Programme continues to be organized around four themes against which schools can be assessed in order to meet specified standards:

- PSHE, including sex and relationship education (SRE) and drug education
- Healthy eating
- Physical activity
- Emotional health and well-being (including bullying)

However, the concept of a whole-school ethos that can promote health relies, inevitably, on the school understanding itself as a resource for children that is located within a broader community framework. It also relies on the school's ability to understand the community from a health perspective by working with other agencies and by combining resources with neighbourhood initiatives that promote child health.

Every school serves a different profile of social, economic and environmental need. For example, the charity Shelter has documented the devastating effects that bad housing alone is having on children's life chances in contemporary England, with four million children living in poverty by 2015. But poor housing is generally clustered in areas of high deprivation and does not affect all school communities equally, thus the need for local school assessments of community-level factors that can affect child health in school (see Mosley and Moorhouse's [2000] example of the Huddersfield profile).

Poor housing alone can impact on a child or young person's ability to learn at school, either because of physical illness, mental health distress or the consequences of accidents* directly linked to poor housing. It is, furthermore, an example of the way in which health-promotion work cannot be divorced from the material and cultural environment in which the school is sited. Understanding the community outside the school gates both broadens understanding of the kinds of health-promotion work that are best designed for any particular school. It is what is meant by a public health approach to health promotion in the school setting.

In other words, child health-promotion work is not simply about lifestyle change. Lifestyle behaviours derive from and are a consequence of social and community cultures. Within a school, for example, the external environment may be such that internal school focus on, for example, obesity or on sexual health may be effectively negated if the child's community and home environment are not factored into the approach. This does not obviate the need for health-promotion interventions focused on lifestyle behaviours but it does demonstrate the need to take the larger social and economic context into consideration.

In 2010, all the major political parties signed up to the target of reducing child poverty to less than 5% by 2020. The figure in early 2015 was nearing 33% of all children. These children have an increased risk of severe ill-health and disability during childhood and early adulthood (Harker 2006, p. 8).

THINKING ABOUT *SOCIAL CAPITAL* IN HEALTH-PROMOTION WORK

It was in studies of rural school community centres in the United States that the notion of social capital as a factor that affects health first emerged. Hanifan (1916, 1920) introduced the term to describe 'those tangible substances [that] count for most in the daily lives of people' (Hanifan 1916, p. 130) and by this he was referring to the cultivation of good will, fellowship, sympathy

---

* Two million children every year are taken to an emergency department as the consequence of accidental injury (Child Accident Prevention Trust 2006). Accidental injury is the single largest cause of death among children after the age of 1 year in the United Kingdom, and the leading cause of disability (Botting 1995).

and social intercourse, signifiers of a healthy community such as the kind that affects child health in the school environment.

The concept of *social capital*, however, has only recently entered the arena of debates about health and it is used elsewhere in this book. Effectively, it can be used here to talk about the school's ability to work within the local community as a social unit, and as a way of describing the internal school community beyond its articulation as simply a group of individual teachers and individual children. This is where the link between an ethos of healthy schools and a concept of health promotion effectively come together.

In other words, lifestyle behaviours derive from and are a consequence of social and community cultures. They are not simply decisions made by individual children alone. Furthermore, health promotion becomes increasingly difficult in the school-age years as the child develops and grows – particularly during adolescence. As the child gains increasing independence over time, the challenges to 'making a difference' in health outcomes actually meant that successful outcomes depend more and more on the health-promotion skills of the adults with whom young people come into contact.

The encouragement towards behaviours that are conducive to personal health and well-being is a complex field (see Lister-Sharp et al. 1999). Success relies on the child's or family's motivation and, particularly, success depends on the child's social, cultural and economic environment. Apart from the many environmental factors (safe play areas, healthy food, access to pleasurable physical activity, safe roads, homes and housing), most health-promoting behaviours are also subject to public agencies' abilities to maximize the opportunities to make healthy personal decisions, and are subject to providing access to accurate information (e.g. the information that young people need in order to make decisions about sexual health). Maximizing the circumstances and opportunities in which these enabling factors are available to children and young people is also a part of the health-promotion map in the school environment.

The interaction between individual behaviours and community-level opportunities for improving health is also complex. The English government policy position on the intersection between school and child health is reflected in *Choosing Health* (Department of Health 2004a) and in *Higher Standards, Better Schools for All* (DfES, 2005). But these do not go far enough alone.

Lister-Sharpe et al. (1999) conducted two systematic reviews of the health-promoting schools approach, and these remain the most comprehensive studies achieved. In their work, they report findings consistent with a concept of social capital:

Overall, a multifaceted approach is likely to be most effective, combining a classroom programme with changes to the school ethos and/or environment and/or with family/community involvement.

(Lister-Sharpe et al. 1999, p. v)

THE SCHOOL HEALTH SERVICE

The end of the twentieth and the beginning of the twenty-first century witnessed the most radical change in school nurse practice and organisation in the whole of its long history, including the virtual disappearance of the school medical officer – a change that removed 'the doctor's handmaiden' role from the activities and planning of school nursing. Furthermore,

There has been a paradigm shift in school nurse practice from a medical model to a social model of working.

(DeBell and Tomkins 2006, p. 18)

Yet, at the same time, the service has not increased in size during the past decade (a maximum of 3000 nurses – most working part-time – for about 11.2 million school-age children in the United Kingdom).

The education and training base for the service has been upgraded development, including questions about service redesign. School nursing was first identified as 'child centred public health' in 2002 in England (Department of Health 2002). Scotland in 2006 announced plans to introduce community healthcare nursing – school nursing, health visiting and district nursing. In other words, the public health practitioner focus is moving the traditional school nurse service towards the introduction of specialist public health practitioners who can provide the school-age child focus that has always been the rationale behind school nursing.

A provision for health within the school environment has been an issue in the British education system since at least the late nineteenth century, a point at which the poor health of recruits to the Boer War revealed harm to the health of boys in England's cities and towns, probably originating in the urban working classes because of the Industrial Revolution (Denman et al. 2002). As a consequence, schools were early identified as an ideal setting to promote child health (Harris 1995). As early as 1882 the Department of Education had issued a policy paper allowing schools to close or to exclude pupils from attending in order to control the spread of infectious disease. These early public health interventions indicated an understanding of the link between school and a child's health (i.e. the school as a gathering point with potential for targeting infection control and later immunization delivery). However, the perceived link between child health and the school environment was not originally so much about the child as about the consequences of poor child health, mainly boys' health, as a national resource to be protected.

Little, however, was formally accomplished until the Board of Education published a handbook, *Suggestions on Health Education* in 1939 (McNalty 1939), when a whole-school approach was first argued. This proposal made little headway until 1968 when the Department of Education and Science published its *Handbook for Health Education* (1968). Still, this document fell short of establishing health as a subject within the curriculum.

From small beginnings (one school medical officer in London in 1890 and one school nurse in 1892), the *Education (Administrative Provisions) Act 1907* recognized the school as a location for child health attention by placing a legal obligation on schools to consider the health of the children in their care with a duty placed on school boards

to provide for the medical inspection of children immediately before, or at the time of, or as soon as possible after, their admission to a public elementary school and on such occasions as the Board of Education direct.

(The *Education [Administrative Provisions] Act 1907*, Section 13[1][b])

Historically, the repeated impetus of attention to child health was triggered by the need for healthy army recruits. For example, in 1904, as many as 60% of boys were found to be unfit for duty because of poor eyesight, dental caries, heart disease and poor growth arising from poor childhood health (Leff and Leff 1959). A range of public health reforms designed to improve child health followed – the *Open Spaces Act 1906*; the *Education (Provision of Meals) Act 1906*; the *Education (Administrative Provisions) Act 1907*; the *Notification of Births Act 1907*; and the *Maternity and Child Welfare Act 1918*.

Until at least the end of the twentieth century, the developing school health services contin-ued to retain as their primary function a screening and surveillance service – the identification of physical health problems, the detection and correction of poor hygiene and malnutrition, and, where possible, the amelioration of the effects of disability. For example, the *Education Act 1918* extended the duties of local education authorities by requiring provision of services for the treatment of minor ailments within primary schools and by extending medical inspections to young people in secondary schools. Despite this largely reactive orientation to health provision, Polnay argued in 1995 that school nurses have continuously linked their service back to its original public health roots by means of their historic support for young people's emotional and well-being needs. As far back as the 1950s it was acknowledged that school nurses supported young people in relation to their emotional health and well-being.

In secondary schools adolescent girls often consult her (the school nurse) … and she can do much to help them and relieve their anxiety.

(Leff and Leff 1959)

In other words, the contemporary school drop-in centres provided by school nurses in order to promote child and adolescent health have a long and surprisingly robust history given the uncertainty that has always surrounded the health-education link.

The school health service in the United Kingdom has also been problematically situated. Until 1974, school nurses and medical officers were employed by local education authorities. This is the pattern of employment for school nursing in most countries across the world (i.e. school nurses tend to be directly employed by schools or school districts). But in 1974, school nursing transferred to the National Health Service (NHS) in the United Kingdom. The aim of this new health service for children was to bring together health professionals (e.g. community and hospital paediatri-cians, clinical medical officers, school nurses, audiologists, speech and language therapists, psy-chologists and community physiotherapists) in order to provide preschool, school health, hospital and specialist services. The success of this integrated approach to child health has always been patchy, and the consequence for school health services has been to create a profile whereby health has been located outside and separate from the education domain. Furthermore, school nursing as the lead health link has not been universally accepted by schools, despite the fact that most schools do rely heavily on school nurses. Where successful, the development of school nursing has had to do with the ability of individual schools to understand the service.

Having said that, it was the Court Report (1976) that caught the sense of radical change in focus to a community-based service. It did this by arguing that child health should be at the centre of planning. Yet, Court drew explicit attention to the inability of 'services to co-operate in the interests of the child' (Court 1976, p. 3). This was a shift of focus, not fully followed up, that understood the community principles that would come to emerge as the health promotion and primary care movements of the 1980s.

By 2013, the function of commissioning plus the transfer of planning to local authorities and to smaller administrative units both appear to continue to echo Court's perceptions of the child at the centre of planning. The *Children and Families Act 2014* provides the operational frame-work to achieve that. Whether the Act achieves this or not will be clearer by 2020.

However, what is striking about the school health service in the early years of the twenty-first century is its commitment to the health of the school-age population rather than its sense of itself as primarily a service for schools. That commitment now takes the form of services delivered at school, in the community, and with families. Scotland, for example, has recognized this with its proposals to incorporate health visiting and school nursing as a common service delivering a public health nursing practitioner role for children and young people. Furthermore, Scotland has specified the functional public health role for school nursing as operating within a community as well as a school setting.

> The national school nursing framework broadens the role of school nursing to include developing health needs assessment for schools, more active involvement in health promotion and supporting schools with the change required to enable mainstreaming of children who require additional support for learning. By 2007, all schools will be expected to become Integrated Community Schools and school nurses will be an integral part of the multi-disciplinary team.

(Scottish Executive 2003, Summary point 11)

This is an agenda that matches the aspirations of school nurses themselves (DeBell and Everett 1997; DeBell and Jackson 2000; DeBell and Tomkins 2006). How Scotland and the rest of the United Kingdom will actually interpret the functions of school nursing within community nursing is yet to be seen.

THE EXTENDED SCHOOLS INITIATIVE

Firmly based in a long tradition of community development within Britain, the Full Service Extended Schools (FSES) initiative was launched in 2001 and became operational in 2003. It was originally part of a government vision for all schools in order to offer a core set of additional activities and services in the school environment by 2010. By 2015, it had become a highly focused investment in extended services within named schools located in the most socially disadvantaged areas of the United Kingdom. Annual investment had reached £12m/annum in 2014/15.

> The FSES initiative seeks to support the development in every local authority (LA) area of one or more schools which provide a comprehensive range of services on a single site, including access to health services, adult learning and community activities as well as study support and 8 a.m. to 6 p.m. wrap-around childcare.

(Cummings et al. 2006, p. ii)

The location of schools within local communities coupled with their estate value (nb., the buildings themselves are not in use much of the day/year) has always raised questions about how better to maximize use of this resource. The FSES initiative was an imaginative and potentially valuable way of bringing together services that need to be delivered locally, by using the school building itself, its resources, its leadership and its location. Furthermore, maximizing the use of the schools estate such that schools can become the locus of enhanced services for children and their families makes good community sense.

The first-year rollout of the initiative (2004–2005) funded Extended Schools located in Behaviour Improvement Programme (BIP) areas (61 projects in year one). This was a way of focusing services on areas with higher deprivation levels. Year-two rollout (25 additional schools in BIP areas and 20 in non-BIP areas) included clusters of schools working together as single FSES sites. By autumn 2006, more than 3000 schools in England had joined the programme (Training and Development Agency for Schools 2006).

The initial short-term goals were linked to improving educational achievement levels but the long-term goals are about the family and community agenda. Project leaders in the first two years sought to embed their work within the *Every Child Matters: Change for Children* (HM Government 2004) agenda. But, significantly, the profile of work is dependent on how well each Extended School is able to develop collaborative, cross-departmental work, and this is at the core of national pressure to find ways to ensure that services work together. This is not an easy agenda. However, there is a long tradition of community-oriented schooling in the United Kingdom, and this initiative builds on that by specifying 'full service schools'.

The head teachers of the pilot schools have been described as 'enthusiasts' by the Universities of Manchester and Newcastle evaluators (Cummings et al. 2006, p. 3). This is unsurprising but it helps to explain the participation rates of schools given the relatively small financial investment in the scheme.

'Reducing health inequalities' is one of many goals within the Extended Schools Initiative. In effect, it comes into play by nature of the focus on attending to family and child needs as a whole, whether these are additional learning opportunities (for adults as well as children), school breakfast schemes; or sustained assistance to children who have behavioural problems (i.e. mental health problems); or to children who are at risk.

What does this mean for health promotion in the school setting? The FSES has a community empowerment agenda, though this is articulated in a variety of ways. The principle message thus far suggests that Extended Schools tend to

1. Make parents feel welcome in the school (open door policy and adult education provision).
2. Engage health and social care professionals in the school environment as a way of assisting families in difficulty.
3. Provide parenting support programmes.
4. Resist the quick route of school exclusions by involving child and adolescent mental health specialists in problem solving.
5. Participate directly in other community activities.

In effect, these are health-promotion interventions that understand the relationship between the family, the school and the child. Not all schools have been equally successful. Some have reported the familiar difficulty of engaging non-education professionals in their extended work. Others, such as rural schools and special schools have reported difficulties arising from poor transport facilities to the school.

However, the determination to involve non-teacher professionals and voluntary workers in the community enhancement agenda of the FSES suggests that

> there is some evidence that this configuration around schools maximizes some opportunities for the delivery of services in disadvantaged neighbourhoods.
>
> **(Cummings et al. 2006, p. 25)**

THE CHILD GROWING UP AT SCHOOL

What is particularly noticeable about the FSES initiative is the interpretation of child health and well-being in terms of those factors that are outside the school gates, factors that can make it difficult for a child to function at school because of the social, cultural and/or family environment in which they live. For these children, health-promotion interventions that rely wholly on health education or health-promotion interventions confined within the school environment can have limited effect.

We have mainly talked about the larger issues, yet it is the child growing up through the school years that is also at issue. Difficulties and needs change during the growing up period. For example, we know that at least two in every ten children and adolescents (Office for National Statistics 2004) experience mental health distress at some point in the school-age years, and the nature of the presenting problem varies with the child's age. These experiences of distress can be brief, prolonged, serious, or time-limited and self-correcting episodes. Teachers do not necessarily find this area of child health easy, and many understandably do not see it as a part of their work profile. In fact, education professionals use a different language. They speak of 'emotional and behavioural problems', not 'mental health problems'.

In addition, consistent reporting over the past decade suggests that about 30% of 16-year-old girls are sexually active. This is a critical health issue because sexual health can affect morbidity, fertility and mental health, and thereby needs to be a target for health promotion and health education.

We also know that contemporary patterns of childhood nutrition and physical activity are in danger of reducing life expectancy, and we know that an entire generation of parents in the United Kingdom has never been taught to cook – school based food technology was removed from the curriculum in the latter part of the twentieth century. Furthermore, we know that too many children arrive at school without breakfast, and that their main meal may well be a school dinner. The nutritional value of school dinners is critical for children who are living in poverty.

The patterns and nature of food consumption, in the home and outside the home, have changed radically in the last decade alone, and the long-term task of improving nutrition and of finding ways to increase physical activity are just that – long-term tasks. A minority of schools in the United Kingdom have begun to provide breakfast for children in need.

Furthermore, weighing and measuring children at school is effective for collecting epidemiological data (see Box 7.1), but this resource investment does nothing to address the underlying causes of poor nutrition. Indeed, height and weight measurement requires resources that might well be better targeted on health-promotion work in the school, the community and at the national regulatory level. These measurement tasks continue to be a source of debate (See DeBell 2014).

We also know that adolescence is a period when risk-taking behaviours increase and, indeed, risk taking is part of growing up. How to help young people think about this is a significant task for the health-promotion approach in school.

Furthermore, we know that the transition periods in school life are critical moments for child health, notably child mental health. These occur when the child enters school, when the child changes from primary to middle school, and particularly, when the child transfers to secondary school. These are periods of uncertainty and anxiety for every child. Health promotion takes on a particular meaning at such points, if only in terms of assisting children to cope with the stress of being young and vulnerable among a new set of peers who are older and who can be frightening. Bullying in UK schools has not decreased, but it can be countered by both the school culture and health and social care professionals if they are integrated within the school itself. It is a factor, for example, when we think about the school as the child's place of work.

And, finally, we have long known that children with disabilities, long-term conditions, and/or complex health needs experience the school years as difficult and problematic.

The profile of necessary skills and competencies that practitioners need to have also changes as the child grows and develops from school entry at the age of 4 or 5 years, through the adolescent period and into transition for adulthood. An understanding of the patterns of ill-health

BOX 7.1: The National Childhood Height and Weight Data Collection Programme

A key component of both influencing and monitoring obesity (and overweight) prevalence is through the establishment of a national Childhood Height and Weight data collection programme. The programme enables local data on childhood obesity to be collected to inform local planning and targeting of local resources and interventions; to enable tracking of local progress against the Public Service Agreement (PSA) target on obesity, and local performance management; and to improve understanding of the pattern, associated factors and causes of the obesity *epidemic* among children.

Primary care trusts and/or school staff have now measured all schoolchildren in the reception year (ages 4 and 5 years) and those in year 6 (ages 10 and 11 years). Height and weight data is used for the calculation of body mass index (BMI) in order to monitor obesity prevalence at a population level (Department of Health 2006).

In England, for example, prevalence rates for overweight/obesity are calculated by deriving every child's BMI plus the child's age and sex following NICE guidelines. The first report from the Department of Health Information Centre specified the categories of overweight and obese children were then used:

- *Healthy weight* is defined as having BMI between the 2nd and 90th centiles
- *Overweight* is defined as having BMI greater than or equal to the 91st and 97th BMI centiles and
- *Very overweight (clinically obese)* is defined as having BMI at or above the 98th centile
- *Underweight* [is] not examined but is specified as below the 2nd BMI centile classification.

Source: DeBell D, in McPherson and Driscoll (eds.), *School Screening Systems*. New York: Nova Publishers, 2014.

and the determinants of health at each stage place singular demands on health-promotion work, and are fundamental for public health practice.

HEALTH EDUCATION IN THE CURRICULUM

Since 2005, schools in England have been encouraged, but not required to use curriculum time for the purpose of developing a more formal role in providing for children's and young people's health. The policy position is that PSHE (the PSHE curriculum) should create a formal structure for the teaching of spiritual, moral and cultural values (Office for Standards in Education [Ofsted] 2005a). The PSHE curriculum, however, is broad, and the concepts within it are open to interpretation by each individual school team. Furthermore, schools face the challenges of finding staff who are sufficiently trained and skilled in order to deliver the curriculum.

To this end, a certification programme (DfES 2002) was created to enable joint skills development for teachers and community nurses such that they could work together in delivering the PSHE curriculum. Its purpose has been to

- Improve the confidence of teachers and community nurses delivering PSHE in schools and out of schools settings
- Provide recognition for individual teachers' and community nurses' experience skills.
- Improve the quality and effectiveness of PSHE provided to children and young people
- Raise the profile of PSHE

- Contribute to the UK's Teenage Pregnancy Strategy's annual goals to reduce the under-18 conception rates
- Address problems relating to health inequalities and social inclusion

The programme was initially devised in response to a report by Ofsted (2002), which highlighted the need for SRE in schools. The SRE curriculum was prompted by the perceived need to establish specialist teams, particularly within secondary schools, that could promote the improvement of young people's sexual health. The certification programme now covers the broader PSHE programme, with a target to achieve at least one trained teacher in every secondary school and one community nurse who can support the school. Again, these are targets – not requirements.

Furthermore, reports from school nurses have repeatedly indicated that teachers often ask healthcare staff to assist them in the classroom when they deliver health education.

This determination to focus joint teacher and community nurse attention on child health was new in 2000 when Ofsted noted the need for extra-curricular subjects that might address children's needs for personal, social, health and economic education (PSHEE). The subject is no longer compulsory but where it exists it is underpinned by a range of initiatives that are designed to build into schools a sense of formal responsibility for child health (see 'The healthy schools programme' and the *Healthy Living Blueprint*, Department of Health 2004b). Because school constitutes the setting for a very significant proportion of a child's life over many years, and because school is the child's place of work, it is an opportune location for promoting health and delivering health messages and health services. Schools are in a position to reach large numbers of children and young people over the highly formative years from early childhood to adolescence (Naidoo and Wills 1998).

The purpose of health education within the curriculum is to provide children and young people with a working knowledge about issues that are important to their health (Stewart-Brown 1998). However, a question immediately arises about the relationship between formal information and its capacity to influence health and health-related behaviours.

What children do with the information they receive at school depends on their personal priorities, resources, their attitudes to and understanding of risk, and their self-perception. Ofsted (2005a) reported support for the concept that education about health subjects and concerns should involve information and knowledge but also argued that this, in itself, is insufficient and added that children also require skill development. In other words, Ofsted called attention to the need for children and young people to have opportunities at school to formulate, develop and explore their own values and attitudes to health.

There is little argument to suggest that the concept of PSHE as a formal part of the curriculum is other than an appropriate direction of travel for schools. Yet it remains a non-statutory subject within the National Curriculum. In March 2013, following a Government review, the subject was specified non-statutory. This does not mean that the subject will remain permanently outside of statute.

By 2005, a framework developed by the Qualifications and Curriculum Authority (Ofsted 2005b) was in place, with the purpose of assisting schools in planning their PSHE* programmes for each age group. There has been considerable debate about whether or not PSHE, like the

---

* Each country refers to the programme differently – Personal and Social Education (PSE) in Wales; Social, Personal and Health Education (SPHE) in Ireland; and it is also known as PSHEE; PSED (Personal, Social and Emotional Development) and PSHCE (Personal, Social, Health and Citizenship Education).

citizenship curriculum and the sex and relationship curriculum (SRE), should become a statutory subject for all children and young people. These debates will continue.

Schools are under pressure to meet government assessment targets, particularly for numeracy, literacy and science. The consequence has been steadily to squeeze curriculum time, thereby leaving little latitude during the school day for contextual subjects in the informal curriculum, such as child health. This means that PSHE can, and often has become marginalized within the curriculum (Naidoo and Wills 1998). In fact, Ofsted reported in 2005a that some schools even at that point were not providing PSHE within the curriculum at all.

Head teachers and their governing bodies are responsible for decisions about the introduction of subjects for study that are additional to core subjects required by statute. There can be a number of reasons for not including formal health-education teaching within the curriculum timetable:

- Lack of staff (education and healthcare staff) with appropriate expertize
- History of not perceiving health matters as a school responsibility apart from special educational needs (SEN) (under statutory requirement)*
- A decision to prioritize other subjects

However, Ofsted (the schools' inspectorate) consistently argues that when schools do not play their part in providing for PSHE, they are assuming an untenable position. Policy direction arising from government position papers such as *Every Child Matters: Change for Children* (HM Government 2004) and *National Healthy School Status: A Guide for Schools* (DfES and Department of Health 2005) also highlighted the responsibilities that schools should assume in order to ensure that children and young people achieve better health outcomes. The *implicit* position is that health status affects ability to learn. The *explicit* position is also that health status affects ability to learn and there is evidence of a high correlation between poor health and low educational achievement.

Arguments in the field suggest that within PSHE, children and young people can gain knowledge, develop life skills, and formulate attitudes that are crucial building blocks for living successfully in social environments, and which thus prepare children and young people for the experiences and responsibilities of later life. Such skills include improved communication skills; interpersonal and decision-making skills; abilities in negotiating, formulating and presenting arguments; skills in comparing and contrasting others' views; team and group skills; as well as skills in independent thinking. These are large claims and, if sustainable, they imply that a curriculum-framed input for health-related work would be of considerable value to children and young people during their school years.

---

* SEN is a statutory identifier referring to learning difficulties and disabilities. 'The term learning difficulties and/or disabilities is used to refer to individuals or groups of learners who have either a learning difficulty in relation to acquiring new skills or who learn at a different rate to their peers. The term is used to cross the professional boundaries between education, health and social services and to incorporate a common language from 0 to 19. The *Disability Discrimination Act* defines that 'a person has a disability if he or she has a physical or mental impairment that has a substantial and long-term adverse effect on his or her ability to carry out normal day-to-day activities'. Physical or mental impairments can include sensory impairments and learning difficulties. The definition also covers medical conditions when they have long-term and substantial effects on pupils' everyday lives. Those designated with SEN under current legislation (education) 'all have learning difficulties that make it harder for them to learn than most learners of the same age' (Ofsted 2005b, p. 3). The *Children and Families Act 2014* will clarify this definition over the next 5 years.

The Independent Advisory Group on Sexual Health and Teenage Pregnancy (2005) recommended that PSHE should become a statutory subject for both primary and secondary schools. The outcomes specified in *Every Child Matters: Change for Children* (HM Government 2004) are required of all statutory bodies working with children and young people. This includes schools. At present, the only curriculum space, as opposed to other school functions and activities, lies within the PSHE specification.

The arguments for statutory inclusion of PSHE within the curriculum have always posited it to be consistent with the larger policy push to improve school inclusion and reduce social inequalities. This is a macro-agenda that affects, in theory, all government departments, including schools. It is, however, a difficult agenda to operationalize, and one that has not been explicitly a school-based responsibility in the past. Some individual schools have always taken these concepts seriously in their work by focusing their attention on the wider community in which the school resides, and by articulating the school itself as an integrated community designed to support the whole of the child's experience at school in an integrated model of learning and health promotion. However, this again is a matter of leadership direction that has historically been left to the discretion of the head teacher.

The profile of expectation about how, and how well the curriculum can improve child health is relatively new (see the discussion of 'The healthy Schools Programme').

A powerful driver for change in schools' attitudes to child and adolescent health remains the Ofsted (2005b, pp. 7–8) *Framework for the Inspection of Children's Services*, which includes schools. The multi-agency inspectors and commissioners responsible for implementing the Framework have the power to specify 'failing schools' and their judgements are articulations of each school's ability to achieve against the *Every Child Matters* framework.

The complex relationship between areas of responsibility for child health has beleaguered debates about the function of education since the introduction of compulsory schooling in the late nineteenth century – now for more than a century – and it continues to produce tension in debates about the function and parameters of responsibility for child health within the school environment. Furthermore, these debates carry a different inflection at different child ages. In other words, primary schools and middle schools tend to have more potential influence over child-health behaviours than do secondary schools. These differences arise from child receptivity to health-education and health-promotion interventions at different ages and stages as the child grows and develops, and they also arise from the very different relationships teachers have with children at each educational stage.

HEALTH-PROMOTION INTERVENTIONS BY PUBLIC HEALTH PRACTITIONERS

Accuracy of information, appropriate to age, and good timing are the three factors that Hall and Elliman (2003) identified as key to good health promotion. This implies that health practitioners are cognizant of age-appropriate interventions as well as precisely accurate about the health information that children receive. Furthermore, health promotion is a matter of staged repetition. For example, sexual health promotion needs to be iterative and age appropriate. It also needs to be context specific. This means that location and timing of service delivery is as important for effectiveness as content (DeBell and Tomkins 2006, p. 12).

These are the skills required of those public health practitioners who conduct health-promotion interventions. The health priorities for such interventions arise from public health data and it takes time to gather, validate and analyse such data.

Health promotion is often thought of in terms of interventions. But, before public health practitioners select an issue for intervention for the purpose of improving an aspect of child or adolescent health, a series of steps will have determined the particular priority areas. First, considerable data will have been collected, validated and analysed at the national level in order to identify (1) the determinants of poor health within the total population; (2) the trends in health behaviours amongst the population that are causing poor health outcomes; and (3) the priorities for health-improvement actions.

At local level (regional and LA levels), similar exercises will be carried out – mainly led by the Public Health Observatories. From these findings (information collection and analysis), priorities for action to improve local health emerge. This, for example, is the way in which childhood obesity emerged as a national priority for health improvement and thus a focus for health-promotion interventions by public health practitioners. *Health Profile of England* (Department of Health 2006) is a recent example. It provides a picture of the 2004 health status of people in England. Similar exercises are conducted within Wales, Scotland and Northern Ireland.

These data and their analysis are not, however, fully comprehensive. The indicators, nevertheless, are used by healthcare commissioners to determine their investment priorities. The actual interventions by public health practitioners tend to develop over time, by means of close analysis of local population needs and in response to the most pressing need (nb., the alarm generated by increasing levels of obesity amongst children).

An example of sophisticated analysis at the local schools population level was conducted by school nurses Mosley and Moorhouse and published in March 2000 for Huddersfield. This work remains the template for identification of how best to conduct an analysis of the health and health needs of the school-age population, based on both local school and health service data. The work also included information from social care and LA derived data.

However, we still need to ask ourselves the question, 'What are the priorities for child health promotion today?' It is probably fair to say that the areas of health-promotion intervention for children of school age by 2015 have become focused on the following needs (not prioritized):

- Nutrition and physical activity
- Child and adolescent mental health (emotional health and well-being, including bullying)
- Accidental and non-accidental injury (including child protection)
- Hygiene and dental health
- Immunizations and protection from communicable disease
- Sexual health and teenage pregnancy
- Risk-taking behaviours, including tobacco, alcohol and illicit substance use
- Long-term conditions, complex health needs and disabilities

Behind these issues for health-promotion interventions lie the key determinants of health: socio-economic inequalities and child poverty; environmental factors such as housing, ethnicity, gender, age and disability profiles; geography; and lifestyle behaviours.

In other words, if we seek to *improve health* or to *promote health,* we do need to ask ourselves what the baseline for *health* is. The epidemiological approach begins from measurements of morbidity and mortality and identifies risk factors. This is the starting point for public health practice and for health promotion in the school environment.

PARENTAL VIEWS ON HEALTH PROMOTION IN THE SCHOOL ENVIRONMENT

Some parents rely wholly on the school to inform their children about basic health issues. This is particularly the case at puberty and adolescence with regard to sexual health matters. At the same time, a minority of parents object to the assertion that schools should teach their children about sensitive health concerns such as sexual health. Anywhere along this spectrum, the questions of health and children's education can become either a collaborative or a dissonant relationship between parents/carers and schools. The repeated policy ideal is that collaborative and consultative approaches between schools and parents, and with other child-orientated agencies, should be the goal. The reality of how to achieve this is challenging.

An initiative to achieve progress towards parent/carer and school collaboration was proposed in the recommendations of *Higher Standards Betters Schools for All: More Choice for Parents and Pupils* (DfES 2005). Parent councils are here recommended in order to assist schools in making decisions relating to health matters such as school meal provision as well as curriculum changes and methods for monitoring parental satisfaction with schools. The policy aspiration is to ensure parental consultation and influence in school decision making. Where child health is concerned, the aspiration is to achieve a collaborative approach whereby parents replicate in the home the health messages provided by the school.

In the 1980s, a parallel approach was attempted with the introduction of parent representation on school governing bodies. The formality of that approach, however, tended inevitably to draw parental involvement from those parents/carers who were most confident and already most involved with their children's education. The new recommendation is for a wider forum of representation that can include the parental voice in decisions about the school curriculum, notably areas that are currently non-statutory elements and that lie within the informal curriculum.

Some parents and carers, for many reasons, require considerably greater levels of practical support in order to improve children's physical health and emotional well-being (see Chapter 10). To meet these needs, the policy aspiration is to put additional activities for parents in place in schools, such as workshops, parenting programmes, behaviour seminars and other related programmes led by health professionals, education staff, Connexions advisers, youth workers and others from the voluntary sector who work with children and young people. In addition, the schools' agenda in England is moving towards transferring greater responsibility for child care and child health to the school environment.

CONSULTING PUPILS

The *Education Act 2002* required all schools to include pupils in the decision making processes about issues that affect them. This is a position that is retained in the *Children and Families Act 2014*. Schools are expected to consult children and young people, and to respond to their needs in order to ensure that, for example, a PSHE programme is relevant and effective, and that the potential for learning is maximized fully (National Children's Bureau 2003). This is in line with the UN Convention on the Rights of the Child 1989 (Chapter 11). A survey published by Ofsted in 2002 found that few schools engaged pupils in planning or evaluation SRE programmes or policies. (SRE is a tandem aspect of the informal curriculum focused on child health.) However, the report also highlighted areas where consultations do take place and, where this does occur, children and young people reported that they value such discussions and that the school gains fresh insights into the curriculum that can assist in long-term development. It needs, however, to be emphasized that such consultations vary considerably in quality and depth. An area of particular concern is the general failure of schools to consult with children who have disabilities, long-term conditions or complex health needs.

The introduction of school councils and the initiation of young people's focus groups have proved to be useful vehicles in gathering such information, including views about personal health and health-related priorities. The Welsh Assembly has taken this approach to a national level in its use of the Funky Dragon initiative, a national approach to consultation focused on participation of all school-age children.

THINKING ABOUT HEALTH-PROMOTION INTERVENTIONS

On the whole, public health practitioners begin to think about health promotion in the school setting from either a perspective of health risk to children (e.g. road safety, reductions in risk taking) or from the perspective of health improvement (e.g. nutrition, sexual health, hand washing and hygiene). However, there is a pre-step that Billingham captured in 1997. She sought to describe public health practice as a way of *seeing* health problems.

> Essentially public health is a distinctive way of seeing health problems: public health nurses and doctors ask different questions about their practice, requiring them to look beyond individuals to populations, such as:
>
> - Why is this happening?
> - How often?
> - What is the social context?
> - Who else should be involved?
> - What works and what doesn't?
>
> They also make different connections: between one individual and another, between individuals and communities, between individuals and social structures, between the stories that people tell them and the epidemiological evidence, between health services and other agencies, between medical and social models of health, and between health and social policies. Public health nurses, moreover, tend to have a commitment to a set of values based on equity, justice and work for social change at local and national levels.

(Billingham 1997, p. 271)

Blair et al. (2003) take this further:

> In practice, many child health workers combine the individual and population perspectives in their day-to-day work and share a similar aim – that of optimizing the health and well-being of all children and young people. Defining common ground, and understanding what those with different backgrounds can contribute to the common cause, is an important objective of child public health.

(Blair et al. 2003, p. 3)

These writers emphasize the point that 'common understanding and cooperation' goes beyond the health sector, thus including teachers, social workers, educational psychologists, school nurses, youth justice teams, youth workers and others who work with children and young people. In other words, public health practitioners do not work alone nor do they work to single-issue agendas.

HEATH PROMOTION AS TARGETED INTERVENTIONS

We have cautioned against the over-simplification inherent in focusing on individual behaviour change and on a definition of health promotion that confines this work to categories of individual interventions. Nevertheless, public health practitioners need to see their work grounded in activities that do link into practical tasks.

To put it another way, the practitioner needs to focus his or her work with children and young people in approaches to health improvement that can make a difference – that produce evidence of change for the better. The school is a location for such work because it is where children gather. In effect, it is an opportunistic location. It is also the child's workplace, and learning to take care of personal health is as critically important to the child's future as is learning to read. Furthermore, the younger the child the more open he/she is to health information, education and health-promotion interventions.

The challenges in the intervention approach, however, are twofold. Individual health risks as a focus for health-promotion activities are themselves susceptible to fashion and change in terms of the attention they demand from public health practitioners. In the 1990s, young people's sexual health was the major public health preoccupation. By the first decades of the twenty-first century, bullying and obesity as well as child protection had moved to centre stage. Sexual health had not been resolved but it had begun to lose sustained media attention and teenage pregnancy numbers had reduced. In fact, we do not have sufficient national evidence to know whether or not sexual health among young people has continued to worsen. For example, full national coverage for chlamydia screening was scheduled for rollout by March 2007. The challenge, of course, is how to capture such information such that it gives us reliable data about young people of school age.

Blair et al. (2003) caught this 'feel' for the way public health practice responds to shifts both in policy pressure and in the relative profiles of health issues, when they included a chapter of practical examples (scenarios) for public health practitioners in child public health (Blair et al. 2003, pp. 193–243). It is probably fair to say that most health-promotion interventions arise from experimental approaches by public health practitioners. This is the case, for example, with many school nurse initiatives. The 'sharing of good practice' that we see in journals, in public policy documents and at conferences is of this kind and is generally under-evaluated or poorly evaluated. The question that arises is how can we know which preventive strategies do work and in what contexts and with what population groups?

For example, a *BMJ Online* study in Scotland (Henderson et al. 2007) reported research that measured the relative effectiveness of conventional school sex education compared with a theoretically based sex education programme (SHARE) by using a follow-up of cluster randomized trial. The SHARE (sexual health and relationships) programme was experimental and considerably more expensive than the conventional school sex education programme because it involved different approaches, more expensive materials and higher levels of investment in staff training by health-promotion departments. Yet 4.5 years after the two interventions (girls followed up at age 20 years), no significant difference was found between the two programmes in the numbers of conceptions and terminations.

The single finding of significance was that

> … effective programmes have to address fundamental socio-economic divisions in society, while the influence of parenting factors on sexual experience points to strategies involving parents.

(Henderson et al. 2007)

Neither the school sex education programme nor the SHARE programme had focused on parental involvement or on socio-economic population profiles as a factor in teenage sexual health, yet these were identified as the highest correlation factors in rates of teenage pregnancy.

In other words, sexual risk taking is closely linked to the socio-economic profile of the particular child population within the school, not merely linked to the school-based health-promotion interventions. This means that family, community and cultural attitudes to early sexual experience and to conception and terminations of conceptions are powerful influences on teenage decision making about sexual behaviour and about teenage pregnancy.

Tabberer et al. (2000) found this to be the case in their study of teenage girls' attitudes to early pregnancy. Their qualitative study of 41 young women in Doncaster found that teenage pregnancy was not planned but was relatively common in the locality under study, and they also found that families, especially the young women's mothers, often played a crucial part in supporting teenagers who gave birth. The health promotion need was for early advice and counselling and early information about abortion. Later studies have found that early access to information about sexual health is a critical need for young people.

Across the United Kingdom, a range of health-promotion interventions by school nurses, health-promotion specialists, and youth workers have together developed precisely these kinds of resources, including access to emergency contraception (DeBell and Tomkins 2006).

Successive studies have consistently reported that about one-third of 16-year-old girls across the United Kingdom are sexually active. This population group needs access to sexual health services that are designed such that young people will find them easy to use and easily accessible.

But it is fair to say that we need far more evidence of the effects of health-promotion interventions than we currently have. The health related choices children and young people make are not merely a consequence of good or poor health education and health-promotion interventions, though these may be a factor for individual children and young people. Choices are powerfully linked to the social environment in which the child lives. This is important for understanding how to select health-promotion interventions during the school-age years. The need is for investment in research that can measure the effects of existing health-promotion interventions.

A task force in the United States was established in the early 1990s to do just this (Zara et al. 2005). In 1996, the Department of Health and Human Services (HHS) established the Task Force on Community Preventive Services with a 15-member panel of experts working with the Centres for Disease Control and Prevention. By 2005, dozens of health specialists and scientists, by working together, had produced *The Guide to Community Preventive Services: What Works to Promote Health?* And this work continues. Its purpose is to answer three key questions about health-promotion interventions that all public health practitioners need to answer:

- What has worked for others and how well?
- How can I select among interventions with proven effectiveness?
- What might this intervention cost, and what am I likely to achieve through my investment?

(Zara et al. 2005, p. xxxv)

These are the primary questions that all public health practitioners need to ask when planning health-promotion interventions for children and young people and for making decisions about such interventions in the school setting.

CONCLUSION

The school is an opportune location for health-promotion work because it is where children and young people gather; where they spend the greatest part of their growing up years outside the home environment; and it is, effectively, their workplace. Historically, in the United Kingdom, there has always been a damaging split between education and health, despite periodic attempts to integrate the two. The twenty-first century, however, has seen a systematic attempt to shift policy and practice to an integrated approach to child health and education, and to do so in terms of a community/neighbourhood perspective. As a social paradigm for health rather than a medical model, this is recognizable and welcoming for the work of public health practitioners.

Every Child Matters: Change for Children (HM Government 2004), which is legally underpinned by the *Children Act 2004*, is the framework that has been designed to define positive child and adolescent health and to specify expected outcomes from services. It is an ambitious direction of travel. It is not, however, an easy agenda because it requires cross-government departmental cooperation and inter-professional working. Particularly since World War II, departmental boundaries (e.g. education, health, social care, the police and housing) have produced, across all four countries of the United Kingdom, diverse ways of working and thinking that are powerfully affected by training cultures. Each professional group articulates its work in its own language and to its own service objectives. Teachers and public health practitioners present us with a useful example of such diversity in working practices and service objectives. Partnership working can be difficult to negotiate for both professions. Having said that, the 'legal duty on local authorities is not to co-operate to improve the well-being of children and young people living in their area' (Evans and Halliday 2006, p. 2). Health promotion is also a complex field. At base, it tends to be articulated in terms of either interventions or changes in regulatory measures designed to improve health and to prevent ill health. These are not merely lifestyle behaviours but also involve attention to those socio-economic, environmental and cultural factors that determine how individual children and young people respond to efforts designed to improve their health or to prevent poor health.

With health promotion work, the public health practitioner finds himself/herself engaged in an activity that demands analysis of the community in which the child lives; attention to the family circumstances; and appropriate response to the individual child. It is this way of *seeing* the whole of the health-improvement agenda and the whole of the child's circumstances and that is demanded of public health practitioners when they think about working with children and young people in the school environment. And where their work is most effective it understands the school as part of a larger community while, at the same time, it involves working with diverse agencies as well as with families themselves.

KEY POINTS

- The history of child health in the school setting in the United Kingdom is not a heartening picture, but policy shift in the twenty-first century across all four countries has provided both the framework (*Every Child Matters: Change for Children*, HM Government 2004) and the legal pressure (the *Children Act 2004* and the *Children and Families Act 2014*) that could enable significant change in this profile.

- A paradigm shift to a social model of health across all departments, agencies, and professions is needed in order to improve child and adolescent health.
- Health promotion, as theorized since the 1980s, can be a powerful tool for public health practitioners. It includes analysis of the determinants of health – the *socio-economic, environmental, psychosocial and cultural* factors that affect child health – and it includes practical interventions.
- Health-promotion interventions require, and do not at present have, a firm evidence base for practice, but public health practitioners tend to think of health promotion, first, in terms of practical interventions.
- Health education is a subset of activities within the health-promotion portfolio. Health education is not a legal curriculum requirement but there is considerable pressure from the school standards authority (Ofsted) for schools to demonstrate that health-improvement measures are integrated into schools' work.
- The NHSP is not a legal requirement but it does represent a pressure on schools to demonstrate their commitment to child and adolescent health.
- Public health practitioners working to health-promotion agendas in the school environment *see* their work in terms of the child, the family, the school and the local community outside the school gates.

REFERENCES

Acheson D. (1998) *Independent Inquiry into Inequalities in Health*. London: Department of Health.

Bartley M. (2003) *Health Inequality: An Introduction to Concepts, Theories and Methods*. London: Blackwell.

Benzeval M, Judge K, Whitehead M. (1997) Tackling inequalities in health: Extracts from the summary. Kings Fund. In: Sidell M, Jones L, Katz J, Peberdy A, eds. *Debates and Dilemmas in Promoting Health: A Reader*. Basingstoke, UK: Macmillan, p. 16.

Billingham K. (1997) Public health nursing in primary care. *British Journal of Community Health Nursing* 2:270

Black D. (1980) *Report of the Working Group on Inequalities in Health. Department of Health*. London: HMSO.

Blair M, Stewart-Brown S, Waterston T, Crowther R. (2003) *Child Public Health*. Oxford, UK: Oxford University Press.

Botting B. (1995) *The Health of Our Children: A Review of the Mid 1990s*. London: Office of Population Census.

Burgher MS, Rasmussen VB, Rivett D. (1999) *The European Network of Health Promoting Schools: The Alliance of Education and Health*. Copenhagen, Denmark: WHO Regional Office for Europe.

Child Accident Prevention Trust. (2006) www.capt.org.uk/allaboutcapt/ main.htm (accessed, 24 January 2007).

Court D. (1976) *Fit for the Future*. London: UK Commission of Enquiry into the Child Health Services.

Cummings C, Dyson A, Papps I, et al. (2006) *Evaluation of the Full Service Extended Schools Initiative, Second Year: Thematic Papers*. London: Department for Education and Skills and Universities of Manchester and Newcastle.

Dahlgren G, Whitehead M. (1991) *Policies and Strategies to Promote Social Equity in Health*. Stockholm, Sweden: Institute for Future Studies.

DeBell D. (2014) Screening for growth and development In McPherson and Driscoll (eds.) *School Screening Systems*. New York: Nova Publishers.

DeBell D, Everett G. (1997) *In a Class Apart: A Study of School Nursing*. Norwich, UK: Norfolk Health Authority.

DeBell D, Jackson P. (2000) *School Nursing within the Public Health Agenda: A Strategy for Practice*. London: McMillan Scott.

DeBell D, Tomkins A. (2006) *Discovering the Future of School Nursing: The Evidence Base*. London: McMillan-Scott.

Denman S, Moon A, Parsons C, Stears D. (2002) *The Healthy Promoting School: Policy, Research and Practice*. London: Routledge.

Department of Education and Science. (1968) *Handbook for Health Education*. London: HMSO.

Department for Education and Skills. (2002) *PSHE Certification Programme for Teachers*. Nottingham: DfES Publications. www.wiredforhealth.gov.uk (accessed, 24 January 2007).

Department for Education and Skills. (2005) *Higher Standards Better Schools for All: More Choice for Parents and Pupils*. Nottingham, UK: DfES Publications.

Department for Education and Skills and Department of Health. (2003) *How the National Healthy School Standard Contributes to School Improvement*. London: Department of Health.

Department for Education and Skills and Department of Health. (2005) *National Healthy Schools Status: A Guide for Schools*. Nottingham, UK: DfES.

Department for Education and Skills and Department of Health. (2006) *Extended Schools and Health Services*. London: DfE.

Department for Education. (2008) *School Food Regulations*. London: DfE.

Department for Education. (2009) *School Food Regulations*. London: DfE.

Department for Education. (2015a) *School Food in England*. London: DfE.

Department for Education. (2015b) *School Food Regulations*. London: DfE.

Department of Education. (2012) *Extended Schools Programme*. www.deni.gov.uk. Accessed 26 August 2015.

Department of Health. (2002) *School Nurse Practice Development Pack*. London: Department of Health.

Department of Health. (2004a) *Choosing Health: Making Healthy Choices Easier*. London: Department of Health.

Department of Health. (2004b) *Healthy Living Blueprint*. London: Department of Health.

Department of Health and Department for Education and Skills. (2004) *National Service Framework for Children, Young People and Maternity Services*. London: Department of Health. www.dh.gov.uk/PolicyAndGuidance/HealthAndSocialCareTopics/ChildrenServices/ChildrenServicesInformation/Childrens ervicesInformationArticle/fs/en?CONTENT_ID=4089111&chk=U8Ecln (accessed, 5 February 2007)

Department of Health. (2006) *Health Profile of England*. London: Department of Health.

Department of Health. (2012) *Getting it Right for Children, Young People and Families*. Gov.uk.

Eisenberg L. (1999) Does social medicine still matter in an era of molecular medicine? *Journal of Urban Health* 76:164–175.

Evans S, Halliday S. (2006) *Indications of Child Health in the East of England: No. 1: Introduction and Overview*. Inpho Briefing Papers on topical public health issues. Issue 20. Cambridge: Eastern Region Public Health Observatory. www.erpho.org.uk (accessed, 24 January 2007).

Flynn P, Knight D. (1998) *Inequalities in Health in the North West*. Warrington: NHS Executive North West. www.nwph.net/nwpho/Publications/inequalities.pdf (accessed, 31 January 2007).

Hall D, Elliman D. (2003) *Health for All Children*. 4th ed. Oxford, UK: Oxford University Press.

Hanifan LJ. (1916) The rural school community center. *Annals of the American Academy of Political and Social Science* 67:130

Hanifan LJ. (1920) *The Community Center*. Boston, MA: Silver Burdett.

Harker L. (2006) *Chance of a Lifetime: The Impact of Bad Housing on Children: Aclives*. Edinburgh, UK: Shelter.

Harris B. (1995) *The Health of the School Child: A History of the School Medical Service in England and Wales*. Buckingham, UK: Open University Press.

Health and Social Care Information Centre. (2013) *National Child Measurement Programme*. London: Health and Social Care Information Centre. www.hscic.gov.uk.ncmp.

Henderson M, Wight D, Raab GM, et al. (2007) Impact of a theoretically based sex education programme (share) delivered by teachers on NHS registered conceptions and terminations: Final results of cluster randomised trial. *BMJ* 334:133.

Heer B, Woodhead D. (2002) *Promoting Health, Preventing Illness: Public Health Perspectives on London CT Mental Health*. London: The King'n Fund.

HM Government. (2004) *Every Child Matters: Change for Children*. Nottingham: DfES Publications. www.everychildmatters.gov.uk/_content/documents/Every%20Child%20Matinserts.pdf (accessed, 21 January 2007).

Hofrichter R (ed.). (2003) *Health and Social Justice: Politics, Ideology, and Inequity in the Distribution of Disease: A Public Health Reader*. San Francisco, CA: Jossey Bass Publication.

Independent Advisory Group on Sexual Health and Teenage Pregnancy. (2005) *Personal, Social and Health Education in Schools: Time for Action*.www.dfes.gov.uk/teenagepregnancy (accessed, 24 January 2007).

Kawachi I, Kennedy B, Wilkinson RG (eds.). (1999) *Income Inequality and Health: The Society and Population Health Reader*. Vol 1. New York: The New Press.

Labonté R. (1993) A holosphere of healthy and sustainable communities. *Australian Journal of Public Health* 17: 4–12

Leff S, Leff V. (1959) *The School Health Service*. London: Lewis.

Lister-Sharp D, Chapman S, Stewart-Brown S, Sowden A. (1999) Health promoting schools and health promotion in schools: Two systematic reviews. *Health Technology Assessment NHS R&D HTA Programme* 3:22. www.ncchta.org/fullmono/mon322.pdf (accessed, 24 January 2007).

Macintyre S, Hart G. (2000) *Synergy No 3. Tackling Health Inequalities in Scotland: A Policy Relevant Research Agenda*. Glasgow, UK: Universities of Glasgow and Strathclyde. www.strath.gla.ac.uk/synergy/policy/3.html (accessed, 24 January 2007).

Marmot M. (2004) *Status Syndrome*. London: Bloomsbury.

Marmot M and Wilkinson R G (eds.). (2006) *Social Determinants of Health*. 2nd ed. Oxford, UK: Oxford University Press.

Mayall B, Bendelow G, Barker S, et al. (1996) *Children University in Primary Schools*. London: The Falmer Press.

McNalty A. (1939) *Suggestions on Health Education. Board of Education for England*. London: HMSO.

Mosley H, Moorhouse J. (2000) *A Profile of the Health and Health Needs of School Age Children in Huddersfield*. Huddersfield, UK: Huddersfield NHS Trust.

Naidoo J, Wills J. (1998) *Health Promotion Foundations for Practice*. London: Baillière Tindall.

National Childrenon Bureau. (2003) *Developing A Whole School Approach to PSHE and Citizenship*. London: National Children Bureau. www.ncb.org.uk (accessed 24 January 2007).

National Audit Office. (2012) *An Update on the Government's Approach to Tackling Obesity*. London: National Audit Office.

National Institute for Health and Clinical Excellence. (2006) Obesity: Guidance on the prevention, identification, assessment and management of overweight and obesity in adults and children. *NICE Clinical Guideline 43: NICE*.

National Institute for Health and Clinical Excellence. (2010) *Clinical Guideline Practice No. CG9*. Eating disorders: Core interventions in the treatment and management of anorexia nervosa, bulima nervosa and related eating disorders. National Collaborating Centre for Mental Health. London: The British Psychological Society and the Royal College of Psychiatrists.

Nicholson W. (2014) *Maximising the School Nursing Team Contribution to the Public Health of School-Aged Children: Guidance to Support the Commissioning of Public Health Provision for School Aged Children 5-19*. London: Department of Health and Public Health England.

Office for National Statistics. (2004) *The Health of People and Young People*. London: Office for National Statistics.

Office for Standards in Education. (2002) *Sex and Relationship Education*. London: HMSO.

Office for Standards in Education. (2005a) *Personal, Social and Health Education in Secondary Schools*. London: HMSO.

Office for Standards in Education. (2005b) *Every Child Matters: Framework for the Inspection of Children on Services*. London: Adult Learning Inspectorate, Healthcare Commission, HMcpsi, Audit Commission, HMIC, HMiP, csci, HM Inspectorate of Prisons, HMiCA.

Pearson P. (2002) Public health and health promotion. In: Cowley S *Public Health in Policy and Practice*. London: Baillière Tindall, pp. 44ll.

Polnay L. (1995) *Report of a Joint Working Party on Health Needs of School Age Children*. London: British Paediatric Association.

Prashar A. (2003) *Key Themes in Supporting Children and Young People in the North West: Public Health Policy and Practice*. Salford, UK: Institute for Public Health Research and Policy.

Rogers LL. (1908) Some Phases of School Nursing. *American Journal of Nursing* 8:966. Reprinted (October 2002) *Journal of School Nursing* 18:253–256.

Royal College of Paediatrics and Child Health. (2009) The UK-WHO growth charts: What is the difference? *UK-WHO Growth Charts – Fact Sheet 2*. www.growthcharts.rcpch.ac.uk.

Sidell M, Jones L, Katz J, Peberdy A. (1997) *Debates and Dilemmas in Promoting Health: A Reader*. Basingstoke, UK: Macmillan.

Scottish Executive. (2003) *A Scottish Framework for Nursing in Schools*. Edinburgh, UK: Scottish Executive.

Stewart-Brown S. (1998) New approaches to school health. In: Spencer N (ed.) *Progress in Community Health*. Vol 2. Edinburgh, UK: Churchill Livingstone, pp. 137–158.

Tabberer S, Hall C, Prendergast S, Webster A. (2000) *Teenage Pregnancy and Choice: Abortion or Motherhood: Influences on the Decision*. York, UK: Joseph Rowntree Foundation.

Training and Development Agency for Schools. (2006) *DfES Announcement – 19 September 2006.*www.tda.gov.uk/remodelling/extendedschools/research-sep06.aspx (accessed, 24 January 2007).

Wales M. (1941) *The Public Health Nurse in Action.* New York, NY: Macmillan.

Wilkinson RG. (1996) *Unhealthy Societies: The Afflictions of Inequality.* London: Routledge.

World Health Organization. (1978) *International Conference on Primary Health Care. Declaration of Alma-Ata.* www.who.dk/AboutWho/Policy/20010827_1 (accessed, 24 January 2007).

World Health Organization. (1986) *First International Conference on Health Promotion. Ottawa Charter for Health Promotion: The Move Towards a New Public health.* Geneva: World Health Organization. www.who.int/hpr/NPH/ docs/ottawa_charter_hp.pdf (accessed, 24 January 2007)

Zara S, Briss PA, Harris KW (eds.). (2005) *The Guide to Community Preventive Services: What Works to Promote Health?* Oxford and New York: Oxford University Press.

ACTS OF PARLIAMENT

All these Acts are published by HMSO in London, and all can be accessed from the UK Parliament website (www.publications.parliament.uk).

Education (Provision of Meals) Act 1906
Open Spaces Act 1906
Education (Administration Provisions) Act 1907
Notification of Births Act 1907
Education Act 1918
Maternity and Child Welfare Act 1918
Health and Social Care Act 2013/2014
Children Act 2004
Children and Families Act 2014

Young people, leisure and health

8

SIMON BRADFORD AND YVONNE McNAMARA

INTRODUCTION AND CONTEXT

European industrialisation and changing family forms in the nineteenth century demarcated childhood and youth from adulthood and created a space – *leisure* – where working class young people were considered beyond the influence of domestic, educational and labour market institutions. Emergent youth leisure organizations during this period were established to discipline and train young people for good citizenship. Regulation of leisure became more overt prior to and during periods of war when concerns for the physical condition of young men and the domestic health of young women were at their highest (Bradford 2006, p. 132). In present-day Europe, leisure is one site where the exigencies of childhood and youth are similarly managed in the attempt to secure young people's responsible citizenship (Department for Education and Skills 2006; Broström 2013). However, various iterations of 'austerity policy' across Europe (Bradford and Cullen 2014) mean that funding for state provision of leisure for young people has been diminished or curtailed. The so-called Big Society promulgated by the Coalition government in the United Kingdom has meant an increased role for the voluntary sector in youth leisure provision (Hilton and McKay 2011, p. 24). Such provision often includes health-oriented objectives. The UK government has continued to pursue a neo-liberal policy framework (especially privileging consumerism, markets, competition, efficiency, private sector involvement in service provision and personal responsibility), but presenting this as increasingly *outcome-led* and shaped by locally determined priorities (Gregory et al. 2012).

This chapter explores young people's leisure and its potential as a location for health interventions. We use the term *young people* broadly to include all children of school age, roughly 4–18. Leisure is a complex concept, not least because of the diversity of definitions of leisure activities in societies where leisure, like all else, is increasingly individualized and commercialized (Beck 2004). However, the exponential rise of commercial leisure opportunities and experiences is mirrored by increasing inequality and poverty in the United Kingdom (Wilkinson and Picket 2009). Young people's leisure experiences are radically shaped by social difference, principally, we argue, by social class, gender and race. In Western knowledge-based societies, leisure is no longer exclusively a domain of *pleasure*, but a setting in which indispensable skills and capacities are transmitted and developed, in the creation of a contemporary neo-liberal identity (Rojek 2010, p. 88). As leisure has also become significant as a site for health interventions aimed at young people (for example, in relation to diet or sexuality), unequal access to leisure opportunities may be reflected in differential consequences for young people's health (Shaw et al. 2005; Department of Health 2005).

Leisure has at least four important dimensions for young people. *First*, it is an institution where they acquire social and cultural capital. Social capital refers to the networks of interpersonal relationships in which young people are situated and in public health terms constitutes social well-being through developing '… the capacity to function as a social being, to form healthy supportive relationships, and to participate positively in community affairs' (Blair et al. 2003, p. 112). Well-being, although a contested idea (Robb 2007, pp. 186–187), minimally depends on positive social networks and the ability to contribute to them. This is particularly relevant to young people as cultural capital, which resides in the forms of knowledge and skill that enable people to become competent members of society, is acquired initially from parents, and its acquisition is gendered, racialized and classed.

Second, leisure provides psycho-social benefits for young people in terms of developing self-esteem, psychological well-being and health (Bradley and Inglis 2012).

Third, leisure defines the symbolic and material spaces ('leisure and pleasure') in which young people engage in the construction of identity, an important component of good health, and where they are, in principle, relatively free from adult intervention. Although all leisure activities seem to have a non-compulsory dimension in common this does not mean that they are necessarily freely chosen. Patterns of leisure activity are shaped by dispositions and capacities, are based on social difference and are inculcated through experience over time.

Finally, in the United Kingdom, leisure has been both managed through organized attempts to influence young people, and simultaneously neglected in circumstances where young people are left to themselves (perhaps increasingly so in times of austerity). Youth leisure has been the location of a range of adult care and control interventions, whether through the nineteenth century ideology of 'rational recreation', the contemporary concept of the 'preventive state' (Parton 2006, p. 164), or policy frameworks like *Every Child Matters* (Chief Secretary to the Treasury 2003), *Youth Matters* (Department for Education and Skills 2005) or *Positive for Youth* (HM Government 2011). Health initiatives targeted on young people have over recent decades been increasingly organized in leisure space, which has become central to public health policy.

PUBLIC HEALTH, POLICY AND YOUNG PEOPLE'S LEISURE

Public health as policy and practice is concerned with identifying and managing social, cultural, institutional and environmental factors that contribute to the health of given populations (Cowley 2002, p. 7). There is debate, however, about what counts as *health* – a fluid, contested and socially constructed concept. But there is even greater debate about *public* health because the concept is multifaceted with complex intersecting psychological, physiological, cultural and social dimensions.

Child public health focuses on the promotion of the 'health and well being of young people in the widest sense' (Blair et al. 2003, p. 1). This encourages a holistic view of young people in the context of their communities and reflects the social, political and economic factors that contribute to health, rather than focusing on individualized medical circumstances. As such, child public health moves beyond issues of mortality, morbidity and the absence of disease, towards a broader concern with communities, patterns of social interaction within them and the impact these may have on health. This places young people's leisure, as a site of social interaction, centre-stage in any consideration of public health.

However, there are tensions here in policy terms. Although, in the United Kingdom, New Labour was influenced by the work of social capital theorists (for example Etzioni 1995; Putnam 1995), it has been suggested that constraints on expenditure mean that *individualizing* health responses has offered government an easier option (Goodwin and Armstrong-Esther 2004). Indeed, health has become a badge of responsible citizenship in, for example, the obesity debate, where bodily slimness is emblematic of 'embodied social fitness' (Monaghan 2005, p. 305) and 'more expansive and intimately connected problems associated with social injustice get hidden' (ibid, p. 308). Indeed, social policy in the United Kingdom, as in other neo-liberal democracies, continues to privilege individual responsibility, especially in relation to obesity, in the attempt to manage the health of the population as a whole (Petersen 1997, p. 197). As part of the obesity debate, the emergence of TV programmes such as *Supersize vs Super Skinny* and *Embarrassing Bodies* have fuelled an individualized culture of blame in which questions of health (and especially aspects of embodiment) are transformed into vicarious entertainment.

We depart from a view of policy-making as a linear practice in which problems are identified, responses formulated, and strategies subsequently implemented. This approach is sometimes referred to as a 'policy cycle' (Parsons 1995, p. 77) but fails to acknowledge the complexity and the contested nature of policy-making and implementation. Policy should be understood as discourse, and the power practices entailed in policy-making actions acknowledged (Ball 1993). Kingdon's model of the 'policy window' (Kingdon 2011) was developed to explain central government *policy action* in which policy windows open and close by the articulation of three figures: '*problems*', '*politics*' and '*policies*'. In relation to young people's health, we take the view that a perpetual policy window exists, framed by *political* definitions of health *problems*. This window frames different problems at different times, invariably influenced by the pragmatic politics of public opinion and moral panic: obesity, substance abuse or teenage pregnancy, for example.

PROBLEMS, *POLITICS* AND *POLICIES* IN YOUNG PEOPLE'S HEALTH

Young people's health in the United Kingdom is shaped by the shifting relationship between problems, politics and policies. Historically, young people have been viewed as a problematic social category (principally a source of social disorder and disruption) and their health problems have been variously defined in a range of legislation and concerns that are continually shifting in the light of wider political developments. For example, concerns about morbidity and mortality from infectious disease have been replaced by the 'morbidities of modern living' (Blair et al. 2003, p. 26) and are reflected in recurrent moral panics about healthy childhoods and healthy leisure.

Current challenges to young people's health – defined as *problems* – include a rise in mental ill health, eating disorders, suicide and self-harm, obesity, substance use (alcohol and drugs), teenage pregnancy, violence and the health effects of poverty (Blair et al. 2003, p. 27; Hagell et al. 2013). In England, Scotland and Wales these concerns continue to form key *policy* strands (HM Government 2010; Scottish Government 2008; Welsh Government 2011). The politics of these initiatives are complex but the dominant current *political* strategy in the United Kingdom is articulated as partnership between the state and others (including young people as partners) and is centred on a range of auditable outcomes (based on, often contested, evidence of 'what works') targeted on so-called *at risk* groups, but with implementation increasingly devolved to private or third sector organizations.

All child public health strategies in the United Kingdom acknowledge, implicitly or explicitly, the importance of leisure. This is a space in which young people can acquire *leisure capital*, which contains three dimensions: economic, social and cultural (Chang 2012). In the context of health, this includes the knowledge, skills and capacities that have the potential to contribute to well-being and that anticipate future life experiences and life chances (Zeijl et al. 2002, p. 381). Like other forms of capital, leisure capital is differentially distributed; therefore *some* young people acquire good knowledge of sexual health, drug and alcohol use and mental health support. Such knowledge or skill (as a form of capital) can be transformed into resilience and the dispositions needed to cope with the exigencies of contemporary life. For other young people, refugees or migrants for example, or looked after young people (Department of Health 2002a, p. 1; National Institute for Health and Care Excellence 2013), the acquisition of leisure capital is more problematic. These groups may be less likely to develop the necessary capacities to deal effectively with challenges arising in their lives, as resilience is also promoted through the development of sensitive, reliable, trusting relationships with adults, through creating opportunities for reflection and through the broader development of social capital (positive social connections outside the home). All of this emphasizes the centrality of leisure. In this context, the Care Leavers Strategy (HM Government 2013) provides an interesting example because its focus is entirely on the accessibility of mainstream and specialist services for care leavers. It recognizes that 'two thirds of looked after children have at least one physical health complaint, and nearly half have a mental health disorder' (ibid, p. 12) yet it fails to make wider links between inequality, leisure and health.

SOCIAL DIFFERENCE, LEISURE AND YOUNG PEOPLE

A characteristic feature of societies like the United Kingdom is that the logic and conviction of social solidarity fostered by class identity has been supplanted by the much less certain, yet increasingly seductive, power of (individualized) consumption, which confers a sense of identity and status (Bauman 2007, p. 53). As a consumed commodity, leisure (activities, fashions, clothes, mobile phones, MP3 players and so on) may have real significance as a source of, albeit, temporary stability and a sense of well-being. However, the 2010 UK census identified a growing divide between rich and poor, with large concentrations of poverty in the post-industrial towns, especially in the North (Office for National Statistics 2011a). This social polarization is significant not just *between* regions, but *within* them, as public sector housing is reduced (about 12% of all rentals), and disadvantaged households have been increasingly clustered together on the fringes of towns and cities (Dorling et al. 2007) raising questions about equitable access to leisure opportunities.

Recent research has demonstrated that societies in which the difference between rich and poor is greatest also have the poorest health indices (Goodwin and Armstrong-Esther 2004, p. 50; Wilkinson and Pickett 2009). The Millennium Survey of poverty and social exclusion in Britain found a bias towards the well-off in leisure service provision, noting that poverty affects children and young people's access to leisure more than any other section of the community (Pantazis et al. 2006, p. 464). This matters because sociability and leisure participation significantly define normal social identities (Hey and Bradford 2006), and poverty is a significant risk factor in acquiring a 'spoiled identity', with the implications this has for health and well-being. Children and young people are particularly vulnerable, as they are targeted by the producers of leisure experiences, yet their capacity to consume leisure is shaped by deepening social inequality. Insofar as leisure offers opportunity for the realization of public health policy, this is clearly important.

Young people's leisure choices and practices are influenced by at least four significant factors. *First*, parents shape young people's leisure choices. Government takes the view that this should be encouraged in the interests of children being helped to make positive '*lifestyle decisions that impact on their health*' (Department of Health 2004, p. 6; HM Government 2011, p. 18). Parents act as role models, for example, by encouraging children to engage in physical exercise and other such activities. Their support consists of a range of cultural and financial resources but social class is an important mediating factor. Such resources include time, energy, money, transport and parental presence at leisure activities. There is contradictory evidence about whether these resources are important for the social reproduction of leisure behaviour and health. United Kingdom studies suggest that a relationship between class and leisure participation can be reproduced over generations (Biddle et al. 2004, p. 686; Roberts 2013, p. 17).

Second, access to physical and social environments matters in shaping children's participation in leisure activities. Urban, rural and suburban locations have different implications for young people's access across a range of potential opportunities. Furthermore, the understanding of built environments, specifically crystallized in parental fears about safety and traffic (Elsley, 2011 p. 105), appears to have resulted in what Biddle et al. (op cit, p. 687) refer to as 'activity toxic environments' where levels of physical activity have diminished. In England and Wales, for example, the Office for National Statistics states that the numbers of children walking to school has remained stable at about 50% despite earlier concerns that the numbers had diminished (Department for Transport 2005, p. 47; Office for National Statistics 2011b, p. 22).

Parental perceptions of risk are important here. More broadly, gender and race also mediate perceptions of what constitutes safe leisure spaces. Brent's (2009) account of communities in Bristol demonstrates the extent to which young people see some settings as unsafe at particular times of the day or week because of the risk of physical and sexual violence. For some children and young people, this perception of risk can result in a sense of alienation from their own neighbourhoods (Morrow 2011, p. 70). Such perceptions, often perpetuated through peer and friendship groups, mean that some leisure activities become impossible to access, exacerbated by physical distance or poor public transport.

Third, the child's age is important in shaping the extent to which leisure can be a vehicle for effective public health interventions. Clearly, there are very significant differences in the leisure interests and practices of, say, five-year-olds and those of sixteen-year-olds. Their personal needs, interests and interface with health issues are quite different. For younger school-age children, though not exclusively, *play* is a principal leisure form and the literature identifies specific health benefits that play provides for younger children in terms of physical and mental health. There is evidence that the earlier children engage in physical leisure activity through play the more likely it is that they will become routinely socialized into such activities, thus increasing the potential health benefits to them (Meltzer et al. 2000). Some evidence indicates that the transition from primary to secondary school in the United Kingdom is particularly influential in children's leisure choices. For example, increased demands from coursework and homework, and growing corporeal self-consciousness (particularly for young women) appear to become barriers to some physical activities (Mulvihill et al. 2000; Hills et al. 2013). Interestingly, there is evidence from Canada suggesting that following the transition to secondary school young people see themselves as too old to begin learning new activity skills (Thompson et al. 2005, p. 435).

Hendry et al. (1993) developed a useful age-based framework for understanding the leisure transitions of children and young people through the school-age years to adolescence. The young people he studied moved from participation in *organized leisure*, predominantly led by adults and typified by the leisure activities of younger children, to *casual leisure* in early adolescence (hanging out with friends) and finally, during later adolescence, to participation in *commercial leisure* (going to pubs, clubs and other commercial sites). Age is suggested as the primary determinant here although Hendry acknowledges gender differences in how boys and girls use leisure opportunities. This work suggests a degree of universalism in leisure patterns and transitions. However, more recent work suggests that leisure has become much more commodified and *individualized* and less attached to or determined by earlier class solidarities (Hendry et al. 2002, p. 12). This does not mean that social class is no longer a contributing factor and some young people obviously have much greater capacity to consume leisure opportunities than others.

Finally, friendship and other peer group relationships are significant in shaping leisure practices because of their impact on the development of personal identity. Many leisure activities are tied to peer and friendship groups: these groups are constituted in leisure spaces and leisure time. Indeed, peer groups appear to provide a basis for *peer education* to which we refer below.

YOUNG PEOPLE, LEISURE AND HEALTH INTERVENTIONS

We consider three settings in which young people engage in leisure and in which leisure capital may be acquired. Importantly, these are contexts where health policy interventions in the lives of young people in the United Kingdom have been developed or are argued by policy-makers and practitioners to be suitable for intervention.

PUBLIC AUTONOMOUS SPACE

The 'street' may be *the* symbol of young people's potential for autonomy, yet young people have always been subjected to surveillance on the street through the institutions of the adult gaze (police, street wardens, youth workers, residents and so on). Arguably, the street (as a metaphor for public space more generally) has always been contested space, with recurrent attempts to sustain it as *adult* space. Nevertheless, it provides an important leisure space for the young and this remains the case despite a persistent historical concern about the imagined relationship between the street, as a dangerous place, and youth and children as either vulnerable or dangerous social categories (Manning et al. 2011, p. 225).

Meeting and being with friends, on the street, in the park, in shopping centres and malls is an alternative to commercial leisure provision and is an important leisure activity for many young people. In a recent UK survey, 60% of 14- to 16-year-olds agreed that 'I often hang about with my friends doing nothing in particular' (Children's Society 2006, p. 14). This confirms research in London (Bradford et al. 2003, pp. 32–33) suggesting this relative autonomy and freedom from adult supervision is the main appeal. The problem for young people is that adults often interpret hanging out as being threatening, dangerous or sinister. In a culture defined by SATs, Key Stages, accredited learning and certificated outcomes, just hanging out seems aimless and unproductive, crying out for adult intervention.

Under the rubric of *community safety* (Squires 2006), the panoptic surveillance of CCTV became ubiquitous in public spaces in the 2000s and was emblematic of New Labour's approach to managing risky social groups, especially youth. Furthermore, anti-social behaviour orders

(ASBOs), introduced in the *Crime and Disorder Act* 1998, criminalized what were, in many instances, civil offences committed by young people in leisure space. Dispersal orders, introduced in the *Anti-Social Behaviour Act* 2003 (preventing young people under 16 years of age from being on the streets unaccompanied by an adult after 9 p.m.) were a further constraint on young people's leisure. Additional legislation, in the *Anti-Social, Crime and Policing Bill* 2013, is currently proceeding through Parliament and promises faster action and prison terms of up to 2 years for under 18s who breach the new orders. The underlying message remains that young people constitute a problem and they are increasingly unwelcome in public space, where they are regarded as being fundamentally 'out of place'.

Despite an often authoritarian and problematizing approach to young people, public spaces have become settings for some health related work. A 2004 UK study noted the significant growth in the number of street-based youth work projects (564 projects in England and Wales that had contact with 65,325 young people) with high-risk groups and working on particular topics. For example, the youth workers interviewed reported that 30% of the young people they were in contact with had health related problems (Crimmens et al. 2004). Street-based or detached youth work appears to offer some potential as a means of working with young people who do not come into contact with other agencies. Its strength seems to lie in youth workers' acceptance of young people as active participants in informal education work. However, under Coalition policy, much of that work has been subject to cuts in local authority and voluntary sector budgets as intervention is targeted on the most vulnerable (National Youth Agency [NYA] 2013).

Proponents argue that detached work has the capacity to contact disaffected or excluded young people and offer information and advice on a range of health-related behaviours. There have been many local projects of this kind in the United Kingdom but hard evidence of long-term effectiveness is difficult to capture. One Scottish report suggested that although this work has potential for helping young people with health matters, evaluation mechanisms are frequently underdeveloped and there is little robust research investigating outcomes (Furlong et al. 1997). More recent work in Northern Ireland indicates that there is evidence of detached youth workers' positive impact on young people's sexual and mental health (Harland et al. 2005, p. 26). In England, some evidence suggests the effectiveness of informal work on health issues in street settings (Merton et al. 2004, p. 10) and others engaged in street-based work report successful engagement with young people in discussing sexual health (Baraitser et al. 2002, p. 21).

There seem to be three points here. *First*, this informal or detached work is based on the assumption that interventions in spaces that young people see as *theirs*, and that are made on their terms are likely to be effective. However, and *second*, there has been little or no rigorous, large scale and long-term research on the effectiveness of street-based work on health issues with young people (Hills et al. 2013, p. 90). *Third*, because of the often brief, informal, person-centred and fluid practices in this work, hard evidence of long-term success in this work is difficult to adduce. Perhaps for these reasons, as Local Authority budgets have reduced, there has been a shift from long-term, area based, open, informal or street-based youth work towards short-term targeted interventions on specific issues or with identified groups (Crimmens et al. 2004).

ORGANIZED LEISURE SPACE

The boundary between leisure and non-leisure is increasingly permeable and distinctions between the two are becoming less meaningful. As part of the *Every Child Matters* agenda that dominated during the latter years of the New Labour government, developments in Extended

Schools meant that increased opportunities for leisure activities focusing on health and well-being and linked to the five ECM outcomes were available to those able to take advantage of them, with 32% of extended schools receiving funding from the health sector (Department for Children Schools and Families 2009, p. 5). Broadly, this meant that young people's leisure time became more structured and increasingly subject to adult control. There are social class variations to this, but as leisure has become perceived to be a source of social and cultural capital, middle class parents, especially, have invested time and personal resources in 'leisure as life-chance'.

Fears about young people's safety have also led to increased supervision of leisure space and activity, particularly for girls and young women (Aapola et al. 2005, p. 115; Cook 2011, p. 281). For example, Extended Schools were seen to provide 'somewhere safe for the child to go' by 36% of parents (Department for Children Schools and Families 2009, p. 51). Increasing parental labour market participation has also led to some children and young people being enrolled in a variety of after-school clubs and groups that provide adult supervision.

Some general patterns of participation in out-of-school sporting activities, the focus for a range of health related interventions, are evident and social class and gender difference are both significant here. More boys than girls (21% and 16%, respectively) participate in sports activities across the age ranges, meeting current UK government guidelines of at least 1 hour of moderately intensive physical activity per day. Participation in physical activities diminishes with age as the percentage of boys meeting those guidelines decreased from 24% for 5- to 7-year-olds to 14% aged 13- to 15-year-olds. Among girls the decrease was more marked, from 23% to 8%, respectively (Health and Social Care Information Centre 2012). However, there is some evidence that young women are increasingly likely to participate in sports that, hitherto, have been associated with young men, for example, football and basketball (Sport England 2003, p. 41; Sport England 2006).

There are complex relationships between other forms of social difference (class, disability and ethnicity) and physical activity. It is clear that social class shapes access to leisure opportunities. Young people from the most deprived areas of the United Kingdom are less likely to be members of sports clubs, youth clubs and other similar organizations. The participation rates of disabled young people are lower than for other young people. Young people from Indian, Pakistani, Bangladeshi and Chinese backgrounds have lower participation rates than white young people (British Heart Foundation 2004, p. 7; Sport England 2006). Insofar as these opportunities have the potential to confer leisure capital on young people, evidence suggests that this is differentially distributed throughout the population.

The most recent reliable figures (and these are dated) suggest that at any given time, 20% of 13- to 19-year-olds participate in youth service activities: clubs, projects and centres (Department for Education 1995). Youth clubs have been the primary focus of youth work, providing a place where young people meet 'that is safe and warm, where they can associate, try out new activities and learn new skills, relate to adults, obtain advice and information, and run things for themselves' (Robertson 2005, p. 3) and they often appeal to younger teenagers. As a 15-year-old young woman in West London said 'when you get to like 14 or 15 you're not going to go down a youth club and get told what to do, you get me? They don't like it' (Bradford et al. 2003, p. 35). Despite this, subsequent research (Bradford et al. 2004, p. 34) found that older teenagers can also be committed to club membership. In this work, one young person identified their youth club as 'a place to have fun, to meet friends, talk with your mates and just mellow out, to get away from schoolwork and parents, a place where you are given a chance'.

In the London-based research, 31% of the total number of young people interviewed belonged to a youth organization; more females than males belonged; 14 was the peak age; and

Case study 8.1: Supportive youth workers

Bradford and colleagues undertook research exploring the impact of supportive and sympathetic youth workers on young people's understandings of health matters and how these contributed to their sense of well-being. The following sequence occurred when one of the interviewers was talking with a group of young women in a youth club in the English midlands.

Interviewer: What do you learn at this club?
Sara: Sex education...
Chloe: Drugs...
Kelly: Yeah, about drugs, safety, sanitary and hygiene...
Interviewer: Periods and stuff? (Kelly nods)

The young women went on to say that these were topics that they wanted information about but the significant thing for them was to receive that information in ways that took them seriously and made them feel valued and respected. This is an example of how skilled and sensitive youth workers can use leisure time activities to provide settings for helping young people to develop their knowledge and capacities in relation to health matters.

there was a significant drop in membership at age 16. The main reason given for belonging to a club was that it provided *'somewhere to meet my friends'* but young people value their experiences in youth clubs for a variety of reasons. Informal access to health information and to informal support is one aspect of these as Case Study 8.1 (from Bradford et al. 2004, p. 38) suggests.

This echoes Baraitser et al. (2002), who point to the value of informal and flexible health-oriented work in leisure settings. In the wider discussion above, the young women identified learning opportunities that fulfilled many of the personal social and health education (PSHE) and citizenship elements of the National Curriculum. They acknowledged a growth in self-esteem and self-worth, as well as important elements of what we understand as social and cultural capital acquired through their youth club membership. This is supported by recent research (Myers et al. 2011) with young people and parents at a club for young people with language difficulties. Parents particularly emphasized the importance of the club in enabling young people to develop socially, this being important in addressing these young people's marginalization.

Broadly, research shows that young people value four aspects of belonging to a leisure time youth organization that may have an important bearing on the capacity of informal health education to support them (Hills et al. 2013):

- The provision of accessible and safe leisure space
- A relevant and interesting combination of leisure and educational opportunities
- Relationships between youth workers (or other adults) and young people that emphasize young people as active participants rather than consumers of services and work that emphasizes the person-centred *process* element of youth work
- The provision of relevant information, advice and informal support or counselling

Youth provision with these characteristics is most likely to articulate with young people's own understanding and interpretation of their health needs. Indeed, the recognition of young people as active agents in the processes involved resonates with current government policy about incorporating user perspectives in public health initiatives (Department for Education and Skills and Department of Health 2004; Greenhalgh et al. 2011).

Ironically, in the context of New Labour's modernization of services this generic, flexible and specifically *leisure-based* youth club work diminished in scale. Targeted work with young people considered to be at risk, as well as work designed to achieve the outcomes specified by *Every Child Matters* dominated the policy agenda of the early and mid-2000s. This trend has largely continued subsequent to the election of the Coalition Government in 2010. Funding for youth provision has reduced by 10.4% between 2010/11 and 2012/13 (NYA 2013). Yet, the headline figure disguises a clear policy trend with expenditure on informal education falling by 17.6%, on substance misuse falling by 16.6% and teenage pregnancy falling by 21.8%, while expenditure on other outcomes led *targeted* work increased by 3.2%. As NYA (ibid, p. 4) indicates '... there is a particular focus on early intervention with vulnerable young people or on targeting limited resources to support the most vulnerable'.

The development of a range of government policy initiatives designed to improve young people's health, often established as partnerships that involved various stakeholders and that aimed at increasing the inclusion of at risk groups, and intended to boost personal responsibility demonstrated some success. Much of this work focused on social problems that achieved a high political profile: for example the Teenage Pregnancy Strategy (Department for Children, Schools and Families 2010) aimed to halve the under-18 conception rate by 2010 (from 46.6 per 1000 in 1998) and to achieve a decline in the rate of conceptions to under-16s. Between 1998 and 2008 the teenage conception rate fell by 13.3% among under-18s and by 11.7% for under-16s (ibid, 2010). Although such initiatives achieved success, some effective informal work may have been lost in the highly prescriptive approaches that now dominate the policy agenda. Programmes like *Positive Futures* (for 10- to 19-year-olds) and *Positive Activities for Young People* (for 8- to 19-year-olds) (2003–2006) were established to work on health issues with marginalized young people during their leisure time. Typically, as the interim evaluation report for *Positive Futures* put it, long-term work is necessary before effectiveness can be identified (Crabbe 2005, p. 119). Ironically, government funding for Positive Futures ceased in March 2013, although some programmes have received continuation funding from police and crime commissioners and other local partners.

Sure Start Plus, another initiative exemplifying similar participative approaches, worked with pregnant teenagers and teenage parents through the use of mentoring, personal advisers and other forms of intensive work in leisure time and spaces. The national evaluation of Sure Start Plus acknowledged innovative work but suggested that the scheme had 'less apparent impact on specific health objectives' (Wiggins et al. 2005, p. 2).

Peer-based education projects also proliferated across the United Kingdom but evidence of effectiveness is ambiguous (sometimes because of poor evaluation strategies and insufficient resources devoted to evaluation) and contested (Mellanby et al. 2000, p. 543; Swann et al. 2003, p. 42). Indeed, qualitative evidence from peer mentor schemes, 'buddy schemes' and other peer-based initiatives that were part of the *National Healthy Schools Standard* suggested that young people often did not use or trust them (Blenkinsop et al. 2004, pp. 11–12). The appeal of peer-based strategies, sometimes stronger for adults than for young people, apparently lies in their claim to empower individuals by encouraging the development of knowledge, skill and individual responsibility.

The Coalition government's *Positive for Youth* (HM Government 2011, p. 64) required every Local Authority in England to provide, for every young person in the Authority's area, access to '... sufficient leisure-time educational and recreational leisure-time activities for the improvement of the wellbeing of 13 to 19 year olds'.

However, there is a lack of clarity over what sufficient provision might be, particularly in the context of a 28% reduction in central government funding to Local Authorities (NYA 2013).

This has clear implications for the provision of leisure activities for children and young people and, in turn, for the deployment of informal health initiatives.

PRIVATE DOMESTIC SPACE AS LEISURE SPACE

Parental fears about their children's vulnerability to traffic, drug abuse, alcohol consumption, violence or paedophiles are particularly acute in contemporary Britain and reflect a generalized culture of social anxiety. These dangers are not necessarily imaginary but the disquiet they provoke is sometimes disproportionate to the extant risks (Furedi 2005). The perceived risks children encounter in public space has, arguably, led to some young people's leisure becoming privatized in a growing 'bedroom culture' (Lincoln 2005, p. 400). This domestication of children and young people's leisure has been accompanied by an expansion in social media, with young people aged 12–15 spending more time online (rising from 14.9 to 17.1 hours a week between 2011 and 2012) and as much time in a week using the Internet as in watching television. They are also more likely than they were in 2011 to use the Internet in their bedrooms: 43% in 2012 and 34% in 2011 (OFCOM 2012). It is estimated that 55% of young people in the United Kingdom have access to and use social networking sites (SNSs) (Karklins and Dalton 2012, p. 206) and that young people's Internet use is increasing faster than any other age group (Quayle and Taylor 2011, p. 45). SNSs enable young people to 'type one-self into being' (Dunne et al. 2010, p. 48), to create social identity and connect with others through the 'profile page'. This is particularly important for young people whose ability to socialize face-to-face is restricted and it may contribute to their social well-being. In the following case study, a carer described the importance of social media and online gaming to a young person with an increasingly debilitating and life-threatening illness.

There are significant gender differences in the way SNSs are used. For example, Subrahmanyam et al. (2008, p. 421) found that young women reported using SNSs to

Case study 8.2: Supportive leisure services

This short case study begins to suggest the contribution that supportive leisure provision can make to the lives of young people.

'I have been visiting a service user with muscular dystrophy for a year. He is 20 years old and has been in a wheelchair for most of his life. He still has the use of his hands and a plethora of technological hobbies. He has a multi-media set up in his bedroom, which incorporates a music system, DJ mixing equipment, a laptop, a television, remote control cars and a computer games console.

The computer games console has access to the Internet, which he utilizes to socialize with his own online community. With a microphone and headphones he can communicate with friends worldwide while engaging with computer games or even watching films. Through this technological medium he engages with a clan to play games and share experiences. Clans are collectives of individuals who engage with a game as a team. He will organize gaming events between his friends and has developed a reliable platform to explore social circles and relationships from the comfort of his own home.

He has a fantastic support network around him and his access to technology provides him with a community that is not always readily available'.

For this young man, leisure has become a space in which he is able to make valuable social connections that support his sense of agency and capacity. Interestingly, social media enables him to move between the private and public aspects of his life-world in a way that might not be possible otherwise, thus making a positive contribution to health and well-being.

reinforce pre-existing friendships whereas boys used them to flirt and make new friends. The impact of SNSs on young women's mental health is, apparently, significant. Girls aged 12–15 are more likely than boys to say they have been bullied online in the past year: 13% compared with 5% (OFCOM 2012). It is suggested that young women are seeking validation through posting images of themselves (on Facebook or Instagram, for example), often focused on their embodied identities: what they look like rather than who they are. These practices may fuel anxieties about body size and shape and for some young people may create the conditions in which eating disorders emerge. There is an apparent growth in the popularity of so-called 'pro-ana' sites that celebrate thinness (Riley et al. 2009, p. 349). Evidence suggests that, despite age restrictions, SNS use is permeating the age range with 14% of all UK children aged 5–15 using a tablet computer (such as an iPad) at home (OFCOM 2012). This has raised concerns about the impact of viewing inappropriate material, grooming for sexual exploitation and cyberbullying, sometimes driven by media reports of tragedies such as young people's suicides associated with bullying on SNSs. A number of youth organizations (for example Childnet) have responded by producing resources on how to address cyberbullying with primary and secondary age children. Although cost is important for public and voluntary sector organizations, some of these are developing expertize in promoting activities and health related messages through using SNSs. Local youth services, for example, often use text messaging to encourage young people to visit web pages or promote positive activities.

The development of smart phone technologies means that young people have access to knowledge and information that is (relatively) uncensored and beyond parental controls. Since 2011, smartphone ownership has increased among all UK children aged 5–15 to 28% in 2014 from 20% in 2011. This is primarily driven by a 21% increase of ownership among children aged 12–15, 62% in 2012 compared with 41% in 2011. From the age of 12 smartphone ownership outstrips ownership of other mobile phones. Half of all 12–15s with a smartphone (52%) say that of all regularly used media, they would most miss using their phone, with the next most-missed medium being using the Internet (18%). Among girls aged 12–15, 15% say their phone is the device they most often use to go online at home (OFCOM 2012).

This level of accessibility raises important questions, including about sexual health and relationship education. Many young men access pornography via the web, although the impact of this on their understanding and expectations of relationships and of their own and young women's bodies is contested (Allen 2007). The ubiquity of SNSs and incidents of young people being recorded so-called 'sexting' and those images being distributed among groups of young people may have damaging effects. However, youth-focused organizations have recognized the value of using the same technologies that young people use to engage with friends around health. For example Brook Advisory Service has established *Ask Brook* web, text and phone services for young people living, studying or working in the London area. Similarly, txtm8 is a sex and relationships text service which promises a response to any enquiry within 30 minutes and is completely free to use (www.livingwellcic.com). Online health projects tend to be area and age specific, which may limit access for some young people. For example www.kooth.com offers information and advice and fully structured counselling services to young people aged 11+ in specified authorities http://www.xenzone.com/kooth.html. For so-called 'hard to reach young people', particularly those who are homeless, or ex-offenders, some youth projects are trying to do more to support young people's access to health information. For example in Liverpool, the Young Persons Advisory Service (YPAS) is part of the GP Champs project supporting young people's access to GPs, and helping to train GPs in talking with young people and providing seamless access to psychological therapies: http://www.youngpeopleshealth.org.uk/5/page/71/

gp-champions-project/. Clearly the Internet has great potential and is being used creatively as a vehicle to engage with young people and to promote well-being.

However, growing adult unease is evident (perhaps fuelling and being fuelled by moral panic) about the perceived risk of web-based predatory paedophiles, the alleged electronic dissipation of children's creativity, empathy and attention span, and the potential for social isolation through the development of increasingly personalized digital technologies (Lewis 2006; Stutz 1996). However, recent research concludes '... there are no exploits or fundamental threats inherent to the social networking setting... rather... (it acts)... as an enabler for existing, long established and well-recognised exploits and activities' (Weir et al. 2011, p. 38). Although the possible risks and potential harms entailed in SNS-based bedroom activities should be acknowledged by young people, parents and policy-makers alike (Livingstone 2013; Livingstone et al. 2012), domestic space is certainly *one* important setting in which there appears to be some potential for positive health interventions as well as the wider acquisition of leisure capital.

For many children and young people, private domestic space, where this exists, is an important feature of growing autonomy. However, for income-poor children, for looked after children, and for other disadvantaged young people, this may present difficulties (Department of Health 2002b, p. 38). Bedroom culture is based principally on the use of electronic media, which may confer capacity and cultural capital on participants. Evidence suggests that large numbers of children are engaged in leisure-based media practices almost from birth (Marsh et al. 2005, pp. 24–25). Children and young people with Internet connections have developed online *virtual* game spaces that provide settings for interactions that contribute to autonomy and agency (Crowe and Bradford 2006) and such access is growing: currently about 83% of UK households (Office for National Statistics 2013). Computer ownership and Internet access are influenced by social difference, but not only by socio-economic status. Levels of family *cultural* capital (e.g. parental post-school educational background) are also important. Middle class young people have higher Internet access and young people in families with less cultural capital tend to own more screen entertainment media. Marsh et al. (op cit) calculated in 2005 that, typically, the young people in their study engaged in screen use (TV, computer games, watching videos, and playing hand held games) for 2 hours and 6 minutes every day. Young people aged 12–15 are spending more time online (rising from 14.9 hours a week in 2011 to 17.1 in 2012) and now devote as much time in a week to using the Internet as to watching television. They are also more likely than they were in 2011 to use the Internet in their bedrooms, 43% in 2012 compared with 34% in 2011 (OFCOM 2012). Although a relatively unexplored setting for public health policy-makers, initiatives and resources exist that draw on young people's information and communication technologies (ICT) competences. Sunderland Voluntary Youth Sector Forum's *Youth Work in a Digital Age* (http://www.svsyf.org) is a good example of working around adult anxieties about digital media and using young people's interests and capacity to maximize the Internet as an educational tool. Similarly, central government has long recognized the potential of digital media in shaping young people's views and capacities. A well-known example of a website focusing on substance and drug use, aimed at young people, parents and carers is *FRANK*, supported by the Department of Health, the Home Office and the Department for Education and Skills (http://www.talktofrank.com/). *FRANK* provides phone and e-mail contacts, a range of health information, and advice in a (presumed) youth-friendly format. The pedagogic assumptions underlying this initiative are partially oriented to a pragmatic discourse of *harm reduction* or *harm minimization* (Rhodes and Hedrich 2010) in which, given appropriate information about risk and reinforcing non-drug use behaviours, young people will make responsible life decisions. *FRANK* also seeks to enable parents and carers to acquire information that will support them in engaging with young people on these matters. This, of course, is a contested and politicized aspect of health policy.

Blogging has become a familiar cultural form and may have health education potential for young people through its capacity to establish online information networks and virtual communities, and to provide easy access and participation in a range of discourse. The popularity of Jack Monroe (http://agirlcalledjack.com) who is emerging as an influential voice in the poverty and healthy eating debate, evidenced by her co-option by the supermarket Sainsbury's and the Guardian newspaper, is indicative of the reach and potential of blogging. Similarly the enormous popularity of Facebook, Instagram, WhatsApp and YouTube suggests that these media remain enormously important in mapping out young people's social lives and identities. Whether their incorporation in health initiatives is quite as engaging for young people remains an open question. These technologies are relatively new and under-researched. However, as social interaction has important health benefits, the outcomes of virtual sociability framed in the context of bedroom cultures is an important area for further research.

CONCLUSIONS: YOUNG PEOPLE, LEISURE CAPITAL AND HEALTH

Leisure is a complex and, intensely, *paradoxical* concept. It designates a limitless range of practices, activities, material and temporal spaces whose only commonality is constituted by being defined and – apparently freely – chosen by participants as leisure. Yet, leisure has a simultaneous designation as a setting in which young people and children, who are often construed as risky social categories, find that they are subjected to invasive, but often obscured, adult surveillance. Leisure, it seems, will always be a vehicle for other interventions. Undoubtedly, leisure spaces exist in which young people can and should engage in critical dialogue about health and well-being, perhaps as part of a wider discussion of citizenship, with sympathetic professionals. In other material and virtual settings, young people should be left to their own devices away from the perpetual adult gaze.

Health, particularly public health, is also a problematic concept. Should health be regarded as a right or a responsibility (or both), *whose* responsibility is health and *who* is entitled to health as a right? To what extent should states be charged with intervening in the private domain (for example, in leisure) in order to encourage happy, productive and healthy citizens? In the United Kingdom and similar neo-liberal states, the responsibility for health and well-being has markedly shifted to the individual and *active* citizen, encouraged in different ways at different times by the state.

We have suggested that the effectiveness of interventions in young people's leisure time and space is difficult to ascertain because the nature of the evidence base is often contested. This is the case because either the existing evidence is insufficiently robust or because of the political nature of policy-making itself and the interests at stake. It is worth remembering that the apparent absence of evidence does not necessarily signal the ineffectiveness of a given intervention.

Although central to the lives of young people in providing relative autonomy, psychosocial well-being, and the acquisition of forms of capital, leisure has also become thoroughly commodified as part of consumer culture. In a society characterized by wide inequality, this has led to the differential distribution of young people's leisure opportunities, determined by social class position and by social difference more widely. Insofar as leisure provides opportunities

Discussion points

This chapter has explored aspects of children's and young people's leisure. It raises many important points about how leisure can make a contribution to children and young people's health. The following questions are worth discussion:

- In your own experience, what is the main contribution that leisure makes to health and well-being (either your own, your family or friends or that of someone you work with)?
- Whose responsibility, in your view, are children and young people's leisure time experiences? Who and which institutions might be involved or should be involved in this?
- One of the characteristics of neo-liberal societies is the growth of inequality. In your experience, how has inequality shaped access to leisure provision and activity? What implications does this have for the health and well-being of children and young people who you know or work with?

for young people to derive enjoyment and acquire and develop *leisure capital* (knowledge, skills and dispositions that can be transformed into resilience and the means for coping with life challenges, including health matters), inequality is of prime significance. The question of *who* acquires leisure capital, and who does not, should be addressed by policy-makers, as increasing privatization and commercialization of leisure in the face of diminishing public provision, coupled with growing inequality compromises the health and well-being of significant numbers of children and young people. However, it seems inevitable that the health of children and young people will continue to be framed in the intersection of problems, policies and politics.

REFERENCES

Aapola S, Gonick M, Harris A. (2005) *Young Femininity, Girlhood, Power and Social Change*. Basingstoke, UK: Palgrave Macmillan.

Allen L. (2007) "Looking at the Real Thing": Young men, pornography, and sexuality education. *Discourse: Studies in the Cultural Politics of Education* 27(1): 69–83.

Ball SJ. (1993) What is policy? Texts, trajectories and toolboxes. *Discourse* 13(2): 9–17.

Baraitser P, Dolan F, Feldman R, Cowley S. (2002) Sexual health work in a playground: Lessons learnt from the evaluation of a small-scale sexual health project. *Journal of Family Planning and Reproductive Health Care* 28(1): 18–22.

Bauman Z. (2007) *Consuming Life*. Cambridge, UK: Polity Press.

Beck U. (2004) *Risk Society towards a New Modernity.* London: Sage Publications.

Biddle SJH, Gorely T, Stensel DJ. (2004) Health-enhancing physical activity and sedentary behaviour in children and adolescents. *Journal of Sports Sciences* 22: 679–701.

Blair M, Stewart-Brown S, Waterston T, Crowther R. (2003) *Child Public Health*. Oxford: Oxford University Press.

Blenkinsop S, Eggers M, Schagen I, et al. (2004) *Evaluation of the Impact of the National Healthy School Standard. Final Report* [online]. http://www.wiredforhealth.gov.uk/PDF/Full_report_2004.pdf

Bradford S. (2006) Practising the double doctrine of freedom: Managing young people in the context of war. In: Gilchrist R, Jeffs T, Spence J, eds. *Drawing on the Past: Studies in the History of Community and Youth Work*. Leicester, UK: NYA: 132–149.

Bradford S, Cullen F. (2014) Positive for youth work? Contested terrains of professional youth work in austerity England. *International Journal of Adolescence and Youth* 19: 1–14. http://dx.doi.org/10.1080/02673843.2013.863733

Bradford S, Kindness L, Hey V, Cullen F. (2003) *"You're Either in or You're out or You're a Saddo…" Report of the Young Agenda Survey Completed in the London Borough of Richmond upon Thames.* London: Richmond Parish Lands Carity in association with Brunel University.

Bradford S, Hey V, Cullen F. (2004) *What Works? An Exploration of the Value of Informal Education Work with Young People.* London: Clubs for Young People in association with Brunel University.

Bradley GL, Inglis BC. (2012) Adolescent leisure dimensions, psychosocial adjustment, and gender effects. *Journal of Adolescence* 35(5): 1167–1176.

Brent J. (2009) *Searching for Community. Representation, Power and Action on an Urban Estate.* Bristol, UK: Policy Press.

British Heart Foundation. (2004) *Couch Kids: The Continuing Epidemic.* London: BHF.

Broström AW. (2013) "Wild Scouts": Swedish scouting preparing responsible citizens for the twenty-first century. *Child and Youth Services* 34(1): 9–22.

Chang YP. (2012) The game generation and its leisure capital: A study in the Taiwan social context. *Westminster Papers in Communication and Culture* 9(1): 133–151.

Chief Secretary to the Treasury. (2003) *Every Child Matters* (Cm 5860). London: The Stationery Office.

Children's Society. (2006) *Good Childhood? A Question for Our Times.* London: Children's Society.

Cook VA. (2011) The teachers seemed a bit obsessive with health and safety: Fieldwork risk and the social construction of childhood. In: Holt L, ed. *Geographies of Children, Youth and Families: An International Perspective.* London: Routledge.

Cowley S. (2002) Public health practice in nursing and health visiting. In: Cowley S, ed. *Public Health in Policy and Practice: A Sourcebook for Health Visitors and Nurses.* Edinburgh, UK: Balliere Tindall.

Crabbe T. (2005) *'Getting to Know You': Engagement and Relationship Building, First Interim National Positive Futures Case Study Research Report.* London: Positive Futures.

Crimmens D, Factor F, Jeffs T, et al. (2004) Reaching socially excluded young people: A national study of street-based youth work. York, UK: Joseph Rowntree Foundation and the National Youth Agency.

Crowe N, Bradford S. (2006) 'Hanging out in Runescape': Identity, work and play in the virtual playground. *Children's Geographies* 4(3): 331–346.

Department for Children, Schools and Families. (2009) *Extended Schools Survey of Schools, Pupils and Parents. A Quantitative Study of Perceptions and Usage of Extended Services in Schools.* Nottingham, UK: DCSF.

Department for Children, Schools and Families. (2010) *Teenage Pregnancy Strategy: Beyond 2010.* Nottingham, UK: DCSF.

Department for Education. (1995) *OPCS Survey of Youth Service Participation.* London: HMSO.

Department for Education and Skills and Department of Health. (2004) *National Service Framework for Children, Young People and Maternity Services.* London: Department of Health Publications.

Department for Education and Skills. (2005) *Youth Matters.* London: DfES Publications.

Department for Education and Skills. (2006) *Youth Matters: Next Steps. Something to Do, Somewhere to go, Someone to Talk to.* Nottingham, UK: DfES Publications.

Department for Transport. (2005) *Focus on Personal Travel.* London: The Stationery Office.

Department of Health. (2002a) *Promoting the Health of Looked After Children*. London: Department of Health Publications.

Department of Health. (2002b) *Children's Homes, National Minimum Standards*. London: The Stationery Office.

Department of Health. (2004) *Choosing Health, Making Healthy Choices Easier*. London: The Stationery Office.

Department of Health. (2005) *Tackling Health Inequalities: Status Report on the Programme for Action*. London: The Stationery Office.

Dorling D, Rigby J, Wheeler B, et al. (2007) *Poverty, Wealth and Place in Britain, 1968–2005*. Bristol, UK: Policy Press.

Dunne A, Lawler M. (2010) Young people's use of online social networking sites: A uses and gratifications perspective. *Journal of Research in Interactive Marketing* 4(1): 46–58.

Elsley S. (2011) Out of the way: Children, young people and outdoor spaces. In: Foley P, Leverett S, eds. *Children and Young People's Spaces, Developing Practice*. Basingstoke, UK: Palgrave Macmillan, 102–115.

Etzioni A. (1995) *The Spirit of Community: Rights and Responsibilities, the Communitarian Agenda*. London: Fontana.

Furedi F. (2005) *Culture of Fear: Risk Taking and the Morality of Low Expectations*. London: Continuum.

Furlong A, Cartmel F, Powney J, Hall S. (1997) *Evaluating Youth Work with Vulnerable Young People*. Glasgow, UK: Scottish Council for Research in Education.

Goodwin M, Armstrong-Esther D. (2004) Children, social capital and health: Increasing the well-being of young people in rural Wales. *Children's Geographies* 2(1): 49–63.

Greenhalgh T, Humphrey C, Woodard F. (2011) *User Involvement in Health Care*. Chichester, UK: Wiley-Blackwell.

Gregory S, Dixon A, Ham C. (2012) *Health Policy Under the Coalition Government. A Mid-Term Assessment*. London: The Kings Fund.

Hagell A, Coleman J, Brooks F. (2013) *Key Data on Adolescence 2013*. London: Association for Young People's Health.

Harland K, Morgan T, Muldoon O. (2005) *The Nature of Youth Work in Northern Ireland: Purpose, Contribution and Challenges*. Belfast, UK: Department of Education.

Health and Social Care Information Centre. (2012) *Health Survey for England, 2012*. Leeds, UK: HSIC.

Hendry LB, Shucksmith J, Love JG, Glendinning A. (1993) *Young People's Leisure and Lifestyles*. Routledge: London.

Hendry L, Kloep M, Espnes G, et al. (2002) Leisure transitions – A rural perspective. *Leisure Studies* 21: 1–14.

Hey V, Bradford S. (2006) Re-engineering motherhood? Sure start in the community. *Contemporary Issues in Early Childhood* 7(1): 53–67.

Hilton M, McKay J. (2011) The ages of voluntarism. An introduction. In: Hilton M, McKay J, eds. *The Ages of Voluntarism. How We Got to the Big Society*. Oxford, UK: Oxford University Press, 1–26.

Hills L, Bradford S, Johnston C. (2013) *Building a Participation Legacy from the London 2012 Olympic and Paralympic Games in Disadvantaged Areas: An Evaluation Report Commissioned by Street Games*. Uxbridge, UK: Brunel University.

HM Government. (2010) *Healthy Lives, Healthy People. Our Strategy for Public Health in England*. CM7985. London: The Stationery Office.

HM Government. (2011) *Positive for Youth. A New Approach to Cross-Government Policy for Young People Aged 13–19*. London: Department for Education.

HM Government. (2013) *Care Leaver Strategy. A Cross-Departmental Strategy for Young People Leaving Care*. London: Department of Education.

Karklins LT, Dalton D. (2012) Social networking sites and the dangers they pose to youth: Some Australian findings. *Current Issues in Criminal Justice* 24(2): 205–222.

Kingdon J. (2011) *Agendas, Alternatives and Public Policies*. 2nd ed. Boston, MA: Longman.

Lewis P. (2006) *Teenage Networking Websites Face Anti-Paedophile Investigation*. http://www.guardian.co.uk/uk_news/story/0,,1811159,00.html

Lincoln S. (2005) Feeling the noise: Teenagers, bedrooms and music. *Leisure Studies* 24(4): 399–414.

Livingstone S, Haddon L, Gorzig A. eds. (2012) *Children, Risk and Safety Online: Research and Policy Challenges in Comparative Perspective*. Bristol, UK: The Policy Press.

Livingstone S. (2013) Online risk, harm and vulnerability: Reflections on the evidence base for child Internet safety policy. *ZER: Journal of Communication Studies* 18(35): 13–28.

Manning R, Jago R, Fionda J. (2011) Socio-spatial experiences of young people under anti-social behaviour legislation in England and Wales. In: Holt L, ed. *Geographies of Children, Youth and Families: An International Perspective*. London: Routledge.

Marsh J, Brooks G, Hughes J, et al. (2005) *Digital Beginnings: Young Children's Use of Popular Culture, Media and New Technologies*. Sheffield, UK: Literacy Research Centre.

Mellanby A, Rees J, Tripp J. (2000) Peer-led and adult-led school health education: A critical review of available comparative research. *Health Education Research, Theory and Practice* 15(5): 533–545.

Meltzer H, Gatward R, Goodman R, Ford T. (2000) *The Mental Health of Children and Adolescents in Great Britain [Summary Report]*. London: National Statistics.

Merton B, Payne M, Smith D. (2004) *An Evaluation of the Impact of Youth Work in England: Research Report RR606*. Nottingham, UK: DfES Publications.

Monaghan LF. (2005) Discussion piece: A critical take on the obesity debate. *Social Theory and Health* 3: 302–314.

Morrow VM. (2011) Researching children and young people's perspectives on place. In: Foley P, Leverett S, eds. *Children and Young People's Spaces, Developing Practice*. Basingstoke, UK: Palgrave Macmillan, 58–72.

Mulvihill C, Rivers K, Aggleton P. (2000) *Physical Activity 'At Our Time': Qualitative Research Among Young People Aged 5 to 15 Years and Parents*. London: Health Education Authority.

Myers L, Davies-Jones C, Chiat S, et al. (2011) "A place where I can be me": A role for social and leisure provision to support young people with language impairment. *International Journal of Language Communication Disorders* 46(6): 739–750.

National Institute for Health and Care Excellence. (2013) *Looked After Children and Young People: NICE Public Health Guidance 28*. Manchester, UK: NICE.

National Youth Agency. (2013) *Youth Services in England: The State of the Nation*. Leicester, UK: NYA.

OFCOM. (2012) *Children and Parents: Media Use and Attitudes Report*. http://stakeholders.ofcom.org.uk/binaries/research/media-literacy/oct2012/main.pdf (accessed on 27 February 2014).

Office for National Statistics. (2011a) *Social Trends 41, Transport*. Newport, UK: ONS.

Office for National Statistics. (2011b) *Who We Are. How We Live. What We Do*. http://www.ons.gov.uk/ons/guide-method/census/2011/index.html (accessed on 7 March 2014).

Office for National Statistics. (2013) *Internet Access, Households and Individuals, 2013*. Statistical Bulletin. London: ONS.

Pantazis C, Gordon D, Levitas R. (2006) *Poverty and Social Exclusion in Britain: The Millennium Survey.* Bristol, UK: Policy Press.

Parsons W. (1995) *Public Policy: An Introduction to the Theory and Practice of Policy Analysis.* Aldershot, UK: Edward Elgar.

Parton N. (2006) *Safeguarding Childhood: Early Intervention and Surveillance in Late Modern Society.* Basingstoke, UK: Palgrave Macmillan.

Petersen A. (1997) Risk, governance and the new public health. In: Petersen A, Bunton R, eds. *Foucault, Health and Medicine.* London: Routledge.

Putnam RD. (1995) Tuning in, tuning out: The strange disappearance of social capital in America. *Political Science and Politics* 28(4): 664–683.

Quayle E, Taylor M. (2011) Social networking as a nexus for engagement and exploitation of young people. *Information Security Technical Report* 16(2): 44–50.

Rhodes T, Hedrich D. (2010) *Harm Reduction: Evidence, Impacts and Challenges. European Monitoring Centre for Drugs and Drug Addiction, Monograph 10.* Luxembourg, Luxembourg: Publications Office of the European Union.

Riley S, Rodham K, Gavin J. (2009) Doing weight: Pro-ana and recovery identities in cyberspace. *Journal of Community and Applied Social Psychology* 19: 348–359.

Robb M. (2007) Wellbeing. In: Kehily MJ, ed. *Understanding Youth: Perspectives, Identities and Practices.* London: Sage Publications, 181–213.

Roberts K. (2013) Social class and leisure during recent recessions in Britain. *Leisure Studies.* http://dx.doi.org/10.1080/02614367.2013.855939

Robertson S. (2005) *Youth Clubs Association, Partnership, Friendship and Fun.* Lyme Regis, UK: Russell House Publishing.

Rojek C. (2010) *The Labour of Leisure. The Culture of Free Time.* London: Sage Publications.

Scottish Government. (2008) *Equally Well, Report of the Ministerial Task Force on Health Inequalities.* Edinburgh, UK: The Scottish Government.

Shaw M, Davey Smith G, Dorling D. (2005) Health inequalities and New Labour: How the promises compare with real progress. *British Medical Journal* 330: 1016–1021.

Sport England. (2003) *Young People and Sport in England Trends in Participation 1994–2002, Research Study Conducted for Sport England by MORI.* London: Sport England.

Sport England. (2006) *Understanding Participation in Sport: What Determines Sports Participation Among 15-19 Year Old Women?* Sport England Research. https://www.sportengland.org/media/141142/15-19-yr-olds-leaflet-final-pdf-1-.pdf

Squires P. (ed.). (2006) *Community Safety. Critical Perspectives on Policy and Practice.* Bristol, UK: Policy Press.

Stutz E. (1996) Is Electronic Entertainment Hindering Children's Play and Social Development? In: Gill T, ed. *Electronic Children: How Children are Responding to the Information Revolution.* London: National Children's Bureau, 59–70.

Subrahmanyam K, Reich SM, Waechter N, Espinoza G. (2008) Online and offline social networks: Use of social networking sites by emerging adults. *Journal of Applied Developmental Psychology* 29(6): 420–433.

Swann C, Bowe K, McCormick G, Kosmin M. (2003) *Teenage Pregnancy and Parenthood: A Review of Reviews, Evidence Briefing.* London: Health Development Agency.

Thompson AM, Rehman LA, Humbert ML. (2005) Factors influencing the physically active leisure of children and youth: A qualitative study. *Leisure Sciences* 27: 421–438.

Weir GRS, Toolan F, Smeed D. (2011) The threats of social networking: Old wine in new bottles? *Information Security Technical Report* 16: 38–43.

Welsh Government. (2011) *Together for Health: A Five Year Vision for the NHS in Wales*. Cardiff, UK: Welsh Government.

Wiggins M, Rosato M, Austerberry H, et al. (2005) Supporting teenagers who are pregnant or parents. *Sure Start Plus National Evaluation: Executive Summary*. London: Social Science Research Unit.

Wilkinson R, Pickett K. (2009) *The Spirit Level, Why More Equal Societies Almost Always Do Better*. Harmondsworth, UK: Allen Lane.

Zeijl E, Du Bois-Reymond M, Te Poel Y. (2002) Young adolescents' leisure patterns. *Society and Leisure* 24(2): 379–402.

Vulnerable children

JANE V. APPLETON

9

INTRODUCTION

The public inquiry into the death of Victoria Climbié, published in 2003, drew significant national and international attention to the failings of public agencies to protect a vulnerable child.

> When Victoria was admitted to the North Middlesex Hospital on the evening of 24 February 2000 she was desperately ill. She was bruised, deformed and malnourished. Her temperature was so low it could not be recorded on the hsopital's standard thermometer. Dr Lesley Alsford, the consultant responsible for Victoria's care on that occasion, said, 'I had never seen a case like it before. It is the worst case of child abuse and neglect that I have ever seen'.

(Department of Health and Home Office 2003, para 1.5)

Victoria was eight years old when she died on the afternoon of 25 February 2000, the victim of sustained and 'almost unimaginable cruelty' (Para 1.1). Lord Laming's Inquiry into her death (Department of Health [DH] and Home Office 2003) identified many occasions when local services had the chance to intervene and protect Victoria, but they failed to do so. His damning report highlighted significant problems in both single agency and multi-agency work and cited 'widespread organisational malaise' (Para 1.21) as the main reason for failing to protect Victoria. The inquiry report resulted in a series of 108 basic good practice recommendations and was closely followed by the publication *Keeping Children Safe* (Department for Education and Skills [DfES], DH and Home Office 2003), the Government's response to the Victoria Climbié Inquiry Report and a Green Paper *Every Child Matters* (DfES 2003).

Yet since 2003 there have been a number of appalling cases of child maltreatment that have been instrumental in bringing vulnerable children to public attention, including Daniel Pelka, Keanu Willams and Hamzah Khan. The tragic death of 17-month-old Peter Connolly on 3 August 2007 in Haringey, London, following repeated injuries by his mother, her boyfriend and another man, prompted an extensive review of child protection arrangements in England. In addition, a number of high profile trials across the United Kingdom and research documents have highlighted that nationally child sexual exploitation is a key issue (Appleton 2014; Barnardos 2012; Berelowitz et al. 2013; DH and Health Working Group Report on Child Sexual Exploitation 2014; Pearce 2014).

Lord Laming's (2009) progress report emphasized the important role that schools and early years settings play in the early identification and intervention with vulnerable children. In June 2010, Eileen Munro was appointed by the government to undertake an independent review of child protection, in England, to address the central question 'what helps professionals make the best judgments they can to protect a vulnerable child'? The final Munro report was published in May 2011, and made a series of recommendations including a revision of the statutory child protection guidance which followed in 2013 (HM Government 2013). Key policy documents emphasize the importance of early identification and the provision of greater support to children living in vulnerable circumstances (Cleaver et al. 2011; HM Government and DH 2011). It is therefore important to consider the needs of the vulnerable school-aged child when addressing public health practice with the school aged population.

This chapter examines the concept of vulnerability and presents key evidence as to why vulnerable school-age children and young people present a significant public health concern. It explores how the adoption of a public health approach is crucial in ensuring that vulnerable school-age children are identified at an early stage and offered the services and support that they need to maximize their health and well-being and potentially to prevent child abuse and neglect.

VULNERABLE CHILDREN AND YOUNG PEOPLE – WHO ARE THEY?

There are many groups of school-age children and young people who may be vulnerable and in need. The phrase vulnerable child is used frequently in health- and social-care practice and has been used interchangeably with disadvantaged child, cause for concern, high dependency, high risk, or child in need. Vulnerable children have been defined as those disadvantaged 'children who would benefit from extra help from public agencies to optimize their life chances and for the risk of social exclusion to be averted' (Blair et al. 2010, p. 16). They include the following:

- Children looked after by local authorities
- Children in public care i.e. hospital or residential care
- Children and young people with disabilities and specific additional needs
- Children with mental health problems
- Children with poor school attendance or who are excluded from education
- Children and young people with behaviour problems
- Young carers
- Homeless young people
- Young offenders

- Children and young people showing signs of engaging in anti-social or criminal behaviour
- Young substance misusers
- Teenage parents
- Children of refugees or asylum seekers
- Children and young people who are separated
- Young people who are victims or at risk of child sexual exploitation
- Young people in secure settings
- Young people in the justice system (Blair et al. 2010; DeBell and Tomkins 2006; HM Government 2013)

The statutory guidance *Working Together to Safeguard Children* (HM Government 2013, p. 12) also stresses that 'professionals should be alert to the potential need for early help for a child who . . . is in a family circumstance presenting challenges for the child, such as substance abuse, adult mental health, domestic violence; and/or is showing early signs of abuse and/or neglect'.

Terminology is often used interchangeably and in some policy, such as the *Common Assessment Framework* (CAF) documentation vulnerable children are referred to as 'children with additional needs' or 'complex needs' (Department for Education [DfE] 2012). Vulnerable children include those at risk of experiencing inequalities, adverse economic situations and suffering poor outcomes (Reed 2012). The term also refers to those children with significant or complex needs which meet the threshold for statutory involvement and are in need of protection (HM Government 2013).

THE CONCEPT OF VULNERABILITY

THE ORIGINS OF THE CONCEPT OF VULNERABILITY

The conceptual basis of much research on vulnerability is seldom clearly specified, but links can often be traced to origins in psychology or sociology. Psychologists in particular have examined the links between vulnerability, stress and health (Selye 1973; Segerstrom and Miller, 2004). Lazarus's (1976) transactional model regards stress as a process in which the person is an active agent who can influence the impact of stress through behavioural, cognitive and emotional strategies. The adoption of such coping mechanisms can be important in reducing the effects of stress and can have a positive influence on health. Sociologists report vulnerability factors leading to ill-health, low self-esteem or an inability to cope particularly when triggered by distressing life events or major difficulties and when protective factors are weakened or absent.

Several authors regard vulnerability as a continuum which is dynamic and constantly changing (Rose and Killien 1983; Lessick et al. 1992; Appleton 1994; Rogers 1997; Purdy 2004; Sabates-Wheeler and Haddad, 2005). Individuals move in and out of vulnerability at various stages of the life trajectory. This appears to be dependent on a complex interplay of internal and external stress factors and coping ability (Rose and Killien 1983; Appleton 1994), with children and young people becoming more vulnerable at times of biological, psychological or social transition, such as during adolescence, school transition, teenage pregnancy and teenage parenthood (Rose and Killien 1983; Rich 1992; Rogers 1997; Dorsen 2010; Cameron 2014). Among the population of homeless adolescents, Dorsen (2010, p. 2825) describes vulnerability 'as the result of multiple layers of influence'. It is widely recognized that there are different levels or degrees of vulnerability. Early assessment of a child or young person's needs is essential to ensure that sources of stress for children within families are identified and appropriate interventions offered (HM Government 2013). Some children are more susceptible to the negative effects of stress than others and are therefore more likely to be vulnerable and suffer health and or social problems.

Vulnerability is often described in terms of, or used interchangeably with the concept of risk. This is a trend which is particularly evident in the mental health, child protection and social work research literature. Rose and Killien (1983, p. 61) have usefully differentiated between the concepts of vulnerability and risk, describing vulnerability as 'personal factors that interact with the environment to influence health' and risk as 'the presence of potentially stressful factors in a person's environment' hazardous to health. Risk factors 'are influences, occurring at any systemic level (i.e. individual, family, community, society), that threaten positive adaptational outcomes' (Waller 2001, p. 292). Rose and Killien (1983, p. 67) suggest that risk and vulnerability are inter-related and 'that one affects the other in a dynamic way' and that characteristics of both the individual and environment may contribute to health, illness and vulnerability.

Research evidence continually illustrates that vulnerability is a complex concept. It is widely acknowledged that a range of predisposing factors can contribute to vulnerability among school-aged children (The Mental Health Foundation 1999; Le Bon and Boddy 2010; Hall and Elliman 2003; Blair et al. 2010). It is often not difficult to explain the causes of or describe the circumstances of a child or young persons' vulnerability. Lists of vulnerability risk factors abound, particularly in relation to child abuse, yet accurately predicting from a research perspective which parents are at risk of abusing their children is fraught with difficulty and potential inaccuracies (Goddard et al. 1999; Sidebotham 2003; Peters and Barlow 2003). Indeed in their systematic review of models of analysing significant harm, Barlow et al. (2012, p. 10) found 'limited evidence about the effectiveness of the available tools'.

However, lists of vulnerability risk factors can be useful in assisting public health professionals to determine whether a child or young person *is* vulnerable, in need or in need of protection. For example, in Section 5 Chapter 2, Rees and Morley highlight risk factors for children suffering mental health problems. Likewise Hall and Elliman (2003, p. 69) describe the following risk factors for the development of psychological and mental health problems among children:

- Poor/inadequate parenting
- Families who are socially deprived
- Living in an inner city area
- Being a boy
- Children with learning difficulties and in young children, delayed language development or other communication difficulties
- Children with other health problems or development
- Adolescence rather than earlier childhood
- Being 'looked after'

Risk factors associated with the wider family and family relationships are also regarded as contributors to children and young people's emotional and mental health problems (Hall and Elliman 2003; Murphy and Fongay 2013; DH 2012a). These include the following:

- Marital discord/parental divorce/volatile relationships
- Family breakdown
- Family violence
- Physical, sexual and/or emotional abuse

- Parental mental health problems
- Lack of warmth/affection/parental coldness or irritability towards the child
- Poor parental supervision/neglect of the child

There is also evidence that a number of resilience factors can enable some vulnerable children to thrive in difficult circumstances and reduce the effects of any risk factors. These are sometimes referred to as a child's *resources* or *protective factors*. For example, many separated children, such as unaccompanied young asylum seekers demonstrate considerable resilience and determination to succeed. There is growing evidence that the act of becoming a young asylum seeker requires great capability and strength of character (Kohli and Mather 2003).

The Mental Health Foundation (1999) has outlined resilience factors for children suffering mental health problems in terms of child, family and environmental characteristics and these are summarized in Table 9.1. In terms of the wider social system, programmes building children's resilience through school-based health promotion and whole school approaches are increasingly recognized as important (Tennant et al. 2007; DH 2012b; Stewart and Wang 2012; NICE 2008, 2009). 'Evidence-based interventions to improve wellbeing and improve resilience include behavioural support, school-based counselling and parenting interventions and provision of evidence informed self-help materials based on the evidence that help guide children and young people as to self-help strategies. This may be particularly important in primary school' (DH 2012d, p. 6).

There are clearly a diverse range of adverse life experiences which may result in a child or young person being vulnerable. Vulnerability itself is a complex phenomenon although it is well recognized that there are particular sets of circumstances which may result in a child being more susceptible to vulnerability. In practice, where it is identified that early help would be of benefit, the child and young person's needs should be assessed on an individual basis, using tools such as the *Framework for the Assessment of Children in Need and their Families* (DH et al. 2000; White et al. 2009; Rose 1984; HM Government 2013), now generally known as the 'Assessment Framework', the *My World Triangle* as part of The Scottish Government's (2012)

Table 9.1 Resilience factors

In the child	In the family	In the environment
Being female	At least one good parent–child relationship	Wider supportive network
Higher intelligence	Affection	Good housing
Easy temperament when an infant	Supervision, authoritative discipline	High standard of living
Secure attachment	Support for education	High school morale and positive attitudes
Positive attitude, problem-solving approach	Supportive marriage/absence of severe discord	Schools with strong academic and non-academic opportunities
Good communication skills		Range of positive sport/leisure activities
Planner, belief in control		
Humour, religious faith		
Capacity to reflect		

Source: Mental Health Foundation, *Bright Futures – Promoting Children and Young People's*, London: The Mental Health Foundation, 1999. With permission.

policy *Getting it Right for Every Child,* the assessment framework in *Understanding the Needs of Children in Northern Ireland* (UNOCINI 2008), or the *CAF* (HM Government 2006). While it may not be difficult to explain the causes of or describe the circumstances of a child or young person's vulnerability, what remains the key challenge is identifying ways to prevent or reduce that vulnerability (DeBell and Tomkins 2006).

VULNERABLE CHILDREN AND THE WIDER SAFEGUARDING AGENDA

So, where does the vulnerable school-aged child fit into the wider safeguarding agenda? Put simply, safeguarding is 'an umbrella term (or spectrum) incorporating all aspects of work with vulnerable children, children in need and children who are suffering, or at risk of significant harm' (Appleton and Clemerson-Trew 2008, p. 265). Safeguarding mirrors the conceptual basis of vulnerability highlighted earlier in the chapter and can be used to illustrate the continuum of needs and children's potential vulnerability. Figure 9.1 illustrates the continuum of needs and services for all children and young people outlined in the CAF documentation. This continuum reflects the different levels of children's needs and vulnerability ranging from children with no additional needs to those with complex difficulties. In the case of Victoria Climbié who was at the acute end of the spectrum, at very high risk and in need of protection, the continuum illustrates the potential for such acute vulnerability to end tragically in death.

Vulnerable children and in particular, the concept of *children in need* has often been conceptualized as a continuum. This perspective emerged from *Messages from Research* (DH and Dartington Social Research Unit 1995), and the subsequent 'refocusing debate'. This debate drew attention to the need to identify ways in which more multi-agency work can be undertaken preventatively with children in need to prevent problems and family breakdown rather than focusing the majority of services on assessment and inquiry into child protection concerns. Viewing vulnerability as a continuum embraces a focus on early needs identification through holistic assessment and an increasing focus on agencies working together to meet the needs of the school-aged child.

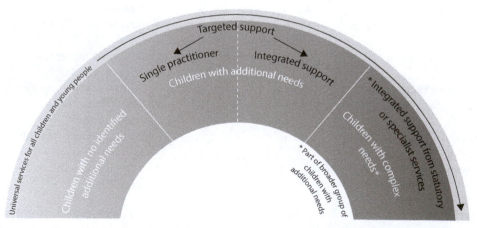

Figure 9.1 Children's needs and services.

SAFEGUARDING CHILDREN

It was *The Children Act (1989)* that first placed a duty on local authorities 'to safeguard and promote the welfare' of vulnerable children (Section 17). At its simplest, safeguarding is about 'keeping children safe from harm, such as illness, abuse or injury' (Children's Rights Director 2004, p. 3). This view was extended in the *Framework for the Assessment of Children in Need and their Families* (DH 2000, p. 5) to incorporate two elements: 'a duty to protect children from maltreatment' and a 'duty to prevent impairment'. This document, developed as part of the Quality Protects Programme and now, replaced by the most recent version of *Working Together to Safeguard Children* (HM Government 2013), provides a model to guide assessment of children and families' needs. It incorporates three key areas:

1. The child or young person's developmental needs
2. The capacity of parents to respond appropriately to those needs
3. The impact of wider family, community and environmental factors on parenting capacity and the child (HM Government 2013)

Widespread use of the Assessment Framework across several agencies, not just social work, has helped to support the broad shift in policy, from one where the central focus has been the identification of child abuse, to the adoption of a broader and more holistic view of children's wellbeing, with impairment identified in the context of a child's development and their current and long-term health and well-being outcomes, with the child very much at the centre (DH et al. 2000; Gray 2002; Cleaver et al. 2004; White et al. 2009; Parton 2014).

This point is illustrated further in the most recent *Working Together to Safeguard Children* (HM Government 2013) guidance which defines 'safeguarding and promoting the welfare of children' as

- Protecting children from maltreatment
- Preventing impairment of children's health or development
- Ensuring that children are growing up in circumstances consistent with the provision of safe and effective care
- Taking action to enable all children to have the best outcomes

(HM Government 2013, p. 7)

The new statutory guidance describes how effective safeguarding arrangements in local areas should be underpinned by two key principles:

- Safeguarding is everyone's responsibility: for services to be effective each professional and organisation should play their full part.
- A child-centred approach: for services to be effective they should be based on a clear understanding of the needs and views of children

(HM Government 2013, p. 8).

Vulnerable school-aged children are increasingly defined as those children where there are concerns about their welfare. Working Together to Safeguard Children (HM Government 2013) acknowledges that promoting children's welfare by providing help early as soon as a difficulty emerges is more effective than reacting later. Safeguarding includes the need for early interventions to proactively identify such children, who, with their families could benefit from early help services, professional input and support (Munro 2011). In schools and Further Education (FE) institutions 'safeguarding responsibilities extend to pupil health and safety, bullying, fulfilling specific statutory requirements together with other issues, for example, arrangements for meeting the medical needs of children with medical conditions, providing first aid, school security, drugs and substance misuse' (DH and DfES 2004, p. 159). The continuum of needs recognizes that there is a potential for any child to be vulnerable and in need of additional support and early intervention. 'The provision of early help services should form part of a continuum of help and support to respond to the different levels of need of individual children and families' (HM Government 2013, p. 14).

CHILD WELFARE CONCERNS, CHILDREN IN NEED AND SIGNIFICANT HARM

Since the mid-1990s there has been a change of focus for much of the work that in the late 1980s and early 1990s would have been considered to be child protection work. Since the publication of *Messages from Research* (DH and Dartington Social Research Unit 1995) and the subsequent 're-focusing debate' it has been widely accepted that child protection must be viewed as a broad concept including all elements of children in need and significant harm. This is further substantiated by the recent policy move to focus on Safeguarding Children.

When a referral is received by a local authority children's social care, a social worker should, within one day decide on the type of response that is needed.

This will include determining whether

- The child requires immediate protection and urgent action is required.
- The child is in need, and should be assessed under section 17 of the *Children Act 1989*.
- There is reasonable cause to suspect that the child is suffering, or likely to suffer, significant harm, and whether enquires must be made and the child assessed under section 47 of the *Children Act 1989*.
- Any services are required by the child and family and what type of services.
- Further specialist assessments are required in order to help the local authority to decide what further action to take

(HM Government 2013, p. 26).

Following, an initial multi-agency assessment, this may indicate that a child is a *child in need* as defined by Section 17 of the *Children Act 1989*.

A child is in need (Part III Sect 17(10)) if his/her vulnerability is such that

- …The child is unlikely to achieve or maintain, or to have the opportunity of achieving or maintaining, a reasonable standard of health or development without the provision of services by the local authority.
- …The child's health or development is likely to be significantly impaired, or further impaired, without the provision of such services, or
- …the child is disabled.

Working Together to Safeguard Children (HM Government 2013) outlines the role that Local Authority Children's Social Care has in coordinating multi-agency children in need assessments where these are outcomes focused. The purpose is to decide which services and support will provide improved welfare to the child and family. The joint agency care plan that is agreed with parents and school-aged child should include practical steps and 'set clear measurable outcomes for the child and expectations for the parents' (HM Government 2013, p. 30).

The care plan should also outline the nature of the support and services provided for the young person and his or her family, and should be clear about which professionals and agencies are providing the service. Some work may be carried out jointly. For example, a school nurse and child and adolescent mental health service (CAMHS) therapist might work with a teenager and their parents in dealing with disruptive school behaviour (Buckland et al. 2005). Such joint working falls within children in need legislation in *The Children Act* (1989 Sect 17). The types of interventions and services which may help school-aged children and their families will vary significantly depending on their particular needs and individual circumstances.

At the acute end of the spectrum, child protection is a key aspect of safeguarding and promoting welfare. In serious or chronic cases where it is suspected that a child is suffering or is likely to suffer significant harm as a result of abuse or neglect, child protection procedures will be needed. The local authority will hold a strategy discussion to decide, with other agencies, whether to initiate enquiries under Section 47 of the *Children Act 1989* (HM Government 2013).

When a child protection conference is convened, the conference members should consider if a child is at continuing risk of significant harm when determining whether the child should be the subject of a child protection plan. Significant harm is the threshold beyond which children in need are regarded as children needing protection and child protection procedures are initiated. A child is in need of protection where there is likely or actual significant harm or he/she is at risk. Yet it is worth noting that neither the *Children Act 1989* nor *Working Together to Safeguard Children* (HM Government 2013) gives a definitive interpretation of the concept of significant harm.

The 2010 version of *Working Together* specified that

> there are no absolute criteria on which to rely when judging what constitutes significant harm. Consideration of the severity of ill-treatment may include the degree and the extent of physical harm, the duration and frequency of abuse and neglect, the extent of premeditation, and the presence or degree of threat, coercion, sadism and bizarre or unusual elements. Each of these elements has been associated with more severe effects on the child, and/or relatively greater difficulty in helping the child overcome the adverse impact of the maltreatment. Sometimes a single traumatic event may constitute significant harm, e.g. a violent assault, suffocation or poisoning. More often, significant harm is a compilation of significant events, both acute and longstanding which interrupt, change or damage the child's physical and psychological development.

(HM Government 2010a, Sect 1(28), p. 36)

That version of the guidance (before it was slimmed down in 2013) highlighted research on sources of stress for children and families which may have an adverse effect on a child's health, development, and well-being which should be taken in to account when assessing children's and families' needs. These sources of stress include social exclusion, domestic violence, mental illness of a parent or carer, parental learning disability and drug and alcohol misuse (HM Government 2010a, Sect 9 (16–66) 262–283).

During the inter-agency child protection conference meeting the safety and welfare needs of the child(ren) should be considered though in an analysis of all relevant information, consideration is given to what action is required and whether a child protection plan should be formulated. 'It is the responsibility of the conference to make recommendations on how agencies work together to safeguard the child in future'. (HM Government 2013, p. 40)

Child protection is defined in the new *Working Together to Safeguard Children* guidance as 'part of safeguarding and promoting welfare. This refers to the activity that is undertaken to protect specific children who are suffering, or are likely to suffer, significant harm' (HM Government 2013, p. 85). Effective child protection is crucially important as part of wider work to safeguard and promote children's welfare.

WHY VULNERABLE CHILDREN AND YOUNG PEOPLE ARE A SIGNIFICANT PUBLIC HEALTH ISSUE

THE EVIDENCE BASE

The key argument for viewing vulnerable school-age children as a public health issue is the negative impact that unidentified or unresolved vulnerability has on the individual child, school community and society (DH 2004). While at one level the United Kingdom government has acknowledged the impact on children's public health of wider social influences such as poverty, unemployment, homelessness and social exclusion (Marmot et al. 2010; Department for Work and Pensions [DfWP] 2012), the publication of *Healthy Lives Healthy People: Our Strategy for Public Health in England* (HM Government 2010b, p. 2) has produced political tensions by focussing attention on a model of early intervention and prevention that seeks to focus on individual responsibility for healthy choices and local community accountability to address needs.

These tensions between the social and the individual causes of vulnerability are exacerbated by the current climate of welfare austerity and hardship for families (Morris and Featherstone 2010; Reed 2012). Identifying problems early or intervening to reduce their initial occurrence or subsequent escalation has been central to the coalition Government's agenda (Allen 2011; Tickell 2011). This focus on prevention and early intervention is reiterated in a number of reports including: *Social Justice: Transforming Lives* (DfWP 2012), C4EO's (2011) report *Grasping the Nettle: Early Intervention for Children, Families and Communities* and Eileen Munro (2011) in her independent review of child protection in England in which she emphasized that early identification and the provision of help and support to vulnerable children and their families is vitally important in contemporary child protection practice.

There is an increasing body of evidence illustrating the adverse consequences for children of a failure to address their needs effectively, linked to negative outcomes in terms of their later social and emotional development (Macdonald 2001; Turner et al. 2006; Bair-Merritt et al. 2006; Davies and Ward 2012). Children living in poverty are more likely to suffer disadvantage including emotional and behavioural problems than are children from more affluent backgrounds (Seccombe 2000; Reed 2012). These children and young people are more likely to experience peer relationship difficulties, suffer depression, social withdrawal, have low self-esteem and self-confidence and do badly at school (Seccombe 2000). The inter-generational cycle of disadvantage is well reported, with children born into disadvantaged or at-risk families, having a greater chance of experiencing similar difficulties to their parents (Social Exclusion Unit 2004).

Cleaver et al. (2011) have, for example, explored parenting capacity and the extent to which 'the toxic trio' of parental mental illness, problem drug and alcohol misuse and domestic violence, as well as parental learning disability can impact on children's safety and parents' ability to meet their children's needs. Recent research conducted by The Centre for Social Justice also illustrates many vulnerable children and young people 'slipping through the net' and being denied appropriate support and care from some statutory services (Eastman 2014, p. 10).

In terms of child protection, the relationships between child rearing problems such as harsh discipline and subsequent childhood behaviour problems, later delinquency, conduct disorders and criminality are well recognized (Farrington 1995; Buchannan 1996; Hosking and Walsh 2005). Farrington (1995) and Silverman et al. (1996) have highlighted the potential long-term mental health difficulties and behavioural problems associated with physical abuse and neglect in childhood. More recently, the US National Survey of Child and Adolescent Well-Being (NSCAW 2012) reported that more than half of young people aged between 11 and 17 years who were reported for child abuse and neglect were also at risk for an emotional or behavioural difficulty (ACF/OPRE 2012b).

Research evidence suggests that there may be a correlation between adult mental health problems, a history of past child abuse or neglect and the child's subsequent ability to parent successfully (Gibbons et al. 1995). Child abuse can result in a child developing poor self-esteem or an inability to form social relationships (Mullen et al. 1996; Bifulco and Moran, 1998). In chronic situations, this may result in childhood behaviour and conduct disorders, anti-social behaviour, substance misuse and later delinquency, violence and imprisonment (Farrington 1995; Kazemian et al. 2011). These are all risk factors.

Child abuse 'is a major contributor to mental health conditions throughout the life course, including depression, anxiety, post-traumatic stress disorder, psychosis and suicide' (DH 2012a p. 23). A recent NSPCC prevalence study (Radford et al. 2011, p. 13) examining the impact of child maltreatment across a sample of 2,275 young people aged 11–17 years and 1,761 young adults aged 18–24 years living in the United Kingdom 'found that all forms of abuse in childhood were generally associated with poorer mental health and elevated delinquent behaviour'.

Lang et al. (2006) reported an association between maternal childhood maltreatment and increased anxiety, depression and illicit drug use during pregnancy and the early post-natal period. Research by Draper et al. (2008) found long-term effects of childhood physical and sexual abuse on health, with study participants at greater risk of both poor physical and mental health. In addition, the Adverse Childhood Experiences (ACE) studies have demonstrated strong links between abuse and neglect in childhood and later health problems, including cardiovascular disease, asthma, diabetes, lung and liver disease and obesity (Felitti et al. 1998; Felitti and Anda 2009; Shin and Miller; Widom et al. 2012).

The influential report *Messages from Research* (DH and Dartington Social Research Unit, 1995) described the long-term negative impacts on children of living in low-warmth/high-criticism environments as far more damaging than a single incident of over-chastisement. Roberts (1996) and Hagell (1998) have also reported the negative effects of children growing up in such environments. An absence of family support mechanisms during childhood may result in high levels of aggression and risk-taking behaviour in later adulthood (Roberts 1996). Reder and Duncan (1999) suggest that a further effect of childhood distress can be seen in family life-cycles, particularly at times of transition such as birth, unemployment or during bereavement. Unresolved childhood vulnerability might affect an adult such that their ability to adjust to changes may be prolonged, or result in relationship difficulties or psychological problems.

Domestic violence can also have a damaging effect on childhood outcomes (Osofsky 2003; Smith Stover 2005; Hosking and Walsh 2005; DH 2006; Holt et al. 2008; Meltzer et al. 2009; Brandon et al. 2012; WHO 2013) and, in particular, children and young people's socio-emotional and behavioural development (Edleson 1999). In Brandon et al.'s (2012) analysis of Serious Case Reviews (SCRS) from 2009 to 2011 nearly two thirds of the cases involved domestic violence. The NSPCC's study of child maltreatment (Radford et al. 2011, p. 11) reported that '12 per cent of under 11s [and] 17.5 per cent of 11–17s and 23.7 per cent of 18–24s had been exposed to domestic violence between adults in their homes during childhood'. The risks to children are further increased when domestic violence occurs alongside parental mental illness or drug and alcohol misuse (Cleaver et al. 1999; Brandon et al. 2012). Violent childhood experiences have also been linked with intimate partner violence in later adulthood relationships (Coid et al. 2001; Whitfield et al. 2003; Afifi et al. 2009).

There is also considerable evidence that certain groups of vulnerable children are more likely to suffer negative outcomes. For example, looked after children and young people are at increased risk of mental health problems (Meltzer et al. 2003; Stanley et al. 2005; Sempik et al. 2008; Hutchinson 2011). They often have poor access to health services and are in greater need of effective health promotion interventions, particularly in relation to emotional wellbeing (DH 2002; Scottish Executive 2004; Fleming et al. 2005; Simpson 2006; DfE and DH 2015; NICE 2010). Likewise there are strong links between being a young carer who lacks adequate professional support and experiencing impaired psychosocial development and low school achievement (Hall and Elliman 2003; DfES 2006; Roberts et al. 2008). 'Almost a third of young carers have serious educational problems or have dropped out of school, with nearly all reporting missing school when the person they care for is having difficulties' (DfES 2006).

While it is clearly well documented that chronic poverty and social disadvantage do increase the likelihood of negative outcomes for children and young people, it is important to stress that not all children growing up in such vulnerable family households will experience poor outcomes (Seccombe 2000, 2002; Barrett 2003). In spite of considerable adversity, young people can and do rise above past abuse, poverty, loss and relationship problems to become mature and well balanced individuals (Bifulco and Moran 1998; Heller et al. 1999; Matsen et al. 1999). Waller (2001, p. 292) has argued that 'resilience is not the absence of vulnerability' but the presence of protective factors and a 'positive adaptation in response to adversity'.

While there is considerable interest in the concept of resilience, as yet there is little understanding of the factors that make some children more resilient than others to child abuse and neglect (Macdonald 2001, NCH/Action for Children 2007). Shaffer (2012) has suggested that in the under-fives a number of protective factors including positive attachment, intelligence, self-esteem, humour, emotion regulation and independence may contribute to an abused child's resilience (Child Welfare Information Gateway 2013).

STATISTICS

Statistical evidence pertaining to the health needs of the school-age population provides further evidence that vulnerable school-age children are a significant public health issue.

VULNERABLE CHILDREN

In 2005, the DfES estimated that of 11 million children in England, 3 million are vulnerable and living in disadvantaged circumstances, with between 300,000 and 400,000 being *children in need* and known to social services at any one time (HM Government 2006b). This is only the second time that the Government has offered an official estimate of the numbers of vulnerable children in England and this is likely to be a significant underestimate of the actual numbers of vulnerable children.

In a more recent study *In the Eye of the Storm*, the research set out to identify the number of families in Britain with children who are vulnerable to the recession and public spending cuts by using a range of different definitions of vulnerability (Reed 2012). The study drew on a number of data sources to make their calculations and defined 'vulnerable families' as those with a least five vulnerability indicators including: poor quality/overcrowded housing, worklessness, maternal mental health problems, parental illness/disability, no qualifications, low income and material deprivation (Reed 2012). In 2008, it was estimated that there were 130,000 vulnerable families with five or more risk indicators, with 310,000 children living in those families. However, if wider definitions of vulnerability are used, 'by 2008 there were nearly three times as many children (885,000) living in families with four or more vulnerabilities, nearly 2 million children living in families with three or more vulnerabilities and 3.9 million with two or more'.

It is also estimated that the numbers of vulnerable families will increase, with the number of children living in extremely vulnerable families (having 6–7 risk factors) estimated to nearly double by 2015, to 96,000 (Reed 2012). As the report stresses, the findings of this work highlight the need to protect children from the impact of adverse economic conditions and 'for particular consideration to be given to the needs of the most vulnerable children and families in our society' (Reed 2012, p. 6).

There are other sources of data which provide an indicator of the extent of children's vulnerability. Regular statistics are collated in the United Kingdom on the numbers of children in need, children looked after and the number of children referred to children's social care and subject to child protection procedures and plans.

CHILDREN IN NEED

Since February 2000, the Office of National Statistics has collected data from local authorities on the numbers of children in need through the Children in Need (CiN) census. The CiN census publishes data on the numbers of children referred to and assessed by children's social services. Data is published at the local authority, regional and national levels on the characteristics of children in need, including numbers of children by type of disability.

At 31 March 2014, it was calculated that there were 378,600 children in need in England, showing an increase of 2.5% from the previous year (DfE 2013).

CHILDREN LOOKED AFTER

Some children and young people who are referred to social services go on to be 'looked after'. Children 'looked after' are a sub-group of children in need and include the following:

- Children accommodated under a voluntary agreement with their parents
- Children who are the subject of an interim or full care order
- Children compulsorily accommodated, including children on remand, those detained or committed for trial and children subject to short-term emergency orders or police protection (DfE 2013a,b)

In England on 31 March 2013, it was estimated that 68,110 children were being looked after by local authorities, 'an increase of 2 per cent compared to 31 March 2012 and an increase of 12 per cent compared to 31 March 2009' (DfE 2013, p. 1). Table 9.2 illustrates the numbers of children looked after by local authorities from 2009 to 2013, by age, gender, category of need and ethnic origin. This table illustrates the increasing numbers of children looked after by local authorities, with only a slight fall in 2011. 'The number of looked after children has increased steadily each year and is now higher than at any point since 1985' (DfE 2013, p. 2). The majority of children 42, 480 (62%) are looked after due to abuse or neglect. The largest category of placement for children looked after on 31 March 2013 was foster care, accounting for 75% of all placements with the numbers of children in foster care placements having increased by 16% since 2009 (DfE 2013a, p. 4). 'The majority of children looked after at 31 March 2013 (74 per cent) are from a White British background. The ethnic breakdown for children looked after has varied little since 2009' (DfE 2013, p. 2).

Table 9.2 Children and young people who were the subject of a Child Protection Plan (CPP) by category of abuse at 31 March

Category of abuse	2009	2010	2011	2012	2013
Neglect	15,800	17,300	18,600	18,220	17,930
Physical abuse	4,400	5,000	4,800	4,690	4,670
Sexual abuse	2,000	2,300	2,400	2,220	2,030
Emotional abuse	9,100	10,800	11,400	12,330	13,640
Multiple	2,900	3,700	5,500	5,390	4,870
Total	34,100	39,100	42,700	42,850	43,140

Sources: Department for Education, *Characteristics of Children in Need in England, 2012–13*, Final, London: DfE, 2013. Table D4 Available online at http://www.gov.uk/government/publications/characteristics-of-children-in-need-in-england-2012-to-2013; NSPCC, *Children Subject to Child Protection plans – England 2009–2013*, London: NSPCC, 2012. http://www.nspcc.org.uk/Inform/research/statistics/child_protection_register_statistics_wda48723.html.

Note: The figures for 2010–2013 relate to the initial category of abuse assigned to the child protection plan rather than the most recent category of abuse.
- Figures may not add due to rounding.
- These figures include unborn children.

Statistics are also collated on vulnerable unaccompanied asylum seeking children. These statistics illustrate that in England at 31 March 2013, there were 1860 unaccompanied asylum seeking children looked after by local authorities, a decrease of 15% on 2012, with 87% being boys and the majority being accommodated in Inner and Outer London (DfE 2013).

Since 2009/2010 outcome data has also been reported for looked after children (DfE 2012) including educational attainment outcomes, special educational needs (SEN), school exclusions, developmental assessments of children below 5 years of age, health (including immunization, dental health and annual health assessment), education and employment after year 11, offending and substance misuse (DfE 2012). The children looked after (CLA) data is also matched to the National Pupil Database.

CHILD PROTECTION STATISTICS

Annual child protection statistics have been collated in England since 1998 on the numbers of children registered on local authority child protection registers, and those subsequently de-registered. These statistics are based on the responses from all local authorities with children's social care service responsibilities. Statistics are available for all four countries of the United Kingdom (see the NSPCC Inform website). In England, annual figures are maintained on the numbers of children referred to and assessed by children's social care services, the numbers of Section 47 enquires and child protection conferences and the numbers of children subject to a child protection plan. The DfE (2013, p. 7–8) reported that in 2013 there were '60,100 initial child protection conferences, up from 56,200 in 2012. These include both conferences resulting from section 47 enquiries and children on existing plans who transferred local authorities'.

Table 9.2 illustrates the number of children who were subject to a child protection plan (CPP) and the category of abuse when the initial protection plan commenced. The *multiple* category indicates that there was more than one abuse category that was relevant to the child protection plan.

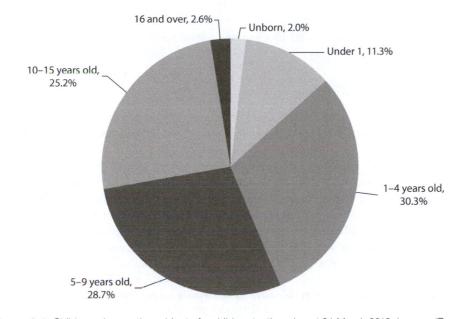

Figure 9.2 Children who are the subject of a child protection plan at 31 March 2013, by age. (From Department for Education, *Statistical First Release*, SFR45/2013, Figure 6, Table A5, p. 17. London: DfE, 2013).

At 31 March 2013 there were 43,140 children and young people who were the subject of a child protection plan in England, 'a small increase of 1.1% on 2012' when the number of children was 42,900 (DfE 2013, p. 8). Of these, 50.3% were male, 47.6% female and 910 2.1% were unborn/unknown gender (DfE 2013). While the largest age group of children subject to a child protection plan was 1–4 years (30.3%), those aged 5 and over accounted for just over 56% of the children (DfE 2013; Figure 9.2).

Since 2009, there has been a year on year rise in the number of children with a child protection plan. As in previous years, 'neglect is the most common initial category of abuse under which children became the subject of a plan, in 41.0% of cases. Emotional abuse is the next most common category (31.7%) followed by physical abuse (11.7%)' (DfE 2013, p. 8).

While these statistics do go some way to demonstrating that vulnerable children are a significant public health issue, caution needs to be maintained when interpreting these figures as they are not a record of all vulnerable children, only vulnerable children who have been officially recognized by children's social care services (Corby 1990). Gilbert et al. (2008) in a review of the evidence of the extent of child maltreatment in high income countries, suggest that official statistics represent less than one tenth of the actual population incidence. They contend that official statistics also provide no indication of the frequency or severity of children's abuse (Gilbert et al. 2008). However, official reports provide some indications as to the demand for child protection services and the burden of dealing with child maltreatment upon other agencies.

Another source of statistical evidence on child abuse and neglect are research studies measuring the prevalence of child maltreatment in a particular sample (Corby 1990). Prevalence rates refer to the proportion of a defined population who have been maltreated during a specified time period such childhood (Cawson 2002; Creighton 2004; Radford et al. 2011). Such research studies, may identify child maltreatment which has not been reported to child protection agencies. Indeed a recent NSPCC report (Radford et al. 2011) estimated that as many as 5% of children under 11 years and 13.4% of those aged 11–17 years may have experienced serious maltreatment by their parents.

SERIOUS CASE REVIEWS

SCRs conducted by Local Safeguarding Children Boards (LSCBs) provide further evidence of children's vulnerability and the extent of serious injury and death. These reviews are conducted, 'for every case where abuse or neglect is known or suspected and either: a child dies; or a child is seriously harmed and there are concerns about how organisations or professionals worked together to safeguard the child' (HM Government 2013, p. 66). The SCR process examines the involvement of agencies and professionals in the child's case to determine if lessons can be learned about the ways in which professionals and organizations work together to safeguard and promote children's welfare (HM Government 2013). There is a requirement for final reports of reports of SCRs to be published (HM Government 2013) and since November 2013, a national repository of published case review reports has been set up through a collaboration between the NSPCC and the Association of Independent LSCB Chairs. Yet until April 2014, no publicly available data was collated on the numbers of SCRS conducted across the United Kingdom. Data from House of Commons Hansard (2014) indicates that of 302 SCR reports commissioned between 10 June 2010 and 31 March 2014, only 114 have been published, 136 are still in progress and others have not been published due to outstanding investigations or serious issues relating to the welfare of the children in the cases (NSPCC 2014). The NSPCC has produced a series of helpful thematic briefings (on topics such as adolescence and disguised compliance) which highlight good practice and learning from some of the SCRs and are published on the NSPCC website.

In terms of obtaining statistics on child deaths, the NSPCC report uses indicators from child homicides (drawing on data from police-recorded crime figures), child mortality statistics and numbers of child suicides (NSPCC 2014). A conservative estimate by the NSPCC suggests that at least 'one child is killed at the hands of another person every week in England and Wales' (NSPCC 2014, p. 4). A recent study of learning from SCRs estimated that there are about 85 (0.77 per 100,000 children aged 0–17) 'violent and maltreatment-related' child deaths per year (Brandon et al. 2012, p. 1). Acquiring accurate child homicide figures for the United Kingdom is problematic (Creighton 1995, 2000; NSPCC 2014) as data is not currently recorded for all fatal child abuse. Mortality statistics 'reflect the number of child deaths where another person was responsible or responsibility is not determined, though their accuracy depends on consistent recording practices' (NSPCC 2014, p. 22). In the United Kingdom in 2012, 'there were 164 suicides of 15 to 19 year olds' (NSPCC 2014, p. 24). The NSPCC (2014, p. 24) note 'information on the number of suicides is an important measure of the safety of children and young people. Suicide may often be the result of a combination of other factors, such as abuse, neglect, family problems or mental health issues'.

While these figures do not offer a complete picture of the numbers of vulnerable children, they do go some way towards demonstrating that the care of vulnerable children is a significant public health issue affecting the child population. There is clearly a continued need for more accurate and reliable official government statistics, in particular around child homicide and SCRs to provide a more effective review of child protection trends. *Working Together to Safeguard Children* guidance (HM Government 2013) has laid down requirements for LSCBs to publish final SCR reports and their response to the review's findings. National overview reports have been commissioned every 2 years, with the most recent focussing on Case Management Reviews being published in Northern Ireland in January 2013 (Devaney et al. 2013) and in

England a review of neglect in SCRs being published in March 2013 (Brandon et al. 2013). In addition, since 1 April 2008 it became compulsory from LSCBs to have Child Death Overview Panels (CDOPs) to review and analyse information on the deaths of any child (under 18 years) resident in the LSCB area (HM Government 2013, see Chapter 5).

What existing figures do highlight, however, is the importance of identifying and working with the vulnerable school-aged population.

WORKING WITH VULNERABLE CHILDREN – ADOPTING A PUBLIC HEALTH APPROACH

A WHOLE POPULATION APPROACH

The need for improved identification of vulnerable children through services that are developed from sound public health principles and a whole population approach was outlined in the *Every Child Matters: Change for Children* programme (DfES 2004), the *National Service Framework for Children, Young People and Maternity Services* (DH and DfES 2004). It is reinforced in the recent Chief Medical Officer (CMO) report (DH 2013) *Our Children Deserve Better.* In the United Kingdom, the Child Health Promotion Programme that is implemented in schools primarily through the work of school nurses working in conjunction with teachers and other professionals, is important because it provides the gateway to identifying school-age children who are experiencing health difficulties and through the provision of a range of services including universal plus and universal partnership plus and beyond (Hall and Elliman 2003; DH 2009; DH and PHE 2010). Such collective approaches are required, at least initially, to ensure that those vulnerable children who are in need (and their families) are reached and offered appropriate services. Individual work with a child and family would only take place once a health, development or learning need has been identified, and this individual focus is not reached unless the whole population has access to such universal provision.

Contemporary concerns about the state of children's health and a widening of health inequalities has focussed attention on intervening early to give every child the best start in life (Marmot et al. 2010; DH 2013). The identification of vulnerable school-aged children must therefore be addressed through public health values and concepts, principally universal access to public health professionals through the Healthy Child Programme (Hall and Elliman 2003; DH 2009), The Healthy Child Programme includes the whole population and should ensure targeted follow-up of children who are missing from school and who, (potentially with their families), do not initially take up interventions or services offered and/or who are hard to reach.

SAFEGUARDING IS EVERYONE'S RESPONSIBILITY

Section 11 of the *Children Act 2004* first emphasized that *'safeguarding children is everyone's responsibility'* (HM Government 2005, p. 9) and placed a statutory duty on key agencies to safeguard and promote the welfare of children. This document has now been replaced by the most recent version of *Working Together to Safeguard Children* (HM Government 2013, p. 8), which states as one of its two core principles that *'safeguarding is everyone's responsibility'*. All public health practitioners working with school-aged children and their families have an important public health role in the identification of vulnerable children and children at risk of significant harm. All staff working in universal services with school-aged children must be trained and knowledgeable about the signs of child abuse and neglect. *Working Together to Safeguard*

Children states that staff 'should receive training to ensure they attain the competences appropriate to their role and follow the relevant professional guidance' (HM Government 2013, p. 50). This is mirrored in other statutory child protection guidance across Wales, Scotland and Northern Ireland. The nationally recognized Intercollegiate Guidance (RCPCH 2014) *Safeguarding Children and Young People: Roles and Competences for Health-Care Staff* has just been revised and this document outlines the competencies (including knowledge, skill, attitudes and values) required of all staff in relation to safeguarding children and young people, including education and training requirements.

All organizations providing children's services must ensure that they have clear policies and procedures for employees about how to safeguard and promote the welfare of children (HM Government 2013). In addition, many public health professionals will have access to practice guidance and child protection supervision, and both single agency training through their organizations and multi-agency training through the LSCB, which will aid in the identification of vulnerable children and young people. Public health professionals will also be supported by named and designated child protection professionals and by designated looked after professionals.

Interestingly the new truncated version of *Working Together to Safeguard Children* (HM Government 2013) has removed much of the detail about the role of individual health professionals who work with children in terms of safeguarding and identifying their welfare needs. Instead the guidance acknowledges that a range of health-care staff play a very important role in child safeguarding. This is detailed as 'understanding risk factors, communicating effectively with children and families, liaising with other agencies, assessing needs and capacity, responding to those needs and contributing to multi-agency assessments and reviews' (HM Government 2013, p. 50). Health professionals should also refer to the clinical guideline *When to Suspect Child Maltreatment* (NICE 2009). The latter provides very useful and practical guidance dividing the alerting features of child maltreatment into when to *consider* or when to *suspect* child abuse and neglect. A new public health.

Staff are also encouraged to adhere to their Local Safeguarding Children's Board (LSCB) procedures and be familiar with the new public health approach to violence prevention for England *Protecting People, Promoting Health* (DH 2012b). Furthermore, public health practitioners should be using the *Assessment Framework* (DH et al. 2000; HM Government 2013) as a structure for guiding their early assessments of vulnerable school-aged children and their families. Indeed many Health-Care Trusts have adapted their health records to incorporate this Framework and use the CAF locally to avoid duplication and repeated assessments of children and families. It is also likely that many public health practitioners will take on the *lead professional role* with some children who have significant or complex needs, to avoid overlap of and reduce inconsistency of services (DfES 2005).

PUBLIC HEALTH ACTIVITY

Thinking back to the continuum discussed earlier in the chapter (see Figure 9.1) a public health professional may be involved in reviewing health needs across the school-age population as part of base-line preventative work or early intervention work to identify vulnerable children. For example, a school nurse should review each school-age child's record at school entry to review the health status of all children. This is important in order to identify health needs early, particularly physical, emotional and social needs so that appropriate interventions can be delivered so that children are better able to reach their potential (DH 2012). The publication of the Child and Maternal (CHiMat) Health Intelligence Network's initial version of the Children and Young People's Health Outcomes Framework, provides important local information for the future planning and commissioning of services for children and young people to improve their health outcomes which will be extremely useful for all public health professionals (see http:// fingertips.phe.org.uk/profile/cyphof).

HELP IDENTIFY AREAS OF NEED

Public health professionals may, following an initial or targeted school-aged child and family health assessment, identify one or more health needs that require short-term targeted intervention. For example, if a child has been bullied a school nurse could work with the teacher, child and parents to increase the child's self-esteem and ability to socialize appropriately with his/her peers. Research evidence has shown that children who are bullied are at risk of low academic achievement, absence from school and school drop-out (Rothon et al. 2011). The school nurse or other professional may also be responsible for referring a school child and his or her family for specialist assessment and input, depending on the nature of the needs identified, possibly involving Children and Adolescent Mental Health services (CAMHs). Further along the continuum, at the medium intervention level, programmes promoting the development of parenting skills may be offered through Extended School projects or Children's Centres, sometime involving psychologists, for parents whose children have additional needs such as behavioural problems.

Still further along the continuum, day or respite care for children might be offered and the provision of services for 'looked after children' (*Children Act 1989*, Part III Sect 22(1) p. 17). At the far end of the continuum, high level intervention will include children who are at continuing risk of significant harm and are the subject of a formal child protection plan and receiving integrated support from statutory and specialist services, with a minority of cases culminating in court proceedings (HM Government 2013). It is important to recognize that multi-agency assessment and care planning could occur at any point along the vulnerability continuum, reinforced through the implementation of the Assessment Framework (DH et al. 2000; HM Government 2013) and the CAF (HM Government 2006).

Shared and joint assessment is a central feature of public health working. Research evidence indicates that inter-agency collaboration during the assessment process of a child referred to Local Authorities Social Care departments has improved since the implementation of the National Assessment Framework (Cleaver et al. 2004), but more recent evidence suggests that further efforts are needed to improve joint working which varies in its nature and quality throughout the country (Francis et al. 2006). This is important in the area of safeguarding and the care of vulnerable children as Lord Laming's Inquiry Report continually exposed the danger to children's health of poor assessments and recording, inadequate information sharing (IS) systems among professionals and a lack of inter-agency working (DH and Home Office 2003). The IS Index in England that held information on all children aged under 18 years, that enabled practitioners working with children to find and contact each other easily and to share information about vulnerable children going missing from school and/or need services and support was closed in 2010, following extensive criticisms of the database around security and privacy issues.

Government policy increasingly recognizes the importance of supporting school-aged children and their families, while emphasizing the need for professionals and their organizations, families, schools, local communities and the voluntary sector to work more closely together to improve outcomes for children and young people (DoH 2013; HM Government 2013). Effective partnership working with both children and their parents and between professionals and their agencies is an essential part of public health working to ensure the needs of vulnerable children are met at all stages of the safeguarding continuum (Appleton et al. 2013; HM Government 2013). It is generally recognized that improved outcomes are more likely to be achieved if the child or young person is focused on as a whole, if services are child-centred and if people work together (HM Government 2013). This latter point was a critical finding of Lord Laming's Inquiry Report:

> I am in no doubt that effective support for children and families cannot be achieved by a single agency acting alone. It depends on a number of agencies working well together. It is a multi-disciplinary task

(Department of Health and Home Office 2003, para. 1.30)

This theme of partnership is continually emphasized in recent policy with calls for better linkages across health services, more effective inter-agency strategies and professionals to work openly together and with children, young people and their families, for example through the 'GP Champions for Youth Health Project' (HM Government 2013; DH 2013). Furthermore, through each area's Children and Young People's Plan (CYPP) there is an increasing emphasis on integrated planning and commissioning to deliver needs based services relevant to vulnerable children in the local community.

CONCLUSION

This chapter has explored the concept of vulnerability, its conceptual origins and its relevance to children and young people's health. It has examined how vulnerable children and young people fit into the UK's wider safeguarding policy agenda and has presented key research evidence as to why vulnerable school-age children present a significant public health concern. Public health practitioners must be knowledgeable about the new legislative and multi-agency practice issues surrounding safeguarding children work and the implications this has for their practice.

The key argument for viewing vulnerable school-age children as a public health issue is the negative impact that unidentified or unresolved vulnerability has on the individual child/young person, their family, school community and wider society. It remains to be seen

KEY POINTS

- The care of vulnerable children and young people is a significant public health issue affecting the child population.
- The term vulnerable child is used to describe children with additional health and social care needs, who would benefit from additional support and services.
- Vulnerability in childhood is inextricably linked to disadvantage and health inequalities.
- A diverse range of adverse life experiences may result in a child or young person being vulnerable. Yet there is also evidence that a number of resilience factors can enable some vulnerable children to thrive in difficult circumstances and reduce the effects of risk factors on health.
- The key argument for viewing vulnerable school-age children as a public health issue is the negative impact that unidentified or unresolved vulnerability has on the individual child, school community and society.
- A public health approach ensures that potentially vulnerable children and young people are identified early and secure the support that they and their families need to promote their health and well-being, to enable them to reach their full potential and to prevent child abuse and neglect.

whether the legislative changes and service developments do start to have an impact on improving the health outcomes of children and young people across the United Kingdom. However, the adoption of a public health approach is important in ensuring that vulnerable school-age children are identified early and offered the services and support that they and their families need to promote their health and well-being. This is crucial to enable these children to reach their full potential and to reduce the risk factors that contribute to child abuse and neglect.

REFERENCES

Administration for Children and Families, Office of Planning, Research and Evaluation (ACF/OPRE). (2012) National Survey of Child and Adolescent Well-Being. Child Well-Being Spotlight. Adolescents with a history of maltreatment have unique service needs that may affect their transition to adulthood. Retrieved from http://www.acf.hhs.gov/sites/default/files/opre/youth_spotlight_v7.pdf. Accessed 18 September 2015.

Afifi T, Macmilan H, Cox B, Asmundson G. (2009) Mental health correlates of intimate partner violence in marital relationships in a nationally representative sample of males and females. *Journal of Interpersonal Violence* 24: 1398–1418.

Allen G. (2011) *Early Intervention: The Next Steps*. London: Cabinet Office.

Appleton JV. (1994) The concept of vulnerability in relation to child protection: Health visitors' perceptions. *Journal of Advanced Nursing* 20: 1132–1140.

Appleton JV. (2014) Editorial: Child sexual exploitation, victimisation and vulnerability. *Child Abuse Review* 23(3): 155–158. DOI: 10.1002/car.2269.

Appleton JV, Clemerson-Trew J. (2008) Safeguarding children: A public health imperative. In: Cowley S, ed. *Public Health in Policy and Practice. A Sourcebook for Health Visitors and Community Nurses*. 2nd ed. London: Baillière Tindall Limited.

Appleton JV, Coombes L, Terletski E. (2013) The use of sociograms to explore collaboration in child protection conferences. *Children and Youth Services Review* 35(12): 2140–2146.

Bair-Merritt MH, Blackston M, Feudtner C. (2006) Physical health outcomes of childhood exposure to intimate partner violence: A systematic review. *Pediatrics* 117: e278–e290.

Barlow J, Fisher J, Jones D. (2012) *Systematic Review of Models of Analyzing Significant Harm: Research Report DFE-RR199*. London: Department for Education.

Barrett H. (2003) *Parenting Programmes for Families at Risk. A Source Book*. London: National Family and Parenting Institute.

Barnardos. (2012) *Cutting Them Free, How is the UK Progressing in Protecting Its Children from Sexual Exploitation*. Ilford Essex: Barnardos.

Berelowitz S, Clifton J, Firmin C, et al. (2013) *'If Only Someone Had Listened' Office of the Children's Commissioner's Inquiry into Child Sexual Exploitation in Gangs and Groups Final Report*. London: OCC.

Bifulco A, Moran P. (1998) *Wednesday's Child*. London: Routledge.

Blair M, Stewart-Brown S, Waterston T, Crowther R. (2010) *Child Public Health*. Oxford, UK: Oxford University Press.

Brandon M, Sidebotham P, Bailey S, et al. (2012) *New Learning from Serious Case Reviews: A Two Year Report for 2009-2011*. London: Department for Education.

Brandon M, Bailey S, Belderson P, Larsson B. (2013) *Neglect and Serious Case Reviews*. London: University of East Anglia/NSPCC.

Buchannan A. (1996) *Cycles of Child Maltreatment: Facts, Fallacies and Interventions.* Chichester, UK: Wiley.

Buckland L, Rose J, Greaves C. (2005) New roles for school nurses: Preventing exclusion. *Community Practitioner* 78(1): 16–19.

Cameron J. (2014) Vulnerability in pregnancy and childbirth. In: Watson G, Rodwell S, eds. *Safeguarding and Protecting Children, Young People and Families. A Guide for Nurses and Midwives.* London: Sage Publications Limited.

Cawson P. (2002) *Child Maltreatment on the Family: The Experience of National Sample of Young People.* London: NSPCC.

Centre for Excellence and Outcomes in Children and Young People's Services. (2011) *Grasping the Nettle: Early Intervention for Children, Families and Communities.* London: C4EO.

Child Welfare Information Gateway. (2013) *Long-Term Consequences of Child Abuse and Neglect.* Washington, DC: US Department of Health and Human Services, Children's Bureau. https://www.childwelfare.gov/pubs/factsheets/sp_long_ term_consequences.cfm. Accessed 18 September 2015.

Children's Rights Director (2004) *Safe from Harm: Children's Views Report.* London: Commission for Social Care Inspection.

Cleaver H, Unell I, Aldgate J. (1999) *Children's Needs – Parental Capacity: The Impact of Parental Mental Illness, Problem Alcohol and Drug Use, and Domestic Violence on Children's Development.* London: The Stationery Office.

Cleaver H, Unell I, Aldgate J. (2011) *Children's Needs – Parenting Capacity: Child Abuse Parental Mental Illness, Learning Disability, Substance Misuse, and Domestic Violence.* 2nd ed. London: The Stationery Office.

Cleaver H, Walker S, Meadows P. (2004) *Assessing Children's Needs and Circumstances. The Impact of the Assessment Framework.* London: Jessica Kingsley Publishers.

The Children Act. (2004) Chapter 31. London: The Stationery Office.

Coid J, Petruckevitch A, Feder G, et al. (2001) Relation between childhood sexual and physical abuse and risk of revictimization in women: A cross-sectional survey. *The Lancet* 358: 450–454.

Corby B. (1990) Making use of child protection statistics. *Children and Society* 4(3): 304–314.

Creighton SJ. (1995) Fatal child abuse – how preventable is it? *Child Abuse Review* 4: 318–328.

Creighton SJ. (2000) Government statistic on child deaths where abuse or neglect may be implicated. In: NSPCC, ed. *NSPCC Out of Sight.* London: NSPCC; 31–33.

Creighton S. (2004) *Prevalence and Incidence of Child Abuse: International Comparisons.* London: NSPCC Inform.

Davies C, Ward H. (2012) *Safeguarding Children Across Services: Messages from Research.* London: Jessica Kingsley.

DeBell D, Tomkins A. (2006) *Discovering the Future of School Nursing: The Evidence Base.* London: McMillan-Scott.

Department for Education. (2013a) *Statistical First Release. Children Looked After in England (Including Adoption and Care Leavers) Year Ending 31 March 2013. SFR 36/2013.* London: Department for Education.

Department for Education. (2013b) *Statistical First Release. Characteristics of Children in Need in England, 2012–13. SFR45/2013.* London: Department for Education.

Department for Education. (2013c) *Statistical First Release. Characteristics of Children in Need in England, 2012–13. SFR45/2013.* London: Department for Education.

Department for Education. (2013d) *Statistical First Release. Children Looked After in England (Including Adoption and Care Leavers) Year Ending 31 March 2013. SFR 36/2013.* London: Department for Education.

Department of Health. (2000) *Framework for the Assessment of Children in Need and Their Families*. London: Department of Health.

Department of Health. (2002) *Promoting the Health of Looked After Children*. London: The Stationery Office.

Department of Health. (2004) *The Chief Nursing Officer's Review of the Nursing, Midwifery and Health Visiting Contribution to Vulnerable Children and Young People*. London: Department of Health.

Department of Health. (2006) *Responding to Domestic Abuse. A Handbook for Health Professionals*. London: Department of Health.

Department of Health. (2009) *Healthy Child Programme: Pregnancy and the First 5 Years of Life*. London: Department of Health.

Department of Health. (2012a) *Report of the Children and Young People's Health Outcomes Forum – Mental Health Sub-Group*. London: Department of Health.

Department of Health. (2012b) *Protecting People, Promoting Health. A Public Health Approach to Violence Prevention for England*. Liverpool, UK: North West Public Health Observatory/ Department of Health.

Department of Health. (2012c) *Getting It Right for Children, Young People and Families. Maximising the Contribution of the School Nursing Team: Vision and Call to Action*. London: Department of Health.

Department of Health. (2012d) *Public Health Outcomes Framework 2013–2016*. London: Department of Health.

Department of Health. (2013) *Our Children Deserve Better: Prevention Pays. Annual Report of the Chief Medical Officer 2012*. London: Department of Health.

Department of Health/Dartington Social Research Unit. (1995) *Child Protection: Messages from Research*. London: HMSO.

Department of Health, Department for Education and Employment and the Home Office. (2000) *Framework for the Assessment of Children in Need and Their Families*. London: HMSO.

Department of Health and DfES. (2004) *National Service Framework for Children Young People and Maternity Services: Core Standards*. London: Department of Health.

Department of Health/Health Working Group Report on Child Sexual Exploitation. (2014) *An Independent Group Chaired by the Department of Health Focusing on: Improving the Outcomes for Children by Promoting Effective Engagement of Health Services and Staff*. London: Department of Health.

Department of Health and Home Office. (2003) *The Victoria Climbié Inquiry. Report of an Inquiry by Lord Laming*. London: HMSO.

Department of Health and Public Health England. (2014) *A Framework for Personalised Care and Population Health for Nurses, Midwives, Health Visitors and Allied Health Professionals: Caring for Populations Across the Lifecourse*. London: PHE.

Department for Work and Pensions. (2012) *Social Justice: Transforming Lives*. London: Department for Work and Pensions.

Devaney J, Bunting L, Hayes D, Lazenbatt A. (2013) *Translating Learning into Action: An Overview of Learning Arising from Case Management Reviews in Northern Ireland 2003-2008*. Belfast, UK: Department for Health, Social Services and Public Safety.

DfES, Department of Health. (2015) *Promoting the Health and Well-Being of Looked-After Children. Statutory Guidance for Local Authorities, Clinical Commissioning Groups and NHS England*. London: DfE and DH. DFE-0010502015.

DfES, Department of Health and Home Office. (2003) *Keeping Children Safe. The Government's Response to the Victoria Climbié Inquiry Report and Joint Chief Inspectors' Report Safeguarding Children.* London: The Stationery Office.

DfES. (2003) *Every Child Matters.* London: The Stationery Office.

DfES. (2004) *Every Child Matters: Change for Children.* Nottingham, UK: DfES Publications.

DfES. (2005) *Lead Professional Good Practice Guidance.* London: DfES.

DfES. (2006) *Targeted Youth Support: Young Carers After School Club.* www.everychild matters. gov.uk/resourcesandpractice (accessed on September 2006).

Dorsen C. (2010) Vulnerability in homeless adolescents: Concept analysis. *Journal of Advanced Nursing* 66(12): 2819–2827. DOI: 10.1111/j.1365-2648.2010.05375.x.

Draper B, Pfaff JJ, Pirkis J, et al. (2008) Long-term effects of childhood abuse on the quality of life and health of older people: Results from the depression and early prevention of suicide in general practice project. *Journal of the American Geriatrics Society* 56(2): 262–271.

Eastman A. (2014) *Enough Is Enough. A Report on Child Protection and Mental Health Services for Children and Young People.* London: The Centre for Social Justice.

Edleson JL. (1999) Children's witnessing of adult domestic violence. *Journal of Interpersonal Violence* 14: 839–970.

Farrington D. (1995) Intensive health visiting and the prevention of juvenile crime. *Health Visitor* 68(3): 100–102.

Felitti V, Anda RF, Nordenberg D, et al. (1998) Relationship of childhood abuse and household dysfunction to many of the leading causes of death in adults. *American Journal of Preventive Medicine* 14: 245–258.

Felitti V, Anda R. (2009) The relationship of adverse childhood experiences to adult medical disease, psychiatric disorders, and sexual behavior: Implications for healthcare. In Lanius R, Vermetten E, Pain C (eds), *The Impact of Early Life trauma on Health and Disease: The Hidden Epidemic.* Cambridge, UK: Cambridge University Press.

Fleming P, Bamford DR, McCaughley N. (2005) An exploration of the health and social wellbeing needs of looked after young people – A multi-method approach. *Journal of Interprofessional Care* 19(1): 35–49.

Francis, J, McGhee J, Mordaunt E. (2006) *Protecting Children in Scotland: An Investigation of Risk Assessment and Inter-Agency Collaboration in the Use of Child Protection Orders.* Edinburgh, UK: School of Social and Political Studies, University of Edinburgh.

Gibbons J, Conroy S, Bell C. (1995) *Operating the Child Protection System: A Study of Child Protection Practices in English Local Authorities.* London: HMSO.

Gilbert R, Spatz Widom C, Browne K, et al. (2009) Burden and consequences of child maltreatment in high-income countries. *The Lancet.* 373(9658): 68–81.

Goddard CR, Saunders BJ, Stanley JR. (1999) Structured risk assessment procedures: Instruments of abuse? *Child Abuse Review* 8: 251–263.

Gray J. (2002) Chapter 8: National policy on the assessment of children in need and their families. In: Ward H, Rose W, eds. *Approaches to Needs Assessment in Children's Services.* London: Jessica Kingsley Publishers.

Hagell A. (1998) *Dangerous Care. Reviewing the Risks to Children from Their Carers.* London: Policy Studies Institute and the Bridge Child Care Development Service.

Hall DMB, Elliman D. (2003) *Health for All Children.* 4th ed. Oxford, UK: Oxford University Press.

Heller SS, Larrieu JA, D'Imperio R, Boris NW. (1999) Research on resilience to child maltreatment: Empirical considerations. *Child Abuse & Neglect* 23(4): 321–338.

HM Government. (2005) *Statutory Guidance on Making Arrangements to Safeguard and Promote the Welfare of Children Under Section 11 of the Children Act 2004.* London: DfES.

HM Government. (2006) *The Common Assessment Framework for Children and Young People: Practitioners' Guide. Integrated Working to Improve Outcomes for Children And Young People.* Nottingham, UK: DfES Publications.

HM Government. (2006b) *Reaching Out: An Action Plan on Social Exclusion.* London: Cabinet Office.

HM Government. (2010a) *Working Together to Safeguard Children: A Guide to Inter-Agency Working to Safeguard and Promote the Welfare of Children.* London: Department for Children, Schools and Families (archived).

HM Government. (2010b) *Reaching Out: An Action Plan on Social Exclusion.* London: Cabinet Office.

HM Government. (2013) *Working Together to Safeguard Children: A Guide to Inter-Agency Working to Safeguard and Promote the Welfare of Children.* London: Department for Education.

HM Government and Department of Health. (2011) *No Health Without Mental Health: A Cross-Government Mental Health Outcomes Strategy for People of All Ages.* London: Department of Health.

Hosking G, Walsh I. (2005) *The WAVE Report 2005. Violence and What to Do About It.* Croydon, UK: Wave Trust.

Holt S, Buckley H, Whelan S. (2008) The impact of exposure to domestic violence on children and young people: A review of the literature. *Child Abuse & Neglect.* 32: 797–810.

House of Commons Hansard. (3 April 2014) Written answers. Children: Protection. Column 786W. www.parliament.uk.

Hutchinson D. (2011) *Looked After Children Talking to ChildLine.* London: NSPCC.

Kazemian L, Spatz Widom, C, Farrington DP. (2011) A prospective examination of the relationship between childhood neglect and juvenile delinquency in the Cambridge study in delinquent development. *International Journal of Child, Youth and Family Studies* 2(1 & 2): 65–82.

Kohli R, Mather R. (2003) Promoting psychosocial well-being in unaccompanied asylum seeking young people in the United Kingdom. *Child and Family Social Work* 8: 201–212.

Lang AJ, Rodgers CS, Lebeck MM. (2006) Associations between maternal childhood maltreatment and psychopathology and aggression during pregnancy and postpartum. *Child Abuse & Neglect* 30: 17–25.

Lazarus R. (1976) *Patterns of Adjustment.* New York: McGraw-Hill.

Le Bon G, Boddy J. (2010) Working with vulnerable primary school aged children and their families: A review of the Australian literature on key principles, issues, and community level approaches. *Journal of Social Inclusion* 1(1): 53–73.

Lessick M, Woodring BC, Naber S, Halstead L. (1992) Vulnerability: A conceptual model applied to perinatal and neonatal nursing. *Journal of Perinatal Nursing* 6(3): 1–14.

Macdonald G. (2001) *Effective Interventions for Child Abuse and Neglect. An Evidence-Based Approach to Planning and Evaluating Interventions.* Chichester, UK: John Wiley & Sons Ltd.

Marmot M, Allen J, Goldblatt P, et al. (2010) *Fair Society, Healthy Lives: The Marmot Review – Strategic Review of Health Inequalities in England Post-2010.* London: UCL. http://www.marmotreview.org.

Matsen A, Hubbard J, Gest S, et al. (1999) Competence in the context of adversity: Pathways to resilience and maladaptation from childhood to late adolescence. *Development and Psychopathology* 11: 143–169.

Meltzer H, Gatward R, Corbin T, et al. (2003) *The Mental Health of Young People Looked After by Local Authorities in England.* London: The Stationery Office.

Meltzer H, Doos L, Vostanis P, et al. (2009) The mental health of children who witness domestic violence. *Child and Family Social Work* 14(4): 491–501.

Mental Health Foundation. (1999) *Bright Futures – Promoting Children and Young People's Mental Health.* London: The Mental Health Foundation.

Morris K, Featherstone B. (2010) Investing in children, regulating parents, thinking family: A decade of tensions and contradictions. *Social Policy and Society* 9(4): 557–566.

Mullen PE, Martin JL, Anderson JC, et al. (1996) The long-term impact of the physical, emotional and sexual abuse of children: A community study. *Child Abuse & Neglect* 20(1): 7–21.

Munro E. (2011) *The Munro Review of Child Protection: Final Report. A Child-Centred System. Cm 8062.* London: Department of Education.

Murphy M, Fonagy P. (2013) Chapter 10: Mental health problems in children and young people. In: Department of Health/Chief Medical Officer, ed. *Our Children Deserve Better: Prevention Pays: Annual Report of the Chief Medical Officer 2012.* London: Department of Health.

National Institute for Health and Clinical Effectiveness. (2008) *Social and Emotional Wellbeing in Primary Education (PH12).* London: NICE.

National Institute for Health and Clinical Effectiveness. (2009) *Social and Emotional Wellbeing in Secondary Education (PH20).* London: NICE.

National Institute for Health and Clinical Effectiveness. (2010) *Looked-After Children and Young People.* London: NICE.

NCH/Action for Children. (2007) *Literature Review: Resilience in Children and Young People.* London: NCH – The Bridge Child Care Development Service/Action for Children.

NSCAW, (2012) Casanueva C, Wilson E, Smith K, Dolan M et al. (2012) *NSCAW II Wave 2 Report: Child Well-Being.* OPRE Report #2012-38. Washington DC: Office of Planning, Research and Evaluation, Administration for Children and Families, US Department of Health and Human Services.

Osofsky J. (2003) Prevalence of children's exposure to domestic violence and child maltreatment: Implications for prevention and intervention. *Clinical Child and Family Psychology Review* 6: 161–170.

Parton N. (2014) *The Politics of Child Protection: Contemporary Developments and Future Directions.* Basingstoke, UK: Palgrave Macmillan.

Pearce J. (2014) 'What's going on' to safeguard children and young people from child sexual exploitation: A review of local safeguarding children boards' work to protect children from sexual exploitation. *Child Abuse Review* 23(3): 159–170.

Peters R, Barlow J. (2003) Systematic review of instruments designed to predict child maltreatment during the antenatal and postnatal periods. *Child Abuse Review* 12(6): 416–439.

Purdy IB. (2004) Vulnerable: A concept analysis. *Nursing Forum* 39(4): 25–39.

Radford L, Corral S, Bradley C, et al. (2011) Child abuse and neglect in the UK today. London: NSPCC.

Reder P, Duncan S. (1999) *Lost Innocents. A Follow-Up Study of Fatal Child Abuse.* London: Routledge.

Reed H. (2012) *In the Eye of the Storm: Britain's Forgotten Children and Families. A Research Report for Action for Children, the Children's Society and NSPCC.* London: Landman Economics.

Rich OJ. (1992) Vulnerability of homeless pregnant and parenting adolescents. *The Journal of Perinatal and Neo-natal Nursing* 6(3): 37–46.

Roberts I. (1996) Family support and the health of children. *Children and Society* 10: 217–224.

Roberts D, Bernard M, Misca G, Head E. (2008) *Experiences of Children and Young People Caring for a Parent with a Mental Health Problem.* Research briefing 24. London: SCIE.

Rogers AC. (1997) Vulnerability, health and health care. *Journal of Advanced Nursing* 26: 65–72.

Rose MH. (1984) The concepts of coping and vulnerability as applied to children with chronic conditions. *Issues in Comprehensive Pediatric Nursing* 7(4/5): 177–186.

Rose MH, Killien M. (1983) Risk and vulnerability: A case for differentiation . . . between personal and environmental factors that influence health and development. *Advances in Nursing Science* 5(3): 60–73.

Rothon C, Head J, Klineberg E, et al. (2011) Can social support protect bullied adolescents from adverse outcomes? A prospective study on the effects of bullying on the educational achievement and mental health of adolescents at secondary schools in East London. *Journal of Adolescence* 34: 579–588.

Royal College of Paediatrics and Child Health. (2014) *Safeguarding Children and Young People Roles and Competences for Health Care Staff. Intercollegiate Guidance.* 2nd ed. London: Royal College of Paediatrics and Child Health.

Scottish Executive. (2004) *Forgotten Children.* Edinburgh, UK: The Stationery Office.

Scottish Government. (2012) *A Guide to Getting It Right for Every Child.* www.scotland.gov.uk/Resource/0045/00458341.pdf. Accessed 13 February 2015.

Seccombe K. (2000) Families in poverty in the 1990s: Trends, causes, consequences, and lessons learned. *Journal of Marriage and the Family* 62(4): 1094–1113.

Seccombe K. (2002) "Beating the odds" versus "changing the odds": Poverty, resilience and family policy. *Journal of Marriage and the Family* 64(2): 384–394.

Segerstrom SC, Miller GE. (2004) Psychological Stress and the human immune system: A meta-analytic study of 30 years of inquiry. *Psychological Bulletin* 130(4): 601–630.

Selye H. (1973) The evolution of the stress concept. *American Scientist* 61: 692–699.

Sempik J, Ward H, Darker I. (2008) Emotional and behavioural difficulties of children and young people at entry to care. *Clinical Child Psychology and Psychiatry* 13(2): 221–233.

Shaffer A. (2012) *Child Maltreatment: Risk and Resilience in Ages Birth to 5. CW360°.* Retrieved from https://www.cehd.umn.edu/ssw/cascw/attributes/PDF/publications/CW360- CEED_Winter2012.pdf.

Shin SH, Miller DP. (2012) A longitudinal examination of childhood maltreatment and adolescent obesity: Results from the National Longitudinal Study of Adolescent Health (AddHealth) Study. *Child Abuse and Neglect* 36(2): 84–89.

Sidebotham P. (2003) Red skies, risk factors and early indicators. *Child Abuse Review* 12(1): 41–45.

Silverman A, Reinherz HZ, Giaconia RM. (1996) The long-term sequelae of child and adolescent abuse: A longitudinal study. *Child Abuse & Neglect* 20(8): 709–723.

Simpson A. (2006) Promoting the health of looked after children in Scotland. *Community Practitioner* 79(7): 217–220.

Smith Stover C. (2005) Domestic violence research what have we learned and where do we go from here? *Journal of Interpersonal Violence* 20(4): 448–454.

Social Exclusion Unit. (2004) *Breaking the Cycle – Taking Stock of Progress and Priorities for the Future.* London: Social Exclusion Unit.

Stanley N, Riordan D, Alaszewski H. (2005) The mental health of looked after children: Matching response to need. *Health and Social Care in the Community* 13(3): 239–248.

Stewart D, Wang D. (2012) Building resilience through school-based health promotion: A systematic review. *International Journal of Mental Health Promotion* 14(4): 207–218.

Tennant R, Goens C, Barlow J, et al. (2007) A systematic review of reviews of interventions to promote mental health and prevent mental health problems in children and young people. *Journal of Public Mental Health* 6(1): 25–32. ISSN 1746–5729.

Tickell C. (2011) *The Early Years: Foundations for Life, Health and Learning—An Independent Report on the Early Years Foundation Stage to Her Majesty's Government.* London: Department for Education.

Turner H, Finkelhor D, Ormrod DR. (2006) The effect of lifetime victimization on the mental health of children and adolescents. *Social Science & Medicine* 62(1): 13–27.

UNOCINI. (2008) *Understanding the Needs of Children in Northern Ireland*. UNOCINI Guidance. Belfast, UK: Department of Health, Social Services and Public Safety, Northern Ireland.

Waller MA. (2001) Resilience in the ecosystemic context: Evolution of the concept. *American Journal of Orthopsychiatry* 71(3): 290–297.

White S, Hall C, Peckover S. (2009) The descriptive tyranny of the common assessment framework: Technologies of categorization and professional practice in child welfare. *British Journal of Social Work* 39(7): 1197–1217.

Whitfield CL, Anda RF, Dube SR, Felitti VJ. (2003) Violent childhood experiences and the risk of intimate partner violence in adults: Assessment in a large health maintenance organization. *Journal of Interpersonal Violence* 18: 166–185.

Widom CS, Czaja SJ, Bentley T, Johnson MS. (2012) A prospective investigation of physical health outcomes in abused and neglected children: New findings from a 30-year follow-up. *American Journal of Public Health* 102(6): 1124–1144.

World Health Organization. (2013) *European Report on Preventing Child Maltreatment*. Copenhagen Denmark: WHO.

5

HEALTH QUESTIONS

Child and adolescent mental health

DAWN REES AND DINAH MORLEY

10

INTRODUCTION

Children are living beings – more living than grown-up people who have built shells of habit around themselves. Therefore it is absolutely necessary for their mental health and development that they should not have mere schools for their lessons, but a world whose guiding spirit is personal love.

Rabindranath Tagore (1933), Calcutta India, Nobel Literature Laureate, 1914

Why does mental health and emotional well-being matter? It is because our children are the adults of the future. That might imply that childhood is merely a necessary pathway to adulthood. It is much more than that. Children are people in their own right and exist in their own time. They make an enormous contribution to the development of the culture and meaning of their own generation and the meaning that parents and society attribute to them (Reder et al. 1993). They have a right to positive advantage which should enhance every aspect of their childhood, and their rights are enshrined in the United Nations Convention on the Rights of the Child 1989.

The context of positive parent – child relationships that scaffold the child's experience of life is an important one. The quality of close and loving personal relationships enhance the sense of self. Over time – and particularly in the early years when the child's sense of belonging, their place in the world, and whether they can rely on someone to be there for them – those close, caring relationships represent a metaphor for the world in a child's eyes. Developing and maintaining continuity and predictability in close, caring relationships enhances positive mental health. Mental health is strengthened by a sense of belonging and, over time, helps the development of a mature and sophisticated range of responses and behaviours. A mix of positive and negative experiences, mediated by good relationships, make it more likely that children will understand themselves and others, and positively manage the inevitable disappointments and discontinuities in life – as well as experiencing fun and enjoyment. Thus being *mentally healthy* can be said to be a key prerequisite for health and success in all aspects of life.

> Children's mental health is the strength and capacity of children's minds to grow and develop with confidence and enjoyment. It consists of the capacity to learn from experience and to overcome difficulty and adversity. It's about physical and emotional well-being, the ability to live a full and creative life and the flexibility to give and take in friendships and relationships. Children who are mentally healthy are not saints or models of perfection but ordinary children making the most of their abilities and opportunities.

(YoungMinds 2006)

However, achieving positive mental health and well-being requires more than simply being cared for. It is enhanced by genetic, family, social and educational circumstances. Children who experience positive responses, where adults nurture and allow them to take reasonable risks, to make friends, and are allowed to make mistakes are more likely to have good mental health, as are children who are not bullied, who do not experience discrimination, who are able to learn and achieve at school. These characteristics are underpinned by a delicate set of interrelated factors and relationships that support the growing child's sense of self, development of empathy for others and physical and emotional resilience.

Being unhappy, isolated or unable to understand what is happening in your life, and experiencing this from a base where adults in the world do not appreciate your stage of development and/or the reasons why you are feeling that way, sets a child on an uncertain trajectory into adulthood and at greater risk of mental health problems (Health Advisory Service 1995; Audit Commission 1999; Meltzer et al. 2005).

The *tabula rasa* of infancy and childhood is profoundly affected by influences on neurological, emotional and cognitive development. Healthy and uninterrupted development is crucial in terms of positive future outcomes. For this reason, the combined impact of social and economic disadvantage can have a profound impact on the developing child, but what appears to mediate these potentially negative factors is the child's self-esteem.

Rutter (2001) argues that poverty makes parenting more difficult, and McLoyd (2001) observes that poverty and economic loss affect parental ability to provide the consistent support and involvement children need. More recently, Field's (2011) report set out the impact of poverty on children's life-chances and social mobility and laid the path for reform in the provision of education in the Foundation Years in the United Kingdom.

THE EVIDENCE

Recent research has built on that of earlier attachment theorists such as Ainsworth et al. (1978); Rutter (1975); Cicchetti and Barnett (1991); Fonagy et al. (1991); Lyons-Ruth (1996); Murray (1992) and reinforces the importance of positive nurturing relationships in infancy and their effect on the development of neurological pathways in the brain (Schaffer 1996; Elliot 1999; Balbernie 2001).

'There is increasing evidence that social interactive experiences affect cognitive growth and entail mutual cooperation of a participant child and a sensitive adult' (Schaffer 1996, p. 99). Infancy sees the most rapid rate of brain growth and hardwiring of neurons, and this process is significantly affected by the child's experience of emotional and physical environments and in particular its experience of nurture.

Childhood is characterized by periods of transition and reorganization, and living in a positive environment (not necessarily a financially rich one) makes all the difference to children's perceptions of themselves. This in turn impacts upon their ability to understand others (Vygotskyi 1978; Fonagy et al. 1991; Schaffer 1996; Balbernie 2001) and to develop sharing and reciprocal relationships with peers. During adolescence we see a further period of significant brain activity. As the frontal cortex develops, there is increased myelination (development of the neuronal sheaths) which speeds up cognitive abilities (Blakemore and Frith 2005). As it develops, the brain is affected by the environment and experience.

The confusion, irrationality and mood changes of adolescence are part of normal development as the brain grows. However, although adolescence is often characterized by these features, discontinuities in development and/or injury can have a significant impact on how a child progresses through the teenage years. Of particular interest is recent research that indicates a correlation between acquired brain injury (ABI), mood changes and involvement in the criminal justice system (Williams et al. 2010).

In 2013, the Harvard Center on the Developing Child produced a number of papers which review the knowledge on childhood brain development and the presence of what is termed toxic stress. There is a response which

can occur when a child experiences strong, frequent, and/or prolonged adversity – such as physical or emotional abuse, chronic neglect, caregiver substance abuse or mental illness, exposure to violence, and/or the accumulated burdens of family economic hardship – without adequate adult support.' This results in 'prolonged activation of the stress response systems (which) can disrupt the development of brain architecture and other organ systems, and increase the risk for stress-related disease and cognitive impairment, well into the adult years.*

The effects of toxic stress can be prevented or reversed where there are supportive relationships with caregivers in early life (see 'Rutter's inoculation theory' below).

CHILDREN'S LIVES TODAY

The lives of twenty-first century children today are complex. They experience the ordinary challenges of childhood which are understood by their parents. But then they also experience the pressures of social media, complex peer relationships, the expectation of achievement and excellence in the school environment, concerns about body image, the potential of gang involvement and sexual exploitation, increasing levels of youth unemployment, homelessness, family breakdown, serial monogamy/blended families and loss of confidence in higher education as a pathway to success. Most of these were neither experienced nor are understood by their parents. These pressures are evident in the increasing prevalence of self-harm among young people.

* http://developingchild.harvard.edu/topics/science_of_early_childhood/toxic_stress_response/.

In studying the social determinants of health and wellbeing of children and young people, the *Health Behaviour of School-Aged Children Survey* (2012) examined the evidence and found that about 30% of English young people reported sub-clinical poor mental health – at least once a week they felt unhappy or 'down'. The study also found that gender inequalities in mental health begin to emerge in adolescence.*

It is important to consider what biological and psychosocial factors *influence* rather than *cause* mental disorder and illness. In addition, it is valuable to re-examine the ways in which children and young people can be helped; the accessibility and utility of local services, and to listen to what children and young people say and how they want people to help.

Equally it is important to reconsider the way in which services are provided so that they have utility, respond to the realities of children's lives and are more accessible and friendly to children and young people.

POLICY CONTEXT

Achieving the good mental health of all children is a key component in the future health of the population and a key factor in the cohesion of families, communities and cultures. *No Health Without Mental Health: A Cross-Government Mental Health Outcomes Strategy for People of All Ages* (2012), supported by *Closing the Gap: Priorities for Essential Change in Mental Health* (2013). These strategies emphasized for the first time the importance of taking a life-course approach to planning and providing mental health services for the population of England and Wales. They included the premise that children and young people's mental health and wellbeing is the foundation on which the health of a population's future adults is built. It also emphasized the importance of positive peri-natal mental health for the developing infant, binding the health care the mother receives to the future health and wellbeing of her baby. A public health approach, combined with other key policy agendas including:

- Targeted support for the most vulnerable families
- Restorative justice in the youth offending population
- A Public Health Outcomes Framework which aims to improve the wider determinants of health, to reduce health inequalities

All these agendas have the potential to protect people's health and to reduce the numbers living with ill health. All have the potential to play a critical role in informing local planning and the delivery of a continuum of services that support positive early childhood experiences and parenting, and respond to the needs of vulnerable young people.

These principles build on earlier initiatives such as *Every Child Matters* (Chief Secretary to the Treasury 2003); *The National Service Framework (NSF) for Children, Young People and Maternity Services* (Department of Health 1999) which were policies brought in under the previous (Labour) administration. In addition, Sure Start, the development of children's centres, and more recent programmes such as *The Healthy Child Programme* (2009) have been key initiatives. Sure Start aims to increase the proportion of young children from birth to age 5 years with normal levels of personal, social and emotional development and to increase the proportion of young children with satisfactory speech and language development at age 2. The *Birth to Three Matters (2005a)* framework supports children in their earliest years, and reinforces the

---

* http://www.hbsc.org/publications/factsheets/pdfs/Mental%20Health/WHO-HBSC%202009-2010%20 International%20Report%20Key%20Findings%20-%20Mental%20Health.pdf.

significance of positive early experiences. Understanding the importance of early childhood development is crucial in that it underpins the components of child and adolescent mental health generally that are discussed in this and other chapters.

The shift of the responsibility in 2013 for delivering public health from the Department of Health to Local Authorities in England and Wales *Healthy Lives, Healthy People* (2010) has determined a leading role for Local Authorities in providing information, advice and services to prevent illness. It also provides assistance to help people minimize any risks to health. The Chief Medical Officer's report *Our Children Deserve Better* (2012*)* highlighted the assertion that early events affect health and wellbeing in later life and that children are the most disadvantaged group with 26.9% of children and young people in or at risk of poverty compared with 22.6% of the total population. Therefore preventative work – a public health approach – is a fundamental need.

The *Health and Social Care Act 2012* introduced a new framework for the NHS in 2013 and set up a national commissioning body – the NHS Commissioning Board – with commissioning responsibility devolved to local Clinical Commissioning Groups and with responsibility to Local Authorities for assessing need and for commissioning and monitoring the effectiveness of health and social care delivery. Multi agency Health and Wellbeing Boards were also set up with a statutory duty to deliver integrated planning and delivery and to incorporate Public Health in planning and delivery.

The Chief Medical Officer's second report* published in 2014 made a clear economic case for promoting early intervention and prevention, integrated planning and delivery, workforce development and refreshed prevalence data. The National Health Service (NHS) England child and adolescent mental health services (CAMHS) Tier 4[†] Report also set out the challenges of delivering comprehensive and age-appropriate inpatient care for children and young people, noting a rise in the number of admissions to adult mental health inpatient care. The Health Select Committee's CAMHS[‡] report, published in 2014 found a deterioration in access to and the range of interventions appropriate for children and young people with mental health problems and emphasized the impact of the recession on families living in poverty and the reduction in CAMHS.

DEFINITIONS OF MENTAL HEALTH IN CHILDREN AND YOUNG PEOPLE

When we talk about mental health we frequently refer to mental illness. But only about 10% of the child population has a mental disorder or illness (Meltzer et al. 2005). We all have the capacity for good mental health, and for most people, when they feel sad or anxious, agitated or mildly depressed, the help and support of friends and families means these symptoms are short-lived.

It is quite clear that there are social as well as health determinants which affect mental health. So what are the components of mental health that we need to build into everyday life to make us mentally healthy?

Mental health is defined as

- The ability to develop psychologically, emotionally, intellectually and spiritually
- The ability to initiate, develop and sustain mutually satisfying personal relationships

---

* Report of the Chief Medical Officer II, 2014.
† https://www.gov.uk/government/uploads/system/uploads/attachment_data/file/351629/Annual_report_2013_1.pdf.
‡ www.england.nhs.uk/wp-content/uploads/2014/07/camhs-tier-4-rep.pdf.

- The ability to become aware of others and to empathize with them
- The ability to use psychological distress as a developmental process so that it does not hinder or impair further development (Health Advisory Service,1995)

To attain good mental health, every child needs an environment where he/she can develop as a rounded, secure person with personal resources that will allow the child to recover safely from bad and sad experiences and to learn and mature from those experiences.

The ability to initiate and sustain good relationships is essential to a fulfilling life, and this includes the capacity to be aware of what is going on in the minds and lives of others. Fonagy (Hartley-Brewer 2005, p. 7) describes this as being able to mentalize or to empathize with others. Failure to acquire this capacity appears to have serious consequences for actions later in life. This is generally referred to as a *theory of mind* (Vygotski 1978; Astington et al. 1988; Schaffer 1996). Put very simply – if you cannot imagine the impact you have on someone and how he or she feels, you are unlikely to be able to modify your own behaviour appropriately in relation to the other person.

It is in all our interests to ensure that the children and young people with whom we come in contact and for whom we have responsibilities are supported to achieve optimum mental health. *Children's mental health is everybody's business and everyone's responsibility.*

Mental health problems, disorders and illnesses of children and young people have only been recognized comparatively recently (Kurtz 1996). Much of the pathological behaviour in children has, in the past, been attributed to inherited defect or lack of control and framed in terms of bad behaviour, illness, madness or social aberration, and sometimes described as irredeemable or requiring punishment. It is only more recently that more flexible levels of public and independent service have been developed across agencies working with children and their families in response to the range of possible presentations and the acknowledged importance of co-ordinated approaches to assessment and treatment for mental disorders in childhood and adolescence.

It is still true to say that many people find it uncomfortable to acknowledge the fact that children can have mental disorders. The Office for National Statistics (ONS) data (Meltzer et al. 2003) asserting that 1 in 10 children between the ages of 5 and 16 years have mental disorders surprised and shocked the public. This public reaction contrasts starkly with other data that shows many adults with mental disorders had their problems diagnosed in childhood but that those problems were often not recognized early enough and sometimes failed to receive appropriate treatment. Young people with mental health problems, even when those difficulties are marked, are also often not recognized as being in difficulty. In two separate studies in Scotland, teachers and general practitioners (GPs) only identified a minority of such young people (Blair 2001; Potts et al. 2001).

In the United Kingdom, The National Institute for Health and Care Excellence (NICE) has published guidance for those working with children and young people on a number of mental health issues, including depression, bi-polar disorder, eating disorder, obsessive compulsive disorder, self-harm, attention deficit hyperactivity disorder (ADHD) and conduct disorder. These guidelines, taken together, make it clear that the responsibility for early diagnosis of children's mental disorders lies with all those involved with this age group.

Opinions differ about whether using the terms mental health or mental disorder in relation to children and young people is stigmatizing and marginalizes young people's experience such that their needs are frequently not recognized and dealt with in a timely way; or at all. Some argue that an alternative and less specific description should be used – such as emotional and psychological well-being – to encompass the broad psychosocial spectrum of both presentation and disorder. Others argue that we should not avoid using the term *mental health* as it is only through accurate assessment, diagnosis and naming–which in turn leads to evidence-based treatment and intervention – that unconscious and conscious behaviours by others that indicate prejudice and lack of understanding about mental illness can be challenged and the resources to provide appropriate local levels of service for the most vulnerable young people can be agreed. In other words, not recognising and naming mental illness diminishes the significance of a diagnosable condition in some children and young people, makes it less likely to be recognized and treated early, and therefore has the potential to restrict access to suitable support and treatment options. This is inevitably a simplification of the complex paradigms of medical and psychosocial models of categorization and public perception.

The language developed by different professions to describe similar types of presentation further adds to the confusion when making real the concept of child and adolescent mental health in multi-agency working. The child with *behaviour problems* in school might be diagnosed with a *conduct disorder* within CAMHS. Within CAMHS, formulating a diagnosis might also include developmental perspectives or neuro-development, some of which might require input from paediatric services or community physicians. For other professionals the same symptoms might be described as being caused by 'misusing' substances and/or being 'involved' in the criminal justice system, by problems with adaption and adjustment, or by ineffective parenting or by all of those factors. It becomes even more complicated when co-morbidity (i.e. having more than one condition at the same time) is present (Table 10.1).

THE DIFFERENCE BETWEEN A PROBLEM AND AN ILLNESS

So what is the difference between a 'problem' and an illness? A mental health *problem* is something that many of us experience. A young person may be sad or anxious for a short period and can be comforted and helped through this time with the support of family, friends and others who are not specialist CAMH professionals.

An illness is when mental health problems become severe and persistent, significantly interfering with the child's ability to function in the world. Those symptoms are similar across all presentations and are used to define illnesses such as depression, psychosis and eating disorders. When disorder and illness are thought to be present there is benefit in taking a clinical approach to formulating a diagnosis and subsequent evidence based interventions and/or treatments within the health system, and in conjunction with other professions and services.

The health classification system most often used is the 10th International Classification of Diseases (ICD-10; World Health Organization 1992). It is anticipated that ICD-11 will be drawn up by 2015 although it is unlikely to come into use for some years after that. Less frequently in the United Kingdom, and usually for specific reasons, which allow a more diverse set of symptoms to be considered during diagnosis, the *Diagnostic and Statistical Manual of Mental Disorders* (DSM V; American Psychiatric Association 2013) will be used. These are the classifications that doctors and clinical psychologists are trained to use in formulating a diagnosis so that the most appropriate evidence based treatments are used.

IDENTIFYING MENTAL HEALTH PROBLEMS AND MENTAL ILLNESS

Mental health exists along a continuum of presentation, description and understanding, and is recognized, categorized, named, diagnosed, and treated in a variety of settings in the United Kingdom and through a range of assessment, treatments and interventions. These are

Table 10.1 Prevalence of specific child and adolescent mental health risk factors and impact on rate of mental disorder

Risk factors	Impact on rate of disorder
In the child	
Physical illness	3 times increase in rate overall
Chronic health problems	4–8 times increase in rate of disorder in
Brain damage	youngsters with cerebral palsy, epilepsy or other disorder above the brainstem
Sensory impairments	2.5–3 times more disorder
Hearing impairment (4 per 1000)	No figures but rate of disorder thought to be
Visual Impairment (0.6 per 1000)	raised
Learning difficulties	2–3 times increase in rate, higher in sever than moderate learning difficulties
Language and related problems (2%, but better methods of identifying required)	4 times rate of disorder
In the family	
Family breakdown (divorce affects 1 in 4 children under 16 years of age); severe marital discord	Associated with a significant increase in disorders (e.g. depression and anxiety)
Family size	Large family size associated with increased rate of conduct disorder and delinquency in boys
Parental mental illness	8–10 times increase in the rate of schizophrenia
Schizophrenia	1.2–4 times increase in the rate of disorder
Maternal psychiatric disorder	2–3 times increase in the rate of delinquency
Parental criminality	
Physical and emotional abuse (of those on child protection registers, 1 in 4 suffer physical abuse and 1 in 8 neglect)	2 times the rate of mental disorder if physically abused and 3 times the rate if neglected
Sexual abuse (6.62% in girls and 3.31% in boys)	2 times the rate of disorder
Environmental risk factors	
Socio-economic circumstances	Gap in applicable evidence base
Unemployment	Gap in applicable evidence base
Housing and homelessness	Gap in applicable evidence base
School environment	9% in grades 1–9 are victims of bullying; 18% of children have self-reported bullying other children themselves
Life events	
Traumatic events	3–5 times rate of disorder. Rises with recurrent adversities

Source: Wallace SA et al., *Child and Adolescent Mental Health*, Abingdon, UK: Radcliff Medical Press, 1997. With permission.

undertaken by different professionals who are, in the main, trained to work with young people and who understand normal and abnormal child development. Some young people are significantly affected by relatively small changes and challenges in their lives, and use various strategies to deal with these difficulties. At the same time, and perversely, other young people appear to defy life-shattering events and sail through, seemingly unscathed.

For those who are in school, managing the problems of behaviour, development, attachment, conduct and/or clinical problems are part of the everyday mix for teachers in the classroom. Sometimes these problems exist in the absence of an obvious cause. How the problem presents will be influenced by family, environmental and genetic factors, along with variations in levels of personal adjustment and function, and social as well as clinical factors may predispose, precipitate or prolong symptoms.

Symptoms may be transitory, ever present and manageable, or they might interrupt a young person's ability to get on with daily life to such a degree that they are both noticed by others and/or referred to a range of professionals. Sometimes symptoms exist but go unnoticed. Young people may then deal with them, with or without informal interventions by others, and grow through them with minimal disruption. In other cases, the ways in which young people function in the world may be profoundly affected, causing them to require intensive support and treatment.

It is important to be able to distinguish between the understandable distress and short-term worries that all children experience, and other problems and disorders that significantly impact upon a child's everyday life and relationships. In such cases, the child may need treatment and/or a range of other supports alongside treatment.

Children with these sorts of problems are often referred to professionals within the education system, for assessment, support, speech and language therapy, behaviour support and management, educational psychology, the school nurse or school counselling service, peer support or to the voluntary sector.

Because the young person's adaptive mechanisms may be more visible in family, social, education, or community settings, their problems are frequently dealt with through a variety of means before the young person is referred to a CAMHS team or another professional.

With mental disorder or illness a child might present in more complicated ways. This presentation is best assessed in the context of the child within the whole family. The family will have attempted to deal with the symptoms for a significant period of time and will have adapted to the behaviour/presentation but often with little understanding of what is wrong, why and how to deal with it. It is the interrelationship between symptoms and their intensity, functional impairment, and the system in which the child lives that, through assessment, a CAMHS team approach will seek to unpick in order to formulate a treatment plan.

CAMHS teams use a variety of assessment tools and statistical manuals including the ICD-10 and DSM V in order to develop a consistent approach to description and categorization. A disorder (or illness) is classed as present if the diagnostic criteria are met as defined by these manuals. The classification of mental disorder and illness is not a simple activity because of considerations about the impact of a child's cognitive and physical development, language skill, and level of ability to verbalize feelings; and sometimes symptoms of illness are confusing.

Age, culture, gender and ethnicity; environment, experience and training will all impact on the way in which a diagnosis is formulated. It will also be influenced by the way in which the problem is described by parents, teachers, social workers and other professionals – all of which can differ. It is not unknown for a child or a young person to be referred to a specialist CAMHS team where there is significant concern but in the absence of an identifiable mental disorder. This is where high quality multi-professional collaboration and respect is essential to reach a decision about what is wrong.

The diagnosis of mental illness in young people is undertaken by a specialist CAMHS team, taking into account the views of the child, the family and other professionals. It is formulated by considering the level and type of symptoms; the intensity of the symptoms; the context of the child's life and the impact of the symptoms on their everyday life. In addition to fulfilling (or not) diagnostic criteria, a supplementary approach is to ask about general symptomatology

Table 10.2 Mental disorders and illnesses

Disorder	Symptoms
Emotional disorders	Phobias, anxiety states and depression. These may be made manifest in physical symptoms such as chronic headache or abdominal pain.
Conduct disorders	Stealing, defiance, fire setting, aggression and antisocial behaviour
Hyperkinetic disorder	Disturbance of activity and attention and hyperkinetic conduct disorder
Developmental disorder	Delay in acquiring certain skills such as speech, social ability or bladder control. They may affect primarily one area of development or pervade a number of areas as in children with autism and those with pervasive developmental disorders
Eating disorders	Pre-school eating problems, anorexia nervosa and bulimia nervosa
Habit disorders	Tics, sleeping problems and soiling
Post-traumatic syndromes	Post-traumatic stress disorder
Somatic disorders	Chronic fatigue syndrome
Psychotic disorders	Schizophrenia, manic depressive disorder or drug-induced psychosis

Source: Kurtz Z, ed. *With Health in Mind: Mental Health Care for Children and Young People*, London: Action for Sick Children, 1992. With permission.

and to describe 'caseness'. This approach means that the person being assessed has enough symptoms to be defined as a clinical case if a certain threshold is reached, irrespective of what the diagnosis is on the classificatory system (Dogra et al. 2003)(Table 10.2).

PREVALENCE OF MENTAL HEALTH PROBLEMS

Prevalence rates for the major disorders have been comprehensively studied by Meltzer et al. (2003) for the ONS. Boys are more likely to have a mental disorder than girls, with 10% of boys and 5% of girls assessed as having a mental disorder between the ages of 5 and 10 years. The proportions change to 13% of boys and 10% of girls between the ages of 11 and 16 years. Meltzer et al. (2005) found that the number of young people in lone-parent families had doubled the rate of disorder compared with those in two-parent families. In reconstituted families, rates were 24% compared with 9% in families with no step children; 17% of children with a parent who had no educational qualifications compared with 4% of those with a parent of degree level qualification; and 20% compared with 8% where parents were not in full-time paid employment. Economic disadvantage, disability benefit receipt, routine occupational groups, living in social housing and in deprived areas all correlated with higher statistics for mental health problems among young people.

Table 10.3 Percentage prevalence of mental disorders in 5–16 year olds by age and sex, as measured for 2004

Type of disorder	5–10 years of age			11–16 years of age			All children		
	Boys	Girls	All	Boys	Girls	All	Boys	Girls	All
Emotional	2.2	2.5	2.4	4.0	6.1	5.0	3.1	4.3	3.7
Conduct	6.9	2.8	4.9	8.1	5.1	6.6	7.5	3.9	5.8
Hyperkinetic	2.7	0.4	1.6	2.4	0.4	1.4	2.6	0.4	1.5
Less common disorders	2.2	0.4	1.3	1.6	1.1	1.4	1.9	0.8	1.3
Any disorder	10.2	5.1	7.7	12.6	10.3	11.5	11.4	7.8	9.6

Source: Meltzer H et al., *The Mental Health of Children and Young People in Great Britain 2004*, London: Office for National Statistics, 2005. With permission.

POSSIBLE CAUSAL FACTORS

There is considerable debate about the causes of mental disorder and illness in children and young people (Hartley-Brewer 2005). Recent analysis has shown a rise in certain types of disorder across the developed countries, although there is now some evidence of a decline in the United States (Hagel 2004). Factors such as changing demography and family patterns in developed countries, pressures of school examinations, and the commercialisation of childhood, changes in diet, obesity, worsening diet, and even the increase in Caesarean section births have all been cited as plausible reasons for this rise in incidence (Table 10.3).

RISK, RESILIENCE AND SELF-ESTEEM

The risk of developing mental health problems and illness is influenced by genetics, the impact of the family and the impact of the environment in which children and young people live. This is combined with their capacity for resilience (which is learned). The risk factors for mental health problems are set out in Box 10.1 and have been arrived at through a synthesis of research outcomes over a considerable time. Each of these risk factors covers a considerable territory. For example, family breakdown and the subsequent separation of the parents has its own specific range of risks (Rutter 1975). These are rooted in the fact that such changes can make problems worse in already troubled children. Younger children may be more affected as they are less able to understand what is happening and may thus be subject to external influences with less ability to process and adapt to stresses and worries. The secure relationship children need with their parents can be disrupted as parents grapple with their own changes and loss and a child's need and wish for parental love and availability can become frustrated. On the other hand, children may exhibit behaviour problems early during the deterioration of a marriage while these decrease when the marriage dissolves (Mooney et al. 2009).

Poverty can affect both child and foetal development as can substance misuse and alcohol misuse, particularly in the pregnant mother (Chasnoff et al. 1980; Cleaver et al. 1999; Harbin and Murphy 2000). Researchers have found that children whose parents are in unskilled manual socioeconomic groups are also more likely to experience serious childhood illness and disability, including mental health problems (Meltzer et al. 2005). Economic disadvantage has also been shown to affect cognitive function as well as some areas of mental health (Kuh et al. 2004). Recent research also suggests that prejudice within the larger social environment can directly affect the mental health of children and young people. For example, lesbian, gay and transgender young people (ages 16–25) have higher levels of mental health problems, self-harm and suicidal ideation (Youth Chances 2014).

The social isolation experienced by some children who frequently use social media has also been found to be associated with reduced feelings of social acceptance and increased feelings of loneliness with conduct disorders (Holder et al. 2009). Bullying is itself associated with a reduced incidence of wellbeing and Childline has recently reported an 87% rise in calls related to online bullying (Childline 2013).

BOX 10.1 Risk Factors for mental health problems

CHILD

- Genetic influences
- Low IQ and learning disability
- Specific development delay
- Communication difficulty
- Difficult temperament
- Physical illness, especially if chronic and/or neurological
- Academic failure
- Low self-esteem

FAMILY

- Overt parental conflict
- Family breakdown
- Inconsistent or unclear discipline
- Hostile and rejecting relationships
- Failure to adapt to child's changing developmental needs
- Abuse: physical, sexual and/or emotional
- Parental psychiatric illness
- Parental criminality, alcoholism and personality disorder
- Death and loss: including loss of friendships

ENVIRONMENTAL

- Socio-economic disadvantage
- Homelessness
- Disaster
- Discrimination
- Other significant life events

Source   Health Advisory Service, *Together We Stand: The Commissioning Role and Management of CAMHS*, London: HMSO, 1995. Crown Copyright material is reproduced with the permission of the Controller of HMSO.

> ### The potential impact of acquired or traumatic brain injury on risk-taking behaviors*
>
> Around 8.5% of the general population at one point in their lives suffer an ABI the most damaging of which is TBI. The condition predominantly occurs in young people resulting predominantly from falls, sports injuries, fights and road accidents, and is a major source of death and disability among this group.
>
> The consequences of brain injury are loss of memory, loss of concentration, loss of awareness of one's own or others emotional state, poor impulse control, and, particularly, poor social judgement. Unsurprisingly, behaviour problems such as conduct disorder, attention problems, increased aggression and impulse control are prevalent with young people with ABI.
>
> Consequently, while those without a TBI are likely to grow out of immature and antisocial behaviour by their mid-twenties, those with TBI are likely to grapple with these issues throughout young adulthood and beyond. Such issues are critical when assessing and managing the long-term effects of brain injury in childhood.
>
> In children the effects of impairments are particularly detrimental, as the cognitive abilities that children rely on to process new information are compromised.*
>
> ---
>
> * Repairing Shattered Lives 2012. p. 11–14 Prof H Williams: Barrow Cadbury Trust

The references to early brain development in the first section of this chapter have significant messages for policy development in child and adolescent health. Policies that deal with adolescent behaviours need to include reference to the nature of physiological change in the brain during the early developmental period and during adolescence as well as the potential for cognitive impairment due to acquired or traumatic brain injury (TBI) For example, should a young person not be punished for actions that might be outside her/his control and where treatment might be available but the clinical disorder has gone unrecognized? This is a difficult policy area in terms of balancing the needs of the individual with the needs of civil society.

Recent research also suggests some links between mental health and diet (Gesch et al. 2002). Walker et al. (2006) reported a link between poor diet and reported psychosocial problems in Jamaican children in findings from a 2-year randomized controlled trial. There is some evidence to show that diets lacking in certain fatty acids and vitamins can have a deleterious effect on mental health and also that certain food additives can adversely affect children's behaviour, particularly those with a precondition such as ADHD (Van de Weyer 2005). This research is in its early days and needs further corroboration, as does research into the impact of substance misuse on mental health (Advisory Council on the Misuse of Drugs 2005), but it suggests that these are areas we might need to be concerned about when assessing risk. A combination of these factors, particularly three or more increases the likelihood of problems.

RESILIENCE

Studies suggest that there are factors which, when in combination, can provide a measure of protection against mental disorders.

The reasons why one child copes in adverse circumstances and another succumbs to mental ill-health are unclear. Many of these resilience factors are linked, and many depend on good early care-giving and continuing secure, confident parenting. This again underlines the importance of support to families when things are not going well. Michael Rutter (2012) talks of a 'steeling' process through which young people who have experienced high levels of stress, and been well supported, appear to have grown stronger through that experience. He refers to this phenomenon as stress-inoculation, i.e. as having the same effect in developing immunity as physical inoculation for diseases such as smallpox.

A consistent approach by professionals who may be involved with less-secure families is a recognized means of providing alternative positive attachment experiences when a child is at risk of mental health distress or illness. This is not an easy objective to achieve in the work environments that many practitioners experience, particularly in the context of the multiple new initiatives and service restructurings that continue to dominate the UK health and social care landscape.

Throughout the literature on child mental health in developed countries we find references to building self-esteem. The repetition of reference to concepts of self-esteem has attracted many proponents in the field of children's mental health, and it needs some explanation. Self-esteem develops through the complex interrelationship between a sense of self, the place of the self in the world, and the relationships and experiences that enhance a strong sense of self. Positive self-esteem is inextricably linked with the development of a concept of the self in these analyses. A positive sense of self is believed to play an important part in confident approaches to new situations, confidence in personal ability and in the likelihood that the world is a safe, not an anxiety-provoking place. It seems self-evident that a child's self-esteem should be developed, *but high self-esteem is not essential to good mental health and achievement. In fact, it can be a limiting factor when the level of self-esteem is inappropriate.*

The most difficult problem in using the term self-esteem is that it is generally over-used and poorly conceptualized. Considerable conceptual work is needed before the term can be applied in a helpful way to public health practice in child and adolescent mental health (Table 10.1).

TREATMENTS AND INTERVENTIONS

The specialist mental health services for children are part of what is referred to as a comprehensive CAMHS. This service has been represented as the four-tiered model (see p. 27) – described as a 'schematic framework' by the Health Advisory Service that first set it out in *Together We Stand* in 1995. A comprehensive CAMHS service encompasses tier 1 – all those practitioners who work with children but who are not mental health specialists – through to tier 4 which describes the highly specialized, usually mental inpatient provision, for those with mental illness. This four-tier approach became a standard model for describing the complexity of provision. As local commissioners and services have responded to more recent policy developments, the tiered model has been adapted to incorporate descriptions of responses and services more likely to be described as *universal* (mild to moderate problems tiers 1–2), *targeted* (moderately severe, severe and complex problems [tiers 2–3] and *specialist* (very severe and possibly life-threatening problems tier 4).

It is not our intention, neither is it within the scope of this chapter, to provide the public health practitioner with a thorough guide to the range of treatments and interventions that might be available in any specific locality for children and young people with mental disorders. Services are in continuous change and development. However, the main areas of treatment are specified in the substantive texts on treatments. Therefore the following section describes the main areas of treatment, but the substantive texts on treatments should be read in more detail.

Most commissioners require that the services and interventions provided are measurable and evidence based. However, although the evidence base of effective intervention and treatment is improving, with the publication of randomized controlled trials (RCTs), as well as advice and guidance from the NICE and the Royal Colleges, in some treatment areas there is still very little solid research on which to make choices. As with physical illness, the type and persistence of the problem dictates the level of response and the most appropriate intervention.

In addition the CAMHS Outcome Research Consortium (CORC) – a collaboration between CAMHS across the United Kingdom – seeks to develop and implement an agreed model of routine outcome evaluation by local services so that the information that is collected about outcomes can be used in meaningful and constructive ways to improve the commissioning and provision of local CAMHS to children, young people and families (CORC 2005).

The emotional health problems experienced by infants are most frequently dealt with by GPs and health visitors but those of older children and young people are most often recognized and dealt with initially, within the school system by classroom teachers, a special education needs co-ordinator (SENCO), the school nurse, an educational psychologist, or the behaviour support team. A GP might be the next port of call and he/she might want to watch and wait, seeing the young person regularly, before possibly referring the child to mental health specialists.

Referrals to school counsellors are common (where such counsellors are commissioned by head teachers) and are popular with children and young people. They find school counselling less stigmatizing and easier to access. In the past, some counsellors were engaged by head teachers but were not trained to work with children and young people and/or not regularly supervised. The British Association of Counselling and Psychotherapy has undertaken research and made recommendations about the efficacy and the quality of school counselling services. It indicates that counselling is one of the most commonly used forms of psychological therapy for young people in the United Kingdom (about 70,000 to 90,000 cases per year). There is also emerging evidence that counselling can be effective in both reducing distress, increasing ability to cope and increasing a young person's ability to engage with study and learning.*

The school or primary healthcare system may also refer the young person to a voluntary organization or to a primary mental health worker before a referral to a specialist CAMHS team is made.

Clinical child mental health specialists are most often involved when there is evidence of a *mental disorder,* (e.g. moderate depression and anxiety, phobias, obsessive behaviours, abnormal, aggressive and hyperactive behaviours and eating disorders) as well as communication disorders such as autism and *mental illnesses* such as bipolar disorders and psychoses. These specialists may be based at a local CAMHS clinic or may be available, for example, in GP surgeries, schools and family centres. Access differs in different localities and depends also on whether or not a multidisciplinary approach is needed or whether treatment from a single CAMHS specialist is felt to be appropriate.

Young Adults Advice & Support Project (YASP) in Manchester.

YASP is part of the Manchester mental health charity HARP and works with children aged 15–25 (HARP is the main charitable organisation for a variety of projects and services for people aged 15 and upwards in Manchester; YASP is the only service within the charity specifically targeted at young people). Based in Levenshulme, a part of central Manchester, and operating within a diverse community, YASP has been established for almost a decade and sees around 300 young people each year. It operates as a "one-stop-shop" providing: welfare rights advice; counselling; a volunteering programme; social activities and an open-access internet café. The counselling service has a particular specialism in working with young refugees and asylum seekers. More information about YASP is available at: http://www.manchestermind.org/projects/project_yasp_about.php.

---

* BACP 2012; School based counselling in secondary schools

Shannon's story

Twelve-year-old Shannon's mum said, 'I just don't know what to do anymore, I can't take this every morning.' Her daughter refused to go to school so she had to take her there and back each day, putting a strain on the family.

Shannon struggled to concentrate in lessons, appeared tearful and anxious, forgot to do her homework and required constant reassurance – sometimes up to ten times a day – from staff in order for her to feel 'secure'.

After referral to Place2Be, Shannon saw a counsellor each Monday and this helped her to come into school after the weekend. As her counselling progressed, she gained confidence that she could talk about her worries and be heard. Her constant need for reassurance lessened.

Shannon's attendance improved from 88.3% to 96.8%. She now has a close group of friends whom she walks to and from school. She has learned to access support from her peers, family, school and Place2Be, as and when she needs it. She has joined the school drama club.

Mum says 'It's amazing not having a daily battle with her about coming into school.'

Source   Place2Be – Shannon's Story: http://www.place2be.org.uk/what-we-do/childrens-stories/shannon/. With permission.

There is a clear evidence base for most common interventions. However, professional opinions can vary about the types of treatments that are effective for particular disorders (Fonagy et al. 2002) especially where co-morbidity exists.

The evidence suggests that behaviour therapies are effective across a range of disorders, and the current trend is for solution-focused therapies that help to develop positive strategies for the future. Some of these approaches are likely to be more effective if combined with other forms of support such as parenting programmes or family therapy. Parenting programmes can work well, notably with the problems of behaviour that are experienced by younger families if manualized programmes are followed carefully.

More recently, the Improving Access to Psychological Treatments (IAPT)* programme for children and young people has been introduced in the United Kingdom. It is built on a similar programme to that which has been in place for the adult population since 2010. *The Children and Young People's IAPT* 2012, aims to improve access to CAMHS, to embed an approach based on partnership between children, young people, families, professional and agencies and to build capability for delivering positive and measurable outcomes for children, young people and families. It increases the choice of evidence based treatments available. Through this programme, local therapists are offered training in Cognitive Behaviour Therapy or Parenting for children aged 3–10 years; or Systemic Family Therapy; or Interpersonal Therapy for Adolescents. The aim is to improve the recognition of problems in the early stages and to improve access to training for non-clinical practitioners and to improve access to appropriate therapies and interventions which will prevent problems getting worse. The programme is supported through the development of outcome measures, higher education learning collaboratives, and an e-learning portal hosted by the Royal College of Paediatrics and Child Health and the English Department of Health, *MindEd*[†].

Many young people with conduct disorders, particularly those with childhood onset, are likely to need access to a CAMHS team on and off throughout their adolescence after an initial treatment – much as anyone with a chronic illness needs continued services. Access to

---

* http://www.iapt.nhs.uk/
[†] http://www.rcpch.ac.uk/minded

appropriate levels of service has often been frustrated by long waiting lists and, to a certain degree, by service requirements to meet specific government targets. More recent changes in NHS architecture, both commissioning and provision, have offered opportunities to re-examine local need and local provision through Joint Strategic Needs Assessments (JSNAs) as well as opportunities to reconfigure both local authority and health provision across the spectrum of need. This increasingly means that CAMHS treatments are offered for a finite number of sessions, usually between 6 and 12. If needs have not been met in that time period, a further referral may become necessary.

There is considerable debate and variable evidence about the efficacy of treatment for conduct disorder. However, a recent health technology assessment by NICE shows effectiveness of parenting programmes for under 12s with conduct disorder (Social Care Institute for Excellence [SCIE] 2011). Multi systemic therapy (MST), an approach which focuses, through the parents/carers, on the totality of the young person's interactions, has been shown to be highly successful with young people with conduct disorders. Research by Butler et al. (2011) shows that 'although both MST and Youth Offending Team (YOT) interventions appeared highly successful in reducing offending, the MST model of service-delivery reduced significantly the likelihood of further non-violent offending during an 18-month follow-up period.' (p. 1220, 2011)

Psychodynamic psychotherapies have a less robust evidence base, but case studies bear witness to their effectiveness with entrenched problems. These treatments tend to be expensive because they can sometimes take many years to complete. However, short-term treatments using these methods are being developed (Baruch 2001). In a randomized control trial conducted by Trowell et al. (2007) to examine the use of individual psychodynamic psychotherapy and family therapy as treatments for moderate and severe depression in children and young people, significant reductions in disorder rates were seen for both individual therapy and family therapy. This study provides further evidence supporting the use of focused forms of both individual psychodynamic therapy and family therapy for moderate-to-severe depression in children and young adolescents.

Pharmacological interventions are an important component of treatment. Antidepressants, although not the treatment of choice, can be useful in stabilizing older adolescents prior to talking therapy. Their use with children has been reviewed by the Medicines and HealthCare Products Regulatory Agency (MHPRA) and contraindications have been identified. Recent NICE (2005) guidelines describe the optimal treatment regime. Drug treatment for ADHD is effective in 70% of cases, but should be combined with behaviour therapy for optimum outcome. In cases of schizophrenia, the evidence is clear that the earlier drug treatment can begin after diagnosis, the less destructive the illness is in terms of the patient's ability to lead a normal life (Birchwood et al. 1997). Patients have traditionally disliked drug treatments because of the unpleasant side-effects, but the newer drugs are better in this respect, making the outcomes for those with this illness much more hopeful than even a decade ago.

WHAT TYPE OF INTERVENTION AND SERVICES ARE HELPFUL IN A PUBLIC HEALTH APPROACH TO CHILD AND ADOLESCENT MENTAL HEALTH

From 1948 to 1997 in the United Kingdom, it is fair to say that child guidance clinics led by child psychiatrists and supported by psychotherapists, social workers and educational psychologists were mainly responsible for child mental health services. Over that period clinics grew in number; demand increased; and waiting times lengthened with concomitant delays in treatment and pressures to prioritize the most severe and longstanding problems.

Little changed in this picture until evidence published in the 1990s suggested a need for policy and practice that could ensure services were able to improve child and adolescent mental health provision (Kurtz 1992; Health Advisory Service 1995; Audit Commission 1999; Mental Health Foundation 1999). Assembling findings of three influential pieces of research (Kurtz 1992, 1996; Health Advisory Service 1995), and combining these findings with new government policy after 1997 enabled the Audit Commission to design a set of guidelines for CAMHS providers (Audit Commission 1999). The Health Advisory Service report (1995) showed that CAMH services, i.e. the whole of the resources available for a particular population which support children's mental health in any way, were being managed and delivered in many formal and informal contexts but without systematic co-ordination. From this the tiered concept of CAMHS provision (tiers 1–4) was initiated.

What appears to help is any service that is easily accessible and non-stigmatising – for example, specific services and helplines for substance misuse, bullying, depression and anxiety. These will include online resources, forums and information, which children and young people find helpful. They also say that they appreciate the anonymity involved. Organisations such as Mindfull (www.mindfull.org) offer online counselling, and YoungMinds (www.youngminds.org.uk) manages Parentline, where parents can seek advice and guidance on understanding and managing their children's problems. Local services, online and telephone support are frequently developed by statutory and voluntary organisations, and young people say they are helpful, but that they are frequently not well advertised or promoted.

DEVELOPING LOCAL RESPONSES BASED ON KNOWN NEED

The current policy context for CAMHS in the United Kingdom emphasizes the need to build CAMH services through a partnership approach involving a range of agencies and including children, young people and their carers in the planning. Good local service planning is now the responsibility of local commissioners and providers who should work in partnership. The *Health and Social Care Act 2012* (Cabinet Office 2012) shifted the locus of control from central government to local health and social care partnerships, intending to inspire and galvanize local systems to better understand and respond to local need. The Act established Health and Wellbeing Boards as a place where key leaders from the health and care system work together to improve the health and wellbeing of their local population and reduce health inequalities.

Health and Wellbeing Boards have strategic influence over commissioning decisions across health, public health and social care. They also strengthen democratic legitimacy by involving democratically elected representatives and patient representatives in commissioning decisions alongside commissioners across health and social care.

Boards bring together clinical commissioning groups and councils to develop a shared understanding of the health and wellbeing needs of the community. They should undertake the JSNA and develop a joint strategy for how these needs can be best addressed, including recommendations for joint commissioning and integrating services across health and social care.

Fiscal austerity has meant that the aspirational element of the policy has been tempered by financial reality. This means that it is crucial to build solid working partnerships to make the best use of resources.

To achieve the complexity of care, specified services for children and young people need to be developed in a systematic way through interagency cooperation. This involves a number of key activities to ensure that services are built on known need and not merely on historical models of service provision. Key components of building a service continuum across agencies,

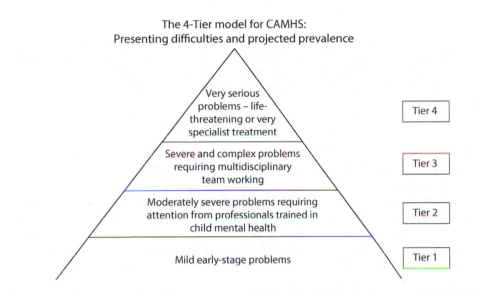

Figure 10.1 Child and Adolescent Mental Health Services (CAMHS): A tiered approach. (Adapted from Kurtz Z, *Treating Children Well: A Guide to Using the Evidence Base in Commissioning and Managing Mental Health Services for Children and Young People*, London: The Mental Health Foundation, 1996.)

and using the specialist skills within each, are predicated on a current needs assessment with an analysis of gaps in service provision. This is particularly important when managing children and young people's transition between services and at particular ages. For example, ensuring clear planning and provision for

- Those children and young people with mental health problems and/or learning disability who are approaching the age of 18
- For children and young people who are in the care of the local authority
- For children and young people in youth custody who might be transferring to the adult estate
- For children and young people approaching the age of 18 who have a mental illness (major disorders, including eating disorder) who thus need planned transitions to adult mental health services

Children and young people should be included in assessments, treatment and care plans – their views are important.

A good public health approach will ensure that, alongside the population based needs assessment, there is a workforce strategy that makes best use of the skills and competencies of the whole children's workforce in order to piece together appropriate services matched by the skills in the workforce in order to ensure better outcomes for children and young people (Figure 10.1).

COMMISSIONING

Local commissioners and public health teams have the complex task of identifying need and commissioning the requisite number and type of services required to deliver to priority areas of need for children with mental health problems and illness. Prior to the enactment of the

Health and Social Care Act of 2012 the CAMHS Grant guidance, the NSF, *Choosing Health* (Department of Health 2004a) and *Commissioning a Patient Led NHS* (Department of Health 2005) all emphasized the need to strengthen the commissioning function by means of structural changes in health and local authorities. Commissioning a *patient-led* NHS and practice-based commissioning together imply commissioning structures that can provide a counterbalance to strong provider organizations. The policy intention at the turn of the century was to encourage choice and contestability and to strengthen partnerships between health, education, local government and non-statutory organizations.

Following the *Children Act 2004*, social services departments merged with education services to become joint children's services departments under a children's services director, moving towards the provision of all children's services, including health, through children's trusts.

New commissioning models required by the 2012 Act offer an inherent challenge to a health dominated model of CAMHS. It re-emphasizes the importance and benefits of collaborative and joint commissioning structures which were intimated in previous legislation, and which could lead to better integration of commissioning and provision. A greater role for local authorities is set out as they resume responsibility for public health and liaise with the other agencies through the Health and Wellbeing Boards.

The strategic planning for CAMHS is a shared responsibility as emphasized in the 2003 Public Service Agreement. This had been further reinforced in 2005 when joint health and local authority performance targets were set for CAMHS and they extended to

- Young people ages 16–17 years
- Provision of 24/7 cover
- Services for children and young people with learning disability
- Services for those children with complex levels of health and social care need

The Health and Wellbeing Boards are charged with the responsibility of undertaking a CAMH needs assessment and a gap analysis, and also responsibility for each local authority to have its own joint CAMH strategy with agreements about levels of investment in CAMHS across all local agencies. The policy aim of all commissioning processes is to improve the performance and management of all children's services; remain outcomes focused; establish clear and sensible care pathways that make sense to the child and their parents; and include children and young people in the planning of those services. This is a formidable and radical change of direction for CAMHS given that no significant policy change had occurred in the quarter century prior to the Health Advisory Service report in 1995.

The principle standard for commissioning CAMHS, as with all children's services in the United Kingdom, is to ensure that the right service should get to the right child at the right time, and in the most appropriate place. For this to happen effectively, agencies are expected to work together to build care pathways that reduce the historic duplication of effort and the need for families to 'tell their story' more than once.

Good local service planning is now the responsibility of local commissioners and providers who should work in partnership. The *Health and Social Care Act 2012* shifted the locus of control from central government to local health and social care partnerships, intending to inspire and galvanize local systems to better understand and respond to local need. *No Health Without Mental Health: A Cross-Government Mental Health Outcomes Strategy for People of All Ages* (2012) provides further impetus for working across agencies and across age boundaries in relation to mental health. Fiscal austerity has meant that the aspirational element of these policies has been tempered by financial reality.

CHALLENGES AND OPPORTUNITIES

There can be no doubt that well-resourced nurture and support for the emotional wellbeing and mental health of children and young people is essential for a stable society. It *is* everybody's business. Over the last two decades there has been increasing interest in, and understanding of, its importance within a burgeoning evidence base that links mental health problems and disorders in young people to increasing levels of problem behaviours. From the mid-1990s, government funds were targeted in order to improve traditional CAMHS.

More recently there has been government recognition of the part played by local authorities in delivering the CAMHS agenda. However the stigma of mental illness remains, and for many children and young people and their families, this is still a potent factor in making much-needed services inaccessible.

The recent Nuffield Foundation Report (2012) found that the shape of the average day for teenagers had changed significantly since 1970 with higher rates of youth unemployment. There are now significantly larger numbers of young people staying on at school but higher concerns about getting a job. The absolute level of alcohol consumption by children aged 11–15 years is higher in the United Kingdom than most other countries with about 25% of UK teens using alcohol by the age of 13. Family size, breakdown and reconstitution affects young people and the rates of conduct disorder in non-intact families tends to be higher than in intact families. The Association for Young People's Health Key Data (2013) expressed concern about the lack of recent national data. However, their report provides helpful figures on a range of topics including self-harm and suicide which make strong assertions about the correlation between self-harm and suicide in groups of vulnerable young people such as those in the youth justice system. Although the trend in suicide figures is downwards, it is concerning that in 2014 The Princes Trust MacQuarie Index* found 1:10 young unemployed people between the age of 16 and 25 felt they had 'nothing to live for'.

Following a consultation with 1600 young people in 2013, YoungMinds has recently established five mini campaigns on the top five issues: sexual pressures, bullying, unemployment, school stress and lack of help. The intention is that young people themselves will run the campaign to improve the situation in all of these five areas. The challenge for CAMHS in the coming period is clearly formidable as services struggle to engage effectively with all those in need, by providing services in the least stigmatizing settings and ensuring that interventions are timely, appropriate and evidence based in the true traditions of using public health theory to inform the design of strong and effective public services based on reliable evidence of need.

CONCLUSION

The mental health and well-being of our children and young people is dependent upon an understanding of the fundamentals of infant and child development and the management of the transitional stages of childhood. Health and local authority economies must build on the assessed needs of the under-18 population, taking a fundamental public health approach to maintaining the best of existing levels of service and reconfiguring others to ensure smooth transition through critical stages of development. Joint CAMH strategies are a key tool with agreed levels of investment against agreed priorities. However, there needs to be much greater

---

* http://www.princes-trust.org.uk/about_the_trust/what_we_do/research/youth_index_2014.aspx.

KEY POINTS

- The mental health of children and young people is everybody's business.
- Support to early parenting helps protect and nurture mental health.
- Attending to the mental well-being of parents is crucial to parents supporting emotionally healthy children.
- The most vulnerable children and young people (hidden populations, those in the criminal justice system, looked after children, children with disabilities, young people approaching adulthood, LGBT etc.) are least likely to receive a level of service appropriate to their needs.
- Commissioning of services should be based on known need and agreed joint priorities between agencies and not on historical patterns of provision.
- Commissioners and providers must demonstrate that they understand the reality of children's lives and develop the sorts of services families say they want to use.
- Commissioners and providers must systematically seek and act upon the opinions of children and young people and their families and develop a quality 'you said, we did' approach.
- The consequences of failing to support vulnerable children, young people and families and failure to understand their mental health needs are highly significant for 'anti-social behaviours' and other negative outcomes for individuals, families and society as a whole.

emphasis on joint policy and service development and how to make the best use of well-trained and experienced staff in order to ensure that there are clear pathways of care for all those requiring a service on the spectrum of services that embrace the concept of child and adolescent mental health.

REFERENCES

Advisory Council for the Misuse of Drugs. (2005) *Further Consideration of the Classification of Cannabis under the Misuse of Drugs Act 1971.* London: Home Office.

Ainsworth M, Blehar M, Waters E, Wall S. (1978) *Patterns of Attachment: A Psychological Study of the Strange Situation.* Hillsdale, NJ: Lawrence Erlbaum Associates In CH008 2/20/07 6:11 PM Page 203–204 Child and adolescent mental health.

American Psychiatric Association. (2013) *Diagnostic and Statistical Manual of Mental Disorders (DSM IV).* Washington, DC: American Psychiatric Publishing Inc.

Association for Young People's Health (2013) *Key Data on Adolescence.*

Astington J, Harris P, Olson D (1988) *Developing Theories of Mind.* New York, NY: Cambridge University Press.

Audit Commission. (1999) *Children in Mind: Child and Adolescent Mental Health.* London: Audit Commission.

Balbernie R. (2001) Circuits and circumstances: The neurobiological consequences of early relationship experiences and how they shape later behaviour. *Journal of Child Psychotherapy* 27: 237–255.

Baruch G Butler S, Hickey N, Fonagy P. (2011) A randomized controlled trial of multisystemic therapy and a statutory therapeutic intervention for young offenders. *American Journal of the Academy of Child and Adolescent Psychiatry* 50 (12): 1220–1235.e2. 10.1016/j. jaac.2011.09.017.

Birchwood M, McGorry P, Jackson H. (1997) Early intervention in schizophrenia (Editorial). *British Journal of Psychiatry* 170: 2–5.

Blair C. (2001) The early identification of risk for grade retention among African American children at risk for school difficulty. *Applied Developmental Science* 5: 37–50.

Blakemore SJ, Frith U. (2005) *The Learning Brain: Lessons for Education*. Oxford, UK: Blackwell Publishing.

Butler S, Baruch G, Hickey N, et al. (2011) A randomized controlled trial of multisystemic therapy and a statutory therapeutic intervention for young offenders. *American Journal of the Academy of Child and Adolescent Psychiatry* 50: 1220–1235.e2.

Cabinet Office. (2012) *The Health and Social Care Act 2012*. London: Stationary Office

Chasnoff IJ, Hatcher R, Burns W. (1980) Early growth patterns of methadone addicted infants. *American Journal of the Disabled Child* 134: 1049–1051.

Chief Medical Officer. (2012) *Our Children Deserve Better*. London: Department of Health.

Chief Secretary to the Treasury. (2003) *Every Child Matters* (Cm 5860). London: Stationery Office. www.everychildmatters.gov.uk/_content/documents/EveryChildMatters.pdf (accessed on 17 January 2007).

Childline. (2013) *Can I Tell You Something? What's Affecting Children*. London: Childline.

Cicchetti D, Barnett D. (1991) Attachment organisation in preschool-aged maltreated children. *Development and Psychopathology* 3: 397–411.

Cleaver H, Unell I, Aldgate J. (1999) *Children's Needs, Parenting Capacity*. London: HMSO.

CAMHS Outcome Research Consortium. (2005) www.corc.uk.net (accessed on 29 January 2007).

Currie C et al. eds. *Social Determinants of Health and Well-Being Among Young People. Health Behaviour in School-aged Children (HBSC) study: International report from the 2009/2010 survey*. Copenhagen, Denmark: WHO Regional Office for Europe, 2012 (Health Policy for Children and Adolescents, No. 6).

Department for Education and Skills. (2005a) *Birth to Three Matters*. Nottingham, UK: DfES Publications.

Department of Health. (2004a) *Choosing Health*. London: Department of Health.

Department of Health. (2009) *Healthy Child Programme*. London: Department of Health.

Department of Health. (2005) *Commissioning a Patient Led NHS*. London: Department of Health.

Department of Health to Local Authorities in England and Wales. (2010) *Healthy Lives, Healthy People*. London: Department of Health.

Department of Health and Department for Education and Skills. (2004) *The National Service Framework for Children, Young People and Maternity Services*. London: Department of Health. www.dh.gov.uk/PolicyAndGuidance/HealthAndSocialCareTopics/ChildrenServices/ChildrenServicesInformation/ChildrenServicesInformationArticle/fs/en?CONTENT_ID_4089111&chk_U8Ecln (accessed on 5 February 2007).

Dogra N, Parkin A, Gale F, Frake C. (2003) *A MultiDisciplinary Handbook of CAMHS for Front Line Professionals*. London: Jessica Kingsley Publishers Ltd.

Elliot L. (1999) *Early Intelligence: How the Brain and Mind Develops in the First Five Years of Life*. London: Penguin.

Field F. (2011) *Think Child, Think Parent, Think Family: A Guide to Parental Mental Health and Child Welfare*. London: HMSO.

Fonagy P, Steele M, Steele H, et al. (1991) The capacity for understanding mental states: The reflective self in parent and child and its significance for security of attachment. *Infant Mental Health Journal* 13: 200–217.

Fonagy P, Target M, Cottrell D, et al. (2002) *A Critical Review of Treatments for Children and Adolescents*. New York, NY: Guilford Publications.

Gesch CB, Hammond SM, Hampson SE, et al. (2002) Influence of supplementary vitamins, minerals and essential fatty acids on the antisocial behaviour of young adult prisoners. *British Journal of Psychiatry* 181: 22–28.

Hagel A. (2004) *Time Trends in Adolescent Well-being*. London: Nuffield Foundation.

Harbin F, Murphy M. (2000) *Substance Misuse and Child Care: How to Understand, Assist and Intervene When Drugs Affect Parenting*. Lyme Regis, UK: Russell House Publishing.

Hartley-Brewer E. (2005) *Perspectives on the Causes of Mental Health Problems in Children and Adolescents*. Report and discussion paper from a YoungMinds Symposium held in association with the Institute for Public Policy Research, March 2005, London. London: YoungMinds.

Harvard University Center on Developing Child: Key Concepts–Toxic Stress Health Advisory Service. (1995) *Together we Stand: The Commissioning Role and Management of Child and Adolescent Mental Health Services*. London: HMSO.

Holder M, Coleman B, Sehn Z. (2009) The contribution of active and passive leisure to children's wellbeing. *Journal of Health Psychology* 14 (3): 378–386.

Kuh D, Power C, Blane D, Bartley M. (2004) Socioeconomic pathways between childhood and adult health. In: Kuh DL, Ben-Schlomo YAA, eds. A *Life Course Approach to Chronic Disease Epidemiology, Tracing the Origins of Ill-Health from Early to Adult Life*. 2nd ed. Oxford, UK: Oxford University Press, 371–398.

Kurtz Z, ed. (1992) *With Health in Mind: Mental Health Care for Children and Young People*. London: Action for Sick Children.

Kurtz Z. (1996) *Treating Children Well: A Guide to Using the Evidence Base in Commissioning and Managing Mental Health Services for Children and Young People*. London: The Mental Health Foundation.

Lyons-Ruth K. (1996) Attachment relationships among children with aggressive behaviour problems – The role of disorganised early attachment patterns. *Journal of Consulting and Clinical Psychology* 64: 64–73.

McLoyd AS. (2001) The impact of economic hardship on black families and children: Psychological distress, parenting and socioeconomic development. *Child Development* 61: 311–346.

Meltzer H, Corbin T, Gatward R, et al. (2003) *The Mental Health of Young People Looked after by Local Authorities in England*. London: HMSO.

Meltzer H, Green H, McGinnity A, et al. (2005) *The Mental Health of Children and Young People in Great Britain 2004*. London: Office for National Statistics.

Mental Health Foundation. (1999) *Bright Futures: Promoting Children and Young People's Mental Health*. London: The Mental Health Foundation.

METRO Youth Chances. (2014) *Youth Chances Summary of First Findings: The Experiences of LGBTQ Young People in England*. London: METRO.

Mooney S, Oliver C, Smith M. (2009) *Impact of Family Breakdown on Children's Well Being: Evidence Review*. London: Thomas Coram Research Unit, Institute of Education, University of London.

Murray L. (1992) The impact of postnatal depression on infant development. *Journal of Child Psychology* 33: 543–561.

National Institute for Health and Clinical Excellence (NICE). (2005) *CG28 Depression in Children and Young People: NICE guideline*. www.nice. org.uk/page.aspx?o_cg028niceguideline (accessed on 11 January 2007).

Nuffield Foundation. (2012) *Social Trends and Mental Health: Introducing the Main Findings*. London: the Nuffield Foundation.

Potts Y, Gillies ML, Wood SF. (2001) Lack of mental well-being in 15-year olds: An undisclosed iceberg? *Family Practice* 18: 95–100.

Public Health England. (2010) *Healthy Lives, Healthy People*. London: Department of Health.

Reder P, Duncan S, Gray M. (1993) *Beyond Blame, Child Abuse Tragedies Revisited*. London: Routledge.

Rutter M. (1975) *Helping Troubled Children*. London and New York: Penguin.

Rutter M. (2001) *Psychosocial Adversity and Child Psychopathology. Research and Innovation on the Road to Modern Child Psychiatry*. London: Gaskell (Royal College of Psychiatrists).

Rutter M. (2012) Resilience as a dynamic concept. *Development and Psychopathology* 24: 335–344# Cambridge, UK: Cambridge University Press.

Schaffer HR. (1996) *Social Development*. Oxford, UK: Blackwell.

Social Care Institute for Excellence (SCIE). (2011) *Think Child, Think Parent, Think Family: A Guide to Parental Mental Health and Child Welfare*. London: SCIE.

Tagore R. (1933) *My School*. (Lecture delivered in America). www.learningnetindia. org/lni/data/publications/revive/vol4/v4-2-m.php (accessed on 29 January 2007) Calcutta India.

Trowell J, Joffe I, Campbell J, et al. (2007) Childhood depression: A place for psychotherapy. An outcome study comparing individual psychodynamic psychotherapy and family therapy. *European Child and Adolescent Psychiatry* 16(3): 157–167.

UNICEF. (1989) *The United Nations Convention on the Rights of the Child*.

Van de Weyer C. (2005) *Changing Diets, Changing Minds*. London: Sustain.

Vygotskyi L. (1978) *Mind in Society: The Development of Higher Psychological Processes*. Cambridge, MA: Harvard University Press.

Walker SP, Chang SM, Powell CA, et al. (2006) Effects of psychosocial stimulation and dietary supplementation in early childhood on psychosocial functioning in late adolescence: Follow-up of randomised controlled trial. *British Medical Journal* 333: 472–476.

Wallace SA, Crown JM, Cox AD, Berger M. (1997) *Child and Adolescent Mental Health*. Abingdon, UK: Radcliffe Medical Press.

Williams WH, Giray G, Mewse AJ, et al. (2010) Traumatic brain injury in young offenders: A modifiable risk factor for re-offending, poor mental health and violence. *Neuropsychological Rehabilitation an International Journal* 20(6): 801–812.

World Health Organization. (1992) *The ICD-10 Classification of Mental and Behavioural Disorders Clinical Descriptions and Diagnostic Guidelines*. Geneva: World Health Organization.

YoungMinds. (2006) London. www.youngminds.org.uk/problems/ (accessed on 29 January 2007).

WEBSITES

Annual CAMH mapping exercise: www.camhsmapping.org.uk

BACP counselling in secondary schools: www.bacp.co.uk/research/publications/School_Counselling.php

CAMHS Outcome Research Consortium: www.corc.uk.net

Care Services Improvement Partnership: www.csip.org.uk

Department for Education and Skills: www.dfes.gov.uk/

Department of Health: www.doh.gov.uk

Every Child Matters: www.everychildmatters.gov.uk/

Faculty for Children and Young People in the British Psychological Society: www.bps.org.uk/dcp-cyp/dcp-cyp_home.cfm

Harvard University – Center on Developing Child: developingchild.harvard.edu/topics/ science_of_early_childhood/toxic_stress_response/

Improving Access to Psychological Treatments (IAPT): www.iapt.nhs.uk/

National CAMHS Support Service: www.camhs.org.uk

National Institute for Health and Clinical Excellence: www.nice.org.uk

National Service Framework for Children, Young People and their Families: www.dh.gov.uk/ PolicyAndGuidance/HealthAndSocialCareTopics/Children

Place2Be – Shannon's Story: www.place2be.org.uk/what-we-do/childrens-stories/ shannon/Services/ChildrenServicesInformation/fs/en

Royal College of Paediatrics and Child Health: www.rcpch.ac.uk/minded

Royal College of Psychiatrists: www.rcpsych.ac.uk

Sure Start: www.surestart.gov.uk

The Princes Trust index: www.princestrust.org.uk/about_the_trust/what_we_do/research/youth_ index_2014.aspx

The Standards Site: www.standards.dfes.gov.uk

World Health Organisation: Health Behaviour in School Aged Children: www.hbsc.org/ publications/factsheets/pdfs/Mental%20Health/WHO-HBSC%202009-2010%20 International%20Report%20Key%20Findings%20-%20Mental%20Health.pdf

YASP: www.manchestermind.org/projects/project_yasp_about.php

YoungMinds (2006) London: www.youngminds.org.uk/problems/

Youth Justice Board: www.yjb.gov.uk

11

The child's perspective and service delivery

TINA MOULES AND NIAMH O'BRIEN

DISCUSSION POINTS

- Are there any risks associated with children's participation?
- What are the barriers to children's participation?
- What do you understand by the term *participation* in your area of work?
- How could you involve children and young people in your work?
- To what extent can we involve all children in a participatory way? Or can we?
- How can we develop systems for the effective monitoring of children's participation?
- How can we know when participation has been achieved? Or can we?
- Consider the idea that non-participation is just as valuable as participation.

CASE STUDIES

Case study 11.1: Children play an active role in decision-making

Children undertaking *You're Welcome* (Department of Health [DH] 2011b) reviews recommended changes to a sexual health clinic. Though they were very positive about the staff and the service, they thought that the reception area was very clinical and could be seen from the road meaning that there was the potential for a lack of privacy and confidentiality. The clinical commissioning group responded by setting aside funds to redesign the reception area and asked the children to help with the design (Blades et al. 2013).

Source: Blades R, Renton Z, La Valle I, et al. (2013) *We Would Like to Make a Change: Children and Young People's Participation in Strategic Health Decision-Making.* London: Office of the Children's Commissioner. http://www.childrenscommissioner.gov.uk/content/publications/content_655 (accessed on 13 January 2014).

Case study 11.2: Children influence the design of toilets in their school

Pupils on the school council in a primary school in Wales raised the need for improvements to be made to their toilets. As a result, the Head teacher and Friends of the School raised funds to pay for the improvements. The pupils helped staff to plan the work and as a result the toilets were transformed into bright, modern and colourful suites. Mirrors were provided as well as soap dispensers and sanitary provision. Pupils now monitor the areas and report any problems immediately. This work has prompted the teachers to improve their toilets (Clarke 2004).

Source: Clarke P. (2004) *Lifting the Lid on the Nation's School Toilets.* Swansea, UK: Children's Commissioner for Wales.

INTRODUCTION

PULSE is a group of young people (aged 12–22 years) who believe that 'children and young people's views about health and wellbeing are important and should be gathered, listened to and acted upon' (PULSE 2013, p. 2). In both the case studies above, that is precisely what happened. Not only were the children and young people* asked for their opinions and views but also they were very clear as to the outcomes of their participation. Since the beginning of the 1990s there has been a drive towards involving children and young people in the development and delivery of services. At no other time in our history has there been so much focus on enabling children and young people to participate in the lives of their communities and the evidence points to a growing recognition of their specific value within society (Department for Education [DfE] 2010; Ahmed et al. 2011; Blades et al. 2013).

What constitutes 'participation' by children is interpreted in many different ways. Often the degree to which they are encouraged or enabled to participate depends largely on the attitude of adults around them and the interpretation those adults place on the term *participation*. As a result, the current focus of the UK government and other bodies on children's participation can run the risk of being implemented in a meaningless way or not implemented at all. In a period of significant reform, however, there is real opportunity for those who work with children and young people to make children's participation in public health decision-making a reality. This chapter begins by examining the case for children's participation in public health service design and delivery and by describing the policy drivers that underpin the situation as it is at the beginning of 2014. The content is then placed firmly in the context of public health, moving on to take a positive approach to enabling participation, presenting ideas for making participation a reality. Then, before concluding, we present a number of case studies to demonstrate examples of good practice.

THE CASE FOR INCLUDING THE CHILD IN SERVICE DESIGN AND DELIVERY

The DfE (2010), in its *Policy paper: Positive for Youth* suggests that embedded in national policy is an assertion that children have a paramount role to play in service provision. One reason

---

* By 'children and young people' we mean all those from birth to 18 years of age. We also use the terms *children* and *young people* interchangeably.

for involving children in service delivery is the potential for services to improve because of their involvement. Involving children in all levels of service planning, delivery and evaluation can lead to services that are more appropriately equipped to meet their specific needs. As Hart and Chesson (1998, p. 1602) argue, 'unless children's perceptions … are known, services cannot respond to their needs and improvements to achieve high quality care cannot be instigated'.

Research studies have shown that the involvement of children and young people can lead to better decision-making, which is more likely to be based on accurate information and therefore more likely to be implemented and subsequently to have beneficial outcomes (Thoburn 1992; Hodgson 1996). Coyne and Gallagher (2011) in their Irish research exploring the experiences of participation in decision-making by children in hospital, report that all of the children in their study (aged 7–18, n = 55) spoke of the need to have information made available to them about their treatment and hospital stay. Some children had a positive experience of being involved in these discussions while others did not. Those children who were actively involved in the decision-making process reported feeling '…valued, happy and less anxious' (p. 2337). In contrast, children who felt less involved reported feelings of confusion, anger, sadness, rejection and betrayal (Coyne and Gallagher 2011).

Aubrey and Dahl (2006) propose that children's perspectives on the services they receive can contribute to the development of new knowledge and to the development of more democratic communities. The children (aged 5–11, n = 21) in their study, which analysed the views of vulnerable children about the significance of the services they received, found that the children held many valid views that related to their relationships with service providers. In addition, Aubrey and Dahl found that the children would have welcomed more involvement in decisions about services that affected them. Importantly, children themselves have indicated that they want to be involved and, more importantly, that they want to be listened to. Primarily they want to be part of decisions about matters that concern them closely, including the education system, public transport, health, education and advice (Borland et al. 2001). Compilation of evidence from a number of consultation documents with children found that with respect to health promotion, children have stated they want to be involved in the design, development and evaluation of both child friendly campaigns and services (LaValle et al. 2012).

Children give a variety of reasons for why they believe they should participate in decision-making about services, including the fact that it offers them new skills, builds their self-esteem and leads to better outcomes, and because they think children have different perceptions from adults (Lansdown 2001; Kirby et al. 2003). Coyne and Gallagher (2011) suggest that the factors promoting participation in hospitals are familiarity with the hospital and staff, the age of the child and professional time.

Moreover, *how* parents include their children in decision-making has an impact on how the children participate. Coyne and Gallagher (2011) conclude that in some cases health professionals and parents underestimate a child's ability to participate in decision-making and do not allow the child adequate time to process the information they have been provided with before they can make a decision. Coyne and Gallagher (2011) call for the development of hospital policies to include the importance of giving children adequate space to make decisions and not to discriminate against children's capabilities based on their age. These authors note that when adults communicate with children in a child-friendly way in accordance with the preferences of the child, it demonstrates to children that adults respect them and take their viewpoints seriously. Indeed Hinton (2008) argues that continuous adult-child communication encourages adults to understand the child's socio-cultural background where language capacity and children's ability are not being confused. Furthermore as the participation of children

....improves the quality of care provided, it is an important investment and one that requires adults to move to a child-centred approach in how they relate to children.

(Coyne and Gallagher 2011, p. 2341)

Social and political arguments for involving children in service delivery rest on the fact that they share the same world as adults, coping with similar factors that affect their lives. As Willow (1997) points out, in her review of local authorities, that failing to involve children or consult with them also fails to take into account their specific views and experiences. It fails to recognize children as future citizens and ignores their *presentness* thereby leaving them without a voice. With no voice, it could be argued that they have no responsibility to contribute to society's norms and rules, which can be 'seen as a form of social exclusion' (Johnson and Ivan-Smith 1998, p. 7).

A society that does not value the contribution of all its members breeds inequality and divisiveness (Willow 1997). Promoting children's participation increases their visibility, brings their needs to the attention of adults and can lead to better decision-making. In a report on effective government structures for children, Hodgkin and Newell (1996, p. 38) argue that if children and young people are given more opportunities to participate in the running of society, 'they will be more willing to engage in the processes of democracy'.

POLICY DRIVERS

Children and young people are key stakeholders of the NHS and their interests must be at the centre of health and local government services.

(Royal College of Paediatrics and Child Health [RCPCH] 2011, p. 2)

Since the first edition of this book was published in 2007, the UK government has undergone major change. In 2010, the United Kingdom came under the leadership of a Coalition Government, the first peacetime Coalition since the 1930s (Brooks 2013). Prior to 2010 New Labour had laid the foundations for the new Coalition's formulation of policies around children that recognized the importance of acknowledging their participation rights (Brooks 2012; Davies 2013).

At the end of 1991 the British Government signed up to the United Nations Convention on the Rights of the Child (UNCRC) (1989). This international treaty gives children a voice, and at the same time presupposes a more socially active role for them. By acknowledging that children still need protection and provision by adults, as well as the right to participate in decisions affecting their lives, the UNCRC recognizes the role of children as social actors. In 2014, the UK Government will report to the committee on the rights of the child on how they have implemented the UNCRC (Children's Rights Alliance for England [CRAE] 2013). The draft report, published for consultation in October 2013, describes the policy changes affecting children yet no analysis of how these changes have impacted on the lives of children themselves is evident (CRAE 2013).

In 2003, the commitment to improving the lives of children, young people and their families was strengthened by the publication of the Green Paper *Every Child Matters* (Chief Secretary to the Treasury 2003), which proposed changes in policy and legislation in England to intensify the focus of services around the needs of children, young people and their families. Support for the proposals was clearly evident in its intention to base services on outcomes identified by children themselves rather than via prescribed organizational change alone. At the beginning of March 2004, the Children Bill was published alongside *Every Child Matters: The Next Steps* (DES 2004) and the Bill received Royal Assent in November 2004. The *Children Act 2004* provides the legal framework for the programme of reform outlined in the Green Paper (Chief Secretary to the Treasury 2003). The Act was an attempt by Parliament to shift the focus from crisis-driven, hard-end-service delivery towards prevention and early detection by the formation of new children's services authorities managed by strategic partnerships that would integrate the planning, commissioning and delivery of services.

The *Children Act 2004* also made provision for the appointment of a Children's Commissioner for England. The devolved administration in Wales established a Children's Commissioner in 2001. A Children's Commissioner was appointed in Northern Ireland in June 2003 and Scotland's Parliament appointed their commissioner in February 2004. Their roles are to ensure that the views of children are heard in the national public arena. Children's wishes to participate in decision-making in relation to the English appointment were evident in July 2002, when more than 150 children and young people went to the House of Commons to question the Minister of State for Children about the proposals for the Commissioner for England. The young people were clear in their message. They wanted the Children's Commissioner for England to be an independent champion for their rights, with equal powers to those already commissioned in Scotland, Wales and Northern Ireland. However, constraints on the post in England meant that the commissioner had limited powers to carry out formal inquiries into individual children's cases. More recently reforms have been made to the role of the Commissioner in England through the Children and Families Bill (2013) with substantial developments towards children's rights (CRAE, 2013). The Bill recommends

...a rights-based mandate, and repeal provisions which allow the Secretary of State to direct the work of the Commissioner.

(CRAE 2013, p. 11)

Although concerns remain about the independence of the Commissioner, CRAE (2013) welcome the proposals made as moving towards independence. CRAE (2013), remain sceptical when they highlight that the secretary of state will preserve the power to appoint and dismiss to the position of Children's Commissioner. The secretary of state will also retain the power to set the budget for the OCC (CRAE 2013).

Brooks (2013) suggests that the Coalition Government has been committed to delivering on its policies with respect to young people as evidenced through the *Positive for Youth: A New Approach to Cross Government Policy for Young People Aged 13–19* (DfE 2010). This policy document outlines the range of measures to be implemented across nine government departments (Brooks 2013; Davies 2013). This was a timely piece of legislation as Davey (2010) found in ascertaining the impact of children's participation in decision-making. She found little consistency across the organizations in how children's involvement in decision-making was monitored or recorded.

Eighteen months after implementation of *Positive for Youth*, the Government produced a document titled *Positive for Youth – Progress Since December 2011* (HM Government 2013). In the forward to this report, MPs Edward Timpson (Minister for Children and Families) and Nick Hurd (Minister for the Civil Society) in commenting on the successes of the initiative suggested

.....if we support young people and give them the appropriate tools, they can innovate, they can collaborate and they can have an impact.

(HM Government 2013, p. 6)

One of the main features in the *Positive for Youth* initiative is the realization that all of those engaged with young people should have a vested interest in the future of young people and that young people themselves should have a valid contribution to informing decisions, shaping provision and inspecting quality (HM Government 2013). Blades et al. (2013) report examples of excellent practice where children have been actively involved in identifying issues and making decisions about how to improve health services alongside adults. However, they suggest this is an exception to the rule and more often children are involved in one aspect of the decision-making process which is often tokenistic, as the decisions have already been made by adults or children are not aware of how they have fed into the overall decision being made. Byrne and Lundy (2013) reiterate this and suggest that when policy and other documents are made available in the public domain children are often reliant on adults to make them aware of the existence of the documents and also to ensure that a child-friendly version of the document is made available.

LEGAL REQUIREMENTS

All providers of services are now legally required to involve service users in every stage of their care and children and young people are included in these provisions (*Social Care Act 2008* [Regulated Activities] Regulations 2010, and the Care Quality Commission [Registration] Regulations 2009 cited in RCPCH 2011). The Royal College (2011) suggests that regular reviews of policies and practices should be undertaken by all health organizations alongside and with children in order to explore where changes and improvements can be made. In addition, these policies should be transparent about how participation activities will contribute to safeguarding and protecting children from harm (RCPCH 2011).

THE PUBLIC HEALTH PERSPECTIVE

Child public health is not simply about providing adult-designed methods for improving child health. Neither is it any longer about screening and surveillance alone. It is, instead, about improving child health and child life chances across whole population groups. At its best, child public health is a social model of medicine incorporating challenges that demand an understanding of the social, economic and psychosocial culture of childhood. The only way we can do that effectively is to hear the child's perspective. Neither health education nor health promotion initiatives will have the positive outcomes we are searching for if the child's perspective is missing. Children and young people have different experiences from adults about their own health and adults would be advised to avoid making assumptions based on their own experiences alone. In a study carried out by the National Children's Bureau (NCB) (Ahmed et al. 2011) to consult young people on the Government Public Health White Paper (*Healthy Lives, Healthy People*) the young participants reported that children and young people need to be involved in planning, designing and implementing public health campaigns. As one young person commented,

> There's a lot of room for the NHS to make things loads better for young people but there's also a lot of room for them to make it quite a bit worse, there's a danger if they don't listen to what we have had to say.

(Ahmed et al. 2011, p. 32)

Children and young people recognize the importance of being healthy but say that they do not always have access to the information and advice that would help them make healthy choices (Morgan 2010; Children's Society 2012; La Valle et al. 2012). In other research children and young people tell us that they feel public health initiatives are too adult focused, designed by adults and that they fail to address the issues that are important for the younger generation (Brady 2008; Ahmed et al. 2011). In a study by O'Brien and Moules (2013) the young people who commissioned the research identified mental health as an important public health issue. Other issues that children and young people identified as being important include stress, bullying, depression, home circumstances and even transport (Cameron 2007; Brady 2008; La Valle et al. 2012).

Vulnerable children face more challenges in relation to their health. For example, children in care identify a lack of information available to them about sexual health, alcohol and drugs (Children and Family Court Advisory and Support Service [CAFCASS] 2008) while children with long-term conditions identified pain management as a key concern (West Bromwich 2011).

The Children and Young People Health Outcomes Forum (CYPHOF) (2012) emphasizes that children should be a major target of public health activity because there is time to establish health routines, behaviours and attitudes to enable them to live healthily for the rest of their lives. The forum goes on to stress the need to include the whole population of children and young people, ensuring that all age groups and all sub-groups with health needs are considered. The report also stresses that

> This is a once in a lifetime chance to make a step change in the way in which public health considers, reflects and includes the voice and meets the health prevention, promotion and protection needs of its child population. It is imperative this chance is not missed. …. Their (children and young people) active engagement is an investment for life and a valuable asset to improve the delivery of public services.

> **(CYPHOF 2012, p. 19)**

If children's 'participation' is to have substance, it will require those who work with children to seek to ensure that children's perspectives are taken into account as the public health reforms (*Health and Social Care Act 2102*) move forward.

PARTICIPATION

What do we mean by participation? Participation, for the purpose of this chapter, is about finding ways of incorporating the views of *all* children and young people in decision-making processes within the context of what is possible both institutionally and culturally (Moules 2005). Participation creates opportunities for children and young people to give their opinions and views and have those views listened to, regardless of how difficult that might be. It is about their opinions being taken seriously in any decision-making process and about them being told exactly how their views have been taken into account. Participation is not an isolated event but is an ongoing process. Children and young people have given their views on what constitutes participation in a number of research studies. First they stress that participation should be respectful with children being treated as persons in their own right, and adults acknowledging that they have something to offer (Neal 2004). Participation should be genuine, useful and focused on change (Stafford et al. 2003) and finally children and young people need access to the necessary information for them to make informed decisions and they emphasize participation as being about 'discussions with adults' (Graham and Fitzgerald 2010).

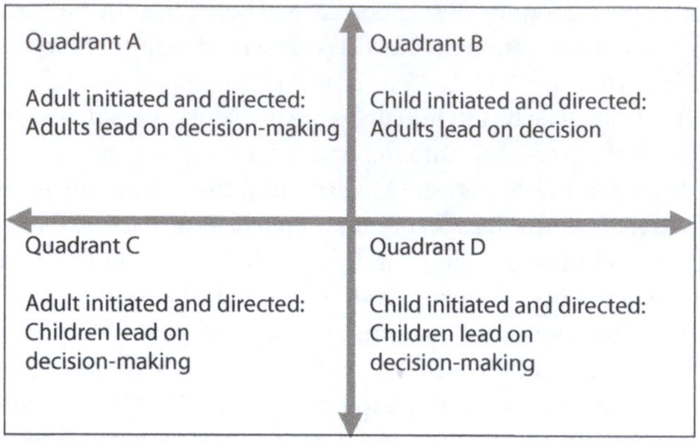

Figure 11.1 Dual axis model of participation.

Coyne and Gallagher (2011), rather than suggesting participation should be 'all or nothing', recommend a continuum of children's participation. These authors found that although children wanted to be involved in discussions about their hospital care, their role was often insignificant and the child's parents and health professionals made the main decisions. They found that most of the 7–18 year olds involved in their study wanted to be involved in some aspects of the decision-making process; some children wanted a large role while others wanted to leave the more 'serious' decisions to adults. A wide range of models of children and young people's participation can be found in the literature (Karsten 2012) including Hart's Ladder of Participation (Hart 1992), Treseder's degrees of participation (Treseder 1997) and Shier's pathways to participation (Shier 2001). One recently developed model is the Dual Axis Model of Participation (Moules and O'Brien 2012). The model starts from the position that participation is happening and adds structure to the various ways in which adults and children can co-operate to achieve the aims of an activity. The model proposes four types of participation all of which can be seen to be present to various degrees and at different times in any one activity/project. These four types of participation are shown in Figure 11.1.

Participation then is about taking part in the decision-making process. In practice though, it is a complex and contextual concept and as such has been described as being multidimensional (Moules and O'Brien 2012) and kaleidoscopic in nature, changing its nature at the 'will of the hands in which it is held' (White et al. 1994) from one moment to another. What has been confirmed though is the fact that participation can evolve, starting with participatory intent and building on this within the limits set by participants and the context (Greenwood et al. 1993; Naylor et al. 2002; Moules and O'Brien 2012).

THE CURRENT SITUATION

By 2015, there have come to be many examples of good practice in relation to the participation of children and young people in decision-making. For example, Davey (2010) reports that since the introduction of the *Children Act* in 2004,

> ...there has been a steady rise in the number of structural mechanisms to enable children to participate in decision-making through student voice and democracy initiatives in schools and youth forums. There has also been a cultural change in the value children, adults and organisations are now placing on children's views.

(Davey 2010, p. 7)

In contrast Davey (2010) suggests the same picture cannot be painted for children's involvement in decision-making in the health service. Historically children were often denied opportunities to contribute to decisions being made about them or to decisions, which influenced policy change. Davey (2010) points to the national surveys on health care and quality of service provision which either usually fail to ask children about their experiences or if these views are sought have little impact on the final decisions made. It seems that there is still a lack of evidence of action and despite a raft of Government policies and guidance, which all stress that every opportunity must be taken to listen to the voices of the young and for their perspectives to be heard, a culture of participation is not commonplace.

In their research paper *We Would Like to Make a Change*, Blades et al. (2013) reviewed local health plans, carried out interviews with local authority health and participation professionals and conducted focus groups with children. This research was carried out to explore children's participation in strategic health decision-making prior to the implementation of the new reforms to the health service in England from April 2013 (Blades et al. 2013). The detailed findings of this report paint a fragmented picture of children's participation in local strategic health decision-making; for example only 28% of the 102 local health plans reviewed showed that children had been meaningfully involved in the development, design or evaluation of the plans (Blades et al. 2013). The authors found that there was

> . . . no coherent national programme of activity to proactively encourage local bodies to include children and young people in strategic health service commissioning or other vital decision-making about NHS provision.

(Blades et al. 2013, p. 2)

Blades et al. suggest that children's participation in local health services has not been fully embedded in everyday practice and there is a reliance on key committed individuals to implement this. Coyne and Gallagher (2011) found that some children reported difficulties in communicating with health professionals and relied on their parents to explain information to them. Cross (2011) reiterates this further and writes that despite changes to policy in the form of children's active engagement to participate in decision-making, vast differences in how practitioners conceptualize participation and equally how they regard participation as relevant in their work is apparent. Limited evidence is available on whether or not children's participation in decision-making improves health and/or social outcomes (Coyne and Gallagher 2011). Indeed, Coyne and Gallagher (2011) acknowledge that for some children participating in decision-making can make situations worse for children in terms of added pressure and responsibility.

In a study exploring the challenges for securing children's rights through policy development in Northern Ireland, Byrne and Lundy (2013) conducted a documentary analysis of policy documents and found that for the most part a child-friendly version of the consultation or the final report was not made available and/or produced. These authors alluded to the fact that consultation with children was often a 'tick-box' exercise. In comparison Davey (2010), in a study commissioned by the OCC to examine children's participation in decision-making in England, found that children were less likely to be involved in setting budgets for services provided for them. Davey (2010) suggests there has been an increase in the number of children involved in the recruitment and selection of staff but there has been little development in the ways in which children are actively involved in decision-making across children's services (Davey 2010).

HEARING CHILDREN'S VIEWS: THE PRACTICE

There has never been as much guidance on the practice of involving children and young people in service design and delivery as now. The literature is awash with principles, reports, booklets, handbooks, charters and standards which have been developed at a national level across a range of sectors (for example *Promoting Children and Young People's Participation through the National Healthy School Standard,* Health Development Agency, 2004*; *Practice Standards in Children's Participation,* Save the Children, 2005†; Quality *Standards for Children and Young People's Participation in CAMHS,* Health and Social Care Advisory Service, 2008‡; *Not Just a Phase: A Guide to the Participation of Children and Young People in Health Services,* RCPCH, 2010§; *Hear by Right in Health Services: Children and Young People's Participation in PCTs, Hospitals and Other Health Settings,* National Youth Agency 2010¶). *Hear by Right in Health Services* (Badham and Wade 2005) is based on the tried and tested standards framework developed by Badham and Wade (2005) for both statutory and voluntary sector organizations to improve their practice and policies on the involvement of children and young people. It is based on the Seven S model of organizational change: shared values, strategy, structures, systems, staff, skills and knowledge and style of leadership. Self-assessment is the key to this model and it is developed across three levels known as *emerging, established* and *advanced* with each level built on the last. By using this approach the active involvement of children and young people is embedded in service delivery and is not just an added extra (Badham and Wade 2005).

Standards have also been developed at a local level, generally only applicable to local agencies. One such example is the Participation Strategy and Charter 2012–2015, *Charter of Participation for Children and Young People in Wirral*** (2006). The Strategy is based on five principles, each with a checklist of things to address to enhance children and young people's ability to participate. It includes an evaluation and action plan for organizations to record what they are doing and to plan for future action. However, operationalizing standards for children's participation in service delivery will depend on many factors including the type of service, the context, the aim of the process and the children involved. Wright et al. (2006, p. 6) propose a 'whole systems approach' that organizations can take to affect a change or improvement in the way in which they implement participation. They identify four aspects of service development that need to be considered namely the *culture, structures, the practice* and *review.*

A *culture* of participation needs to be established where there is a shared commitment to the involvement of children. Senior management support is important and their backing is important for ensuring participation initiatives are agreed and moved forward and for ensuring children's voices are acted on (Oldfield and Fowler 2004). Indeed a lack of commitment by senior management is still seen as one of the barriers to effective participation (Davey 2010). Identifying leaders for change, building capacity and effective partnership working are all essential on the pathway to a culture of participation. In developing a culture and to make participation by children meaningful, organizations need to be clear about what they want to achieve and the values that underpin their work. The barriers to participation need to be identified and steps are needed to break them down. In particular, it may be necessary to promote attitudinal change among adults (Oldfield and Fowler 2004; Cross 2011).

---

* http://www.nice.org.uk/niceMedia/documents/promoting_participation_nhss.pdf.
† http://www.savethechildren.org.uk/sites/default/files/docs/practice_standards_participation_1.pdf.
‡ http://www.hascas.org.uk/pdf_files/HASCASselfassessCAMHSparticipation.pdf.
§ http://www.rcpch.ac.uk/system/files/protected/page/RCPCH_Not_Just_a_Phase_0.pdf.
¶ http://www.ayph.org.uk/publications/100_hbr%2022.4.10[4].pdf.
** http://www.teenwirral.com/downloads/18.

In an organization with a culture of participation, involvement of children and young people is an integral part of the way in which it operates, participation is meaningful and sustainable and is everyone's responsibility (RCPCH 2010). In a survey by Davey (2010), many professionals and organizations were positive about the involvement of children and young people in participation work and the majority supported the view that there are no decisions in which children cannot be involved. More than two thirds of organizations surveyed stated that they had policies/strategies in place to support participation. However, while this is a positive finding, the study also found that participation was limited in some areas – notably health services where children's opportunities to be involved in decision-making were limited or had little impact. There is some limited evidence of children participating in strategic decisions but again it is patchy (Coad and Shaw 2008; Burke 2010; Coyne and Gallagher 2011).

As the culture changes so too does the importance of developing and planning the *structures* and systems to support it. The structures to be considered include staff, resources and the processes for decision-making and planning. Funding is vital in order to provide the resources needed to implement effective and sustainable participation activities. The need for long-term funding of participation work was top of the list of suggestions by front-line workers and organizations for promoting better children's involvement (Davey 2010). Evidence does point to an increase in resources to support participation (Davey 2010) with increased evidence of training for staff. However, Davey (2010) also reports that there is a lack of training for senior staff and that this needs to be remedied if participation is to be embedded in all parts of an organization. Participation workers reported that senior staff tend to have a lack of understanding about the resources required to fully support children's participation (Davey 2010).

Putting participation into *practice* requires the involvement of all children, regardless of their age, culture and ethnic origin. It means accessing the perceptions of children in hard to reach groups like Traveller children and the children of asylum seekers. It means hearing the voices of disabled children and those with learning difficulties. The environment must be child friendly and one in which they can express their views without fear of feeling intimidated. Different approaches to participation, involving creative and flexible methods, are required and should be appropriate to the context and to the children involved. Importantly children must be given the choice to participate or not, depending on their own personal and contextual situation (Coyne and Gallagher 2011).

For example, Davey (2010) found children in secondary school were more likely to be involved in decision-making than those in primary school with participation by children under the age of 8 years scarce. In childhood research, McNamee and Seymour (2012) suggest there is an over-representation of children aged 10–12 years who are either actively involved in the process of research or as data sources. This they argue is potentially down to the competence-based approach where researchers tend to group children in terms of their ages rather than level of understanding. As detailed above, guidance about the 'how' of participation abounds in the literature. One such document is *Putting Children at the Centre: A Practical Guide to Children's Participation** published by Save the Children (2010). This online resource provides practitioners with clear, easy to use practical guidance regarding the 'how' of participation under the following headings:

- Advance preparation
- Qualities of a good facilitator
- Tailoring your approach to the evolving capacities of children and young people
- How children and young people learn

---

* http://www.savethechildren.org.uk/sites/default/files/docs/Putting_Children_at_the_Centre_final_%282%29_1.pdf.

- Creating a child-friendly environment
- Planning a session or activity with children and young people
- Ensuring non-discriminatory practice
- Ensuring the health and safety of children and young people
- Trouble-shooting and dealing with difficult situations
- Involving children and young people in facilitation

(Save the Children 2010, p. 26)

Last, it is important that a *review* of all the above is carried out in order to make judgments about the effectiveness of the participation process and the impact it has on service design and delivery. Regular review helps to identify the benefits of involvement for the children and for the services they use. Feedback to children enables them to see the impact they have and strengthens the value adults place on children's perceptions (RCPCH 2012). Even though health services have improved to some degree, the overwhelming evidence points to a lack of monitoring and evaluation in many participatory activities with children (Oldfield and Fowler 2004; Davey 2010). In the survey by Davey (2010), only 37% of organizations evaluated the impact of participation. In the focus groups conducted by Davey (2010), children who had been involved in the decision-making process criticized adults for not providing them with feedback about how their opinions had influenced the decisions made. They argued that 'having the means to voice an opinion was only the first stage in engaging children in decision-making' (p. 11). Coad and Shaw (2008) in their scoping review of children's choices in health care found that although children want more input into planning and developing appropriate services, there is limited evaluative research on whether these choices are acted upon and whether they inform any positive future changes in service delivery.

FEEDBACK TO CHILDREN

The RCPCH (2011) emphasizes that children must receive feedback about how their participation has influenced decisions made in service delivery and design. The RCPCH stress that when children see where their participation has made a difference this can be empowering for children. The RCPCH (2011) suggest that children, like adults, are not a homogenous group and different children will want to be engaged in different ways (if at all). Practitioners need to understand the individuality of each child and recognize when it is an appropriate time to engage them. An example offered by the RCPCH (2011) is that some children might only want to become involved in decision-making, or have ideas for change after they have experienced the service on offer.

A review of the process of participation can be carried out using many of the various models of participation available. Using the Dual-Axis Model (Figure 11.1) participation can be plotted in the different quadrants during different parts of the activity/event or at the end. The plotting ought to be carried out by both participating children and practitioners and then compared. The result of plotting participation will be to identify how the balance of decision-making, initiation and direction fluctuates during the life of an activity/project. Evaluation of the process can help to improve individual or organizational performance in children's participation and also helps to identify skills or knowledge gaps and develop appropriate training.

CASE STUDIES

The following examples show how children and young people of different ages and abilities can participate at a range of levels in the area of public health from strategic design through to local interventions.

SCHOOL NURSE REFORM – CONSULTATIONS WITH CHILDREN AND YOUNG PEOPLE

In 2011, the DH set up the School Nurse Development Program and recognized the importance of seeking the views of children and young people in shaping the profession for the future. As a result the development team invited the British Youth Council (BYC), NCB and the North West Regional Youth Work Unit (NWRYWU) to seek the views of children and young people. Between them the projects aimed to find out children's and young people's experiences of the existing school nurse system, the priorities for school nursing and more broadly the health service in schools and to ascertain the things that school nurses could do to help children keep healthy. The findings were reassuringly similar across the three projects (Figure 11.2).

Young people were identified as being key partners in the development and their views were said to be 'central to the School Nurse Programme of Development' (DH 2012, p. 37). The DH states that the key issues raised by the children and young people were accessibility, visibility and confidentiality and that these 'views and ideas were fed directly into the DH's School Nursing Development Plan' (DH 2012, p. 37). Children and young people and their families are cited as being 'advisors to the programme' and 'champions for improving local services and health outcomes' (DH 2012, p. 7) and in a programme co-produced with children, there is a commitment to involving in ongoing service review.

BYC (2011)

Method 1: Online survey
Sample: 1599; 11–18 age group.

Method 2: Focus groups at BYC Conventions:
Sample: 202.
Findings:
1. School nurses need to:
   • Be visible and well known
   • Offer early help
   • Offer choice
2. Young people want to offer their views about the service they receive.

NWRYWU (Moxon 2011)

Method: Future focused consultation exercise
Sample: 50 aged 13–19.
Significant findings:
   • Confidentiality – need for a discrete and trusted independent service
   • Identified attributes of a 'good' school nurse service
   • School nurse should be known and visible.
   • Would like access to a range of services in school

NCB (2011b)

Method: Survey mixture of closed and open questions on two pages.
Sample: 293 children aged 6–11 in eight schools across England.
Key findings:
   • School nurses need to be visible and introduced to children
   • Most of those who had seen the school nurse had positive experience
   • School nurses should be kind, caring, friendly, helpful and someone who would listen
   • Children want help with healthy eating, bullying, problems at home

Figure 11.2 Findings from three schools nurse projects.

CYBER-BULLYING – RESEARCH COMMISSIONED BY YOUNG PEOPLE

One of the responsibilities of the NCB is to promote the involvement of children and young people in the work of the Public Health Research Consortium (PHRC). In 2006, the NCB set up The Young People's Reference Group, which, with further funding from the PHRC and the Wellcome Trust, was able to continue in the form of the PEAR* (Public health, Education, Awareness, Research) Project. PEAR consisted of two reference groups, one based in London and the other based in Leeds with a total of 20 young people aged 13–18. As part of their work with the PHRC, PEAR identified mental health and bullying as two of the main public health issues for young people. The young people decided that they would like to commission a research project to explore the impact of cyber-bullying on young people's mental health. They had not found much research on this new form of bullying, and thought that it might still be relatively invisible or inaccessible to adult researchers. The group also felt that, as most of the research on bullying and mental health starts from an adult perspective, they wanted to commission their own research project. As a result they commissioned researchers from Anglia Ruskin University to carry out this project with them (O'Brien and Moules 2013).

PEAR and the Anglia Ruskin researchers decided on a participatory design using a mixture of quantitative and qualitative methods meaning that the young people were actively involved in all aspects of the research. Prior to the research taking place, PEAR alongside the NCB researchers decided on the topic for investigation, helped write the project specification and short-listed the proposals. PEAR also drafted the questions for possible candidates and contributed to the final commissioning decision. The methods used included an online survey using SurveyMonkey aimed at all young people aged 12–18 across England. The survey was followed up with two focus groups. In total 490, young people took part in the study and the key findings are shown in Figure 11.3. PEAR made a number of recommendations for practice and policy (Figure 11.4.)

The PEAR project (process and impact) was reviewed following its completion in 2010 (Davey 2011) using a number of methods including an online survey, interviews, focus groups

---

The key findings:

- Overall twice the number of girls than boys said they had experienced cyber-bullying in some way.

- Of those who said they had been affected by cyber-bullying the most common effect was to their confidence, self-esteem and mental and emotional well-being.

- A quarter of those who had been cyber-bullied (28.8%, $n = 23$) stayed away from school and over a third (38.9%, $n = 31$) stopped socialising outside school.

- Of those who had been cyber-bullied, over half had sought support mainly from parents and friends.

- Most of the young people thought that cyber-bullying is as harmful as traditional bullying but some feel it does not exist and is down to the victims ability to cope with it.

Figure 11.3 PEAR Project: Cyber-bullying and mental health. (From O'Brien and Moules, *The Impact of Cyber-Bullying on Young People's Mental Health. Final Report.* Chelmsford, UK: Anglia Ruskin University and NCB, 2010. http://www.ncb.org.uk/media/111007/cyber-bullying_report.pdf).

---

* http://www.ncb.org.uk/pear.

Develop educational programmes around awareness for young people, parents/carers and schools.

Deliver education that brings together young people and their families to enhance communication in relation to online media.

Educate young people about what constitutes acceptable behaviour online.

Support young people to report incidents of cyber-bullying through other young people who could help change attitudes and provide a source of support to young people.

Develop policies that take a holistic approach and which stress the importance of developing values of care and kindness among young people.

Figure 11.4 Recommendations for practice and policy. (From O'Brien and Moules, *The Impact of Cyber-Bullying on Young People's Mental Health. Final Report.* Chelmsford, UK: Anglia Ruskin University and NCB, 2010. http://www.ncb.org.uk/media/111007/cyber-bullying_report.pdf).

and data collected in formal evaluations during the life of the project. Members of PEAR gave feedback on research proposals being submitted for funding and as one researcher states:

> The PEAR group gave us useful advice and feedback about the proposal, the basic research idea, and also advice about the research design and appropriate methods, ethical issues in working with young people, and involving young people in research.

(Davey 2011, p. 20)

In addition public health researchers, who had worked with the PEAR group, said they would be more likely to involve young people in future projects as a result of the PEAR model (Davey 2011). Impact on the young people was also evident and included a sense of achievement, seeing progress and a feeling of being valued (following input from National Institute for Health and Care Excellence [NICE] at one of their conferences) and an advanced understanding of research and evaluation. With regard to the process, the evaluation identified a number of challenges facing practitioners and researchers who want to involve children and young people. These are mainly time constraints, the need for sufficient resources and support for the young people and researchers, and the need for feedback.

SEXUAL HEALTH SERVICES

McCarthy et al. (2012) set out to explore whether using the Internet as a way of educating young people about sexual health would be feasible. The research team carried out 21 focus groups and 6 one-to-one interviews with a total of 67 young people aged 16–22 years. The participants all supported the creation of a website that had been developed with the input of young people and they felt that existing sites did not address their needs. They identified a range of features that such a website should have, which included the following:

- Content needs to be straightforward, honest and accurate with the use of uncomplicated words, especially in relation to sexual pleasure, communication, sexually transmitted diseases, pregnancy and emotional issues. Youth speak should not be used
- Look and feel of the website – images should reflect diversity of UK young people, with a clear website name and pages limited in textual content. Content should be updated

and new information uploaded every week. Young people wanted social interaction (anonymous) to be possible with videos (real-life situations with good actors).

The researchers were able to develop a website*, which met the needs of young people and which combines the views if young people with theory-based interactive elements. However McCarthy et al. (2012) highlight the challenges experienced during the project the main one being technical and budgetary constraints within which they had to work. Some of the ideas the young people had, for example the use of discussion boards and regular updating, were impossible to implement for financial and ethical issues. McCarthy et al. conclude that consulting with young people is valuable and allows them to offer key insights to influence interventions for sexual health promotion.

ENABLING DISABLED CHILDREN'S PARTICIPATION

The views of disabled children are no less important than those of other children especially as they are bound to experience significant contact with health services. Though government policy regarding participation by children and young people applies to all children regardless of their ability, participation by disabled children, and in particular by those who rely on technology to communicate, is limited (Franklin and Sloper 2009). This is more than likely due to a number of practical problems including communication difficulties, time constraints and the need to potentially access disabled children through a range of gatekeepers (Franklin and Sloper 2009). Traditional methods of data collection are not necessarily appropriate for use with disabled children and young people and so a range of non-traditional methods is becoming available. One example of involving disabled children and young people is the consultation by Turner (2003) who carried out a consultation in Wales to inform the National Children's Framework. One hundred and five disabled children and young people, between the ages of 5–25, were spoken to.

> The sample included children and young people with: autism, cerebral palsy, attention deficit hyperactivity disorder (ADHD), learning disabilities and difficulties, Down's syndrome, mobility and access difficulties, sensory disabilities (primarily speech and hearing impairments), mental health difficulties and chronic illness.

(Turner 2003, p. 4)

The methods used to collect data were developed with guidance from a group of disabled children and young people and included a focus on activities and games, ranking exercises, draw and write (Horstman et al. 2008), and Makaton. Further guidance on appropriate methods to use with disabled children is available on the Internet (Figure 11.5).

One of the key conclusions was that disabled children and young people want to have an opportunity to give their views both on service design and provision as the following quote from one of the children shows:

> Disabled children and young people should be involved in helping to make services better. We should be asked about what we would like to see happen to us. Our views should be taken into consideration.

(Turner 2003, p. 28)

* http://www.sexunzipped.co.uk/home.

National Children's Bureau. (2008). *How to Involve Children and Young People with Communication Impairments in Decision-Making*. London: NCB.

http://www.participationworks.org.uk/files/webfm/shop_files/howto_Communication.pdf [accessed 20 February 2014].

Making Ourselves Heard – A national project to ensure disabled children's views are heard. Has a wide range of resources.

http://www.councilfordisabledchildren.org.uk/what-we-do/networkscampaigning/ making-ourselves-heard [accessed 20 February 2014].

Disability Toolkit – Up-to-date information on resources, policies, research, examples of good practice.

http://sites.childrenssociety.org.uk/disabilitytoolkit/ [accessed 20 February 2014].

Figure 11.5 Guidance for involving disabled children.

ASKING YOUNG CHILDREN FOR THEIR VIEWS

Even very young children deserve to have their views listened to and it is up to practitioners to learn how to tune in to what babies and young children are saying. The Young Children's Voices Network (YCVN)*, under the auspices of the NCB, promotes the participation of babies and children up to 5 years old. Listening is the first step in enabling participation, a listening culture values children's involvement. YCVN (Blades and Kumari 2011, p. 8) defines listening as

> An active process of receiving (hearing and observing), interpreting and responding to communication – it includes all the senses and emotions and is not limited to the spoken word.

Much of the published work around the participation of young children (especially those under 5) is in the field of early years education. However, health practitioners have much to learn from exploring the different ways used by early years practitioners to gather young children's views. An interesting example here is from a daycare nursery in Leeds who wanted to find out what the babies and children (aged 3 months to 5 years old) thought about their staff 'uniform' of a T-shirt with the nursery's name on it, referred to below as the 'BB T-shirt'. To include all the children, the staff devised a 'listening' activity, which could be adapted to each age group. They placed various pieces of clothing, fabric and staff T-shirts into a large basket. The children were then helped by familiar carers to explore the contents of the basket. Staff observed the children, took photographs, recorded verbal comments and gave the older children the option of drawing pictures. Figure 11.6 shows what they found.

Staff concluded that the children did not like the staff T-shirts but instead preferred colour and texture. They stopped wearing the T-shirts.

This example may seem to be dealing with a small issue. However it indicates that if you use the right methods and listen carefully to young children, even babies, you can learn much that could influence not only small areas of practice but also larger policy issues. Other resources available to help encourage listening to babies and young children are shown in Figure 11.7.

* http://www.ncb.org.uk/areas-of-activity/early-childhood/networks/young-childrens-voices-network.

Babies of 3–16 months loved the different textures, bracelets and beads. They did not explore the BB T-shirts.

Children of 16–24 months explored the basket and chose items they wanted to wear, which did not include the BB T-shirts.

Children of 24–36 months selected and discussed favourite items; they showed no preference for the BB T-shirts.

Children of 36–60 months dressed a member of staff to make her beautiful. The only two items they did not select were the BB T-shirts.

Figure 11.6 Findings from the nursery project.

Listening as a Way of Life—A set of eight leaflets on a range of topics, containing details of research, practice and methods that work with young children from birth to eight. http://www.ncb.org.uk/areas-of-activity/early-childhood/resources/publications/listening-and-participation [accessed 21 February 2014].

2010. *Let's Listen Young Children's Voices – Profiling and Planning to Enable Their Participation in Children's Services.* London: NCB. http://www.participationworks.org.uk/files/webfm/files/rooms/early_years/Let'slisten.pdf [accessed 20 February 2014].

Clarke and Moss (2011).

Figure 11.7 Guidance for listening to young children.

CONCLUSION

This chapter has provided an overview of the case for participation by children of all ages in service design and delivery. The benefits to children and to the services they use are well documented and the increase in participatory initiatives to hear their voices is evident across all voluntary and statutory organizations, at both a local and national level. The policy background clearly spells out a commitment to listen to the views of children and young people on behalf of the Government. However, the reality is not always as effective as it might be and many barriers still exist which mitigate against children's voices being heard and listened to. These barriers stem mainly from the fact that participation is not embedded into organizations and because there is a vast difference between how practitioners perceive participation. The opportunities to involve children, however, are there for practitioners to take up. Participation by children in service delivery will not happen without planning but it is also important to recognize that participation is a dynamic process that develops over time and needs input from all levels including staff, management, children, parents and external organizations.

KEY POINTS

- Involving children and young people in service design and delivery provides benefits for services, for children and young people, recognizes children and young people as citizens.
- The *Positive for Youth* initiative acknowledges that all of those engaged with young people should have a vested interest in the future of young people and that young people themselves should have a valid contribution to informing decisions, shaping provision and inspecting quality.
- Child public health is a social model of medicine incorporating challenges that demand an understanding of the social, economic and psychosocial culture of childhood. The only way we can do that effectively is to hear the child's perspective.
- Participation creates opportunities for children and young people to give their opinions and views and have those views listened to, regardless of how difficult that might be.
- Organizations need to take a *whole systems approach* when changing or improving the way they enable children and young people to participate. Four aspects of service development need to be considered namely the *culture, structures, the practice* and *review*.

REFERENCES

Ahmed A, Adams B, Kertesz C, et al. (2011) *Healthy Lives, Healthy People: Young People's Views on Being Well and the Future of Public Health.* London: NCB. http://www.ncb.org.uk/media/37997/vss_publichealth_report.pdf (accessed on 23 January 2014).

Aubrey C, Dahl S. (2006) Children's voices: The views of vulnerable children on their service providers and the relevance of services they receive. *British Journal of Social Work* 36: 21–39.

Badham B, Wade H. (2005) *Hear by Right: Standards for the Active Involvement of Children and Young People.* London: The NYA/Local Government Association. www.nya.org.uk/hearbyright

Blades R, Renton Z, La Valle I, et al. (2013) *We Would Like to Make a Change: Children and Young People's Participation in Strategic Health Decision-Making.* London: Office of the Children's Commissioner. http://www.childrenscommissioner.gov.uk/content/publications/content_655 (accessed on 13 January 2014).

Blades R, Kumari V. (2011) *Putting Listening Practice at the Heart of Early Years Practice: An Evaluation of the Young Children's Voices Network.* London: NCB. http://www.ncb.org.uk/media/61764/evaluation_of_ycvn_final_report.pdf (accessed on 20 February 2014).

Borland M, Hill M, Laybourne A, Stafford A. (2001) *Improving Consultation with Children and Young People in Relevant Aspects of Policy Making and Legislation in Scotland.* Glasgow: University of Glasgow.

Brady L-M. (2008) *Young People's Public Health Reference Group (2008) Pilot Project – Executive Summary.* London: National Children's Bureau. http://phrc.lshtm.ac.uk/papers/PHRC_YPPHRG_Final_Report.pdf (accessed on 22 January 2014).

Brooks R. (2013) The social construction of young people within education policy: Evidence from the UK's coalition government. *Journal of Youth Studies* 16(3): 318–333.

Burke T. (2010) *Anyone Listening? Evidence of Children and Young People's Participation in England.* London: National Children's Bureau.

Byrne B, Lundy L. (2013) Reconciling children's policy and children's rights: Barriers to effective government delivery. *Children and Society* 1–11. doi: 10.1111/chso.12045.

Cafcass. (2008) *Cafcass Health and Wellbeing Review: The Experiences of Young People in Care.* London: Cafcass.

Cameron C. (2007) Access to health services: Care leavers and young people in difficulty. *ChildRight* 238: 22–25.

Cavat J, Sloper P. (2004) The participation of children and young people in decisions about UK service development. *Child: Care, Heath and Development* 30: 613–621.

Chief Secretary to the Treasury. (2003) *Every Child Matters* (Cm 5860). London: Stationery Office. www.everychildmatters.gov.uk/_content/documents/EveryChildMatters.pdf (accessed on 17 January 2007).

Clarke, A, Moss P. (2011) *Listening to Young Children: The Mosaic approach.* London: NCB.

Clarke P. (2004) *Lifting the Lid on the Nation's School Toilets.* Swansea, UK: Children's Commissioner for Wales.

Children and Young People's Health Outcomes Forum. (2012) *Report of the Public Health and Prevention sub-group.*https://www.gov.uk/government/uploads/system/uploads/attachment_data/file/216854/CYP-Public-Health.pdf (accessed on 14 January 2014).

Children's Rights Alliance for England. (2013) *State of Children's Rights in England: Review of Government Action on United Nations' Recommendations for Strengthening Children's Rights in the UK.* http://www.crae.org.uk/media/64143/CRAE_England_Report_WEB.pdf (accessed on 7 January 2014).

Children's Society. (2012) *The Good Childhood Report 2012: A Review of Our Children's Well-Being.* London: Children's Society.

Coad JE, Shaw KL. (2008) Is children's choice in health care rhetoric or reality? A scoping review. *Journal of Advanced Nursing* 64(4): 318–327.

Coyne I, Gallagher P. (2011) Participation in communication and decision-making: Children and young people's experiences in a hospital setting. *Journal of Clinical Nursing* 20: 2334–2343.

Cross B. (2011) Becoming, being and having been: Practitioner perspectives on temporal stances and participation across children's services. *Children and Society* 25: 26–36.

Davey C. (2010) *Children's Participation in Decision-Making. A Summary Report on Progress Made Up to 2010.* London: NCB. http://www.participationworks.org.uk/files/webfm/files/npf~/npf_publications/A%20Summary%20Report_jun10.pdf (accessed on 13 January 2014).

Davey C. (2011) *Evaluation of the PEAR Project.* London: National Children's Bureau. http://www.ncb.org.uk/media/111188/pear_evaluation_report_0211.pdf (accessed on 17 February 2014).

Davies B. (2013) Youth work in a changing policy landscape: The view from England. *Youth and Policy* 110: 6–32.

Department for Education. (2010) *Policy Paper: Positive for Youth: The Statement.* https://www.gov.uk/government/publications/positive-for-youth-a-new-approach-to-cross-government-policy-for-young-people-aged-13-to-19/positive-for-youth-the-statement#contents (accessed on 5 February 2014).

Department for Education and Skills. (2004) *Every Child Matters: The Next Steps.* Nottingham, UK: DfES Publications. www.everychildmatters.gov.uk/_content/documents/EveryChildMattersNextSteps.pdf (accessed on 17 January 2007).

Department of Health. (2011a) *Healthy Lives, Healthy People: Update and Way Forward*. https://www.gov.uk/government/publications/healthy-lives-healthy-people-update-and-way-forward (accessed on 13 January 2014).

Department of Health. (2011b) *You're Welcome – Quality Criteria for Young People Friendly Health Services.* Crown Copyright.

Department of Health. (2012) *Getting it Right for Children, Young People and Families. Maximising the Contribution of the School Nursing Team: Vision and Call to Action.* London: DH.

Franklin A, Sloper P. (2009) Supporting the Participation of Disabled Children and Young People in Decision-making. *Children & Society* 23(1): 3–15.

Graham A, Fitzgerald R. (2010) Progressing children's participation: Exploring the potential of a dialogical turn. *Childhood* 17(3): 343–359.

Greenwood DJ, Whyte WF, Harkavy I. (1993) Participatory action research as a process and as a goal. *Human Relations* 46(2): 175–192.

Hart R. (1992) *Children's Participation. From Tokenism to Citizenship*. Florence, Italy: UNICEF International Child Development Centre.

Hart C, Chesson R. (1998) Children as consumers. *British Medical Journal* 316: 1600–1603.

Hinton R. (2008) Children's participation and good governance: Limitations of the theoretical literature. *International Journal of Children's Rights* 16: 285–300.

HM Government (2013) *Positive for Youth: Progress Since December 2011*. https://www.gov.uk/government/uploads/system/uploads/attachment_data/file/210383/Positive-for-Youth-progress-update.pdf (accessed on 21 January 2014).

Hodgson D. (1996) *Young People's Participation in Social Work Planning: A Resource Pack.* London: National Children's Bureau.

Hodgkin R, Newell P. (1996) *Effective Government Structures for Children.* London: Calouste Gulbenkian Foundation.

Horstman M, Aldiss S, Richardson A, Gibson F. (2008) Methodological issues when using the draw and write technique with children aged 6 to 12 years. *Qualitative Health Research* 18(7): 1001–1011.

Johnson V, Ivan-Smith E. (1998) Children and young people's participation: The starting point. In: Johnson V, Ivan-Smith E, Gordon G, et al. eds. *Children and Young People's Participation in the Development Process.* London: Intermediate Technology Publications; 5–8.

Karsten A. (2012) *A Potpourri of Participation Models.* http://www.youthpolicy.org/library/documents/a-potpourri-of-participation-models/ (accessed on 1 February 2014).

Kirby P, Lanyon C, Cronin K, Sinclair R. (2003) *Building a Culture of Participation. Involving Children and Young People in Policy, Service Planning, Delivery and Evaluation.* London: DeFS Publications.

La Valle I, Payne L, Gibb J, Jelicic H. (2012) *Listening to Children's Views on Health Provision: A Rapid Review of the Evidence.* http://www.ncb.org.uk/media/723497/listening_to_children_s_views_on_health_-_final_report_july__12.pdf (accessed on 22 January 2014).

Lansdown G. (1995) *Taking Part. Children's Participation in Decision Making.* London: IPPR.

McCarthy O, Kenneth Carswell K, Murray E, et al. (2012) What young people want from a sexual health website: Design and development of sexunzipped. *Journal of Medical Internet Research* 14(5): e127.

McNamee S, Seymour J. (2012) Towards a sociology of 10–12 year olds? Emerging methodological issues in the 'new' social studies of childhood. *Childhood* 20(2): 156–168.

Morgan R. (2010) *Children on Rights and Responsibilities: A Report of Children's Views by the Children's Rights Director for England.* London: Ofsted.

Moules T. (2005) *Whose Quality Is It? Children and Young People's Participation in Monitoring the Quality of Care in Hospital: A Participatory Research Study.* Unpublished PhD Study: Anglia Ruskin University.

Moules T, O'Brien N. (2012) Participation in perspective: Reflections from research projects. *Nurse Researcher* 19(2): 17–22.

Moxon D. (2011) *Someone You Know and Can Trust. Consultation with Young People on the Future of School Nurses.* Mersyside: NWRYWU. http://www.nwrywu.org.uk/wp-content/uploads/2011/08/School-Nurse-report.pdf (accessed on 10 January 2014).

Naylor PJ, Wharf-Higgins J, Blair L et al. (2002) Evaluating the participatory process in a community-based heart health project. *Social Science & Medicine* 55(7): 1173–1187.

NCB. (2011) *School Nurses Survey Results.* London: NCB. http://www.ncb.org.uk/media/686035/school_nurses_report_final.pdf (accessed on 10 January 2014).

Neal B. (2004) *Young Children's Citizenship: Ideas into Practice.* York: Joseph Rowntree Foundation.

O'Brien N, Moules T. (2010) *The Impact of Cyber-Bullying on Young People's Mental Health. Final Report.* Chelmsford: Anglia Ruskin University & NCB. http://www.ncb.org.uk/media/111007/cyber-bullying_report.pdf (accessed on 10 January 2014).

O'Brien N, Moules T. (2013) Not sticks and stones but tweets and texts: Findings from a national cyberbullying project. *Pastoral Care in Education: An International Journal of Personal, Social and Emotional Development* 31(1): 53–65.

Oldfield C, Fowler C. (2004) *Mapping Children and Young People's Participation in England.* Research Report No 854. London: National Youth Agency.

PULSE. (2013) *Young People's Views on the Lancashire Health and Wellbeing Strategy.* Lancashire: Lancashire County Council. http://council.lancashire.gov.uk/documents/s18524/Children%20Young%20Peoples%20response%20to%20Health%20and%20Wellbeing%20Strategy%20Pulse.pdf (accessed on 29 April 2014).

Royal College of Paediatrics and Child Health (RCPCH). (2010) *Not Just a Phase. A Guide to the Participation of Children and Young People in Health Services.* London: RCPCH.

Royal College of Paediatrics and Child Health (RCPCH). (2011) *Involving Children and Young People in Health Services.* London: NHS Confederation. http://www.rcpch.ac.uk/system/files/protected/page/Involving%20CAYP%20in%20Health%20Services.pdf (accessed on 5 February 2014).

Shier H. (2001) Pathways to participation: Openings, opportunities and obligations. *Children and Society* 15: 107–117.

Stafford A, Laybourn A, Hill M, Walker M. (2003) Having a say: Children and young people talk about consultation. *Children & Society* 17(5): 361–373.

Street C, Herts B. (2005) *Putting Participation into Practice: Working in Services to Promote the Mental Health and Well-Being of Children and Young People.* London: Young Minds.

Thoburn J. (1992) *Participation in Practice – Involving Families in Child Protection.* Norwich, UK: University of East Anglia.

Treseder P. (1997) *Empowering Children & Young People: Promoting Involvement in Decision-Making.* London: Save the Children.

Turner C. (2003) *What Disabled Children and Young People in Wales Think About the Services They Use.* Cardiff, UK: Barnardos & NCH Wales. http://www.barnardos.org.uk/cymru_are_you_listening_eng.pdf (accessed on 2 February 2014).

West Bromwich. (2011) *Adolescent Health & Teenage Pregnancy Peer Research Report April 2011.* Changing Young Lives. Western Cheshire, UK: NHS.

White SA, Sadanandan NK, Ashcroft J, eds. (1994) *Participatory Communication: Working For Change And Development.* New Delhi, India: Sage Publications.

Willow C. (1997) *Hear! Hear! Promoting Children and Young People's Democratic Participation in Local Government.* London: LGIU.

Wright P, Turner C, Clay D, Mills H. (2006) *The Participation of Children and Young People in Developing Social Care.* London: SCIE. http://www.scie.org.uk/publications/guides/guide11/files/guide11.pdf (accessed on 28 January 2014).

Index